Radiotheranostics – A Primer for Medical Physicists I

This book covers scientific, clinical, and educational aspects of radiotheranostics in cancer control. Setting the framework, the first volume defines *radiotheranostics* and describes the history of radionuclide therapy and theranostics, and the biology of cancer. It examines the clinical applications of unconjugated radionuclides, such as ^{131}I and ^{223}Ra, and of radionuclide-conjugated cancer-specific vectors: peptides, small molecules, antibodies, and nanoparticles; introduces clinical trials and drug development; and reviews epidemiological studies and the adverse effects of radionuclide therapy – both radiation injuries and chemical toxicity.

It presents the chemistry and physics of radionuclide production, discusses radioactivity measurements and traceability, and addresses important instrumentation aspects: calibration, quantitative imaging, and quality control.

Volume I concludes with guidance on the education, training, and competence of a radiotheranostic multidisciplinary team and summarizes the principal physics characteristics of *theranostics* today – including many to be expanded in the second volume – while offering a glimpse into tomorrow.

This volume provides the foundations for the more advanced second volume, which explores dosimetric and radiation safety, aiming to empower medical physicists and demonstrate to the cancer community how to improve cancer control and yield increased patient survival times.

It will be a valuable reference for medical and health physicists with basic knowledge of nuclear medicine.

Key Features

- Provides a comprehensive introduction to the topic, presenting readers with thorough treatment in a cohesive two-volume book.
- Presents a rigorous approach while remaining accessible to students and trainees in the field.
- Contains consistent and extensive references to allow readers to delve deeper into the subject.

Cari (Caridad) Borrás is a certified medical physicist in Washington, DC, USA, where she works as an international consultant and has an adjunct faculty position at the George Washington University School of Medicine and Health Sciences. She obtained a Doctor of Science (Physics) degree from the University of Barcelona, Spain, having done a thesis research project on the dosimetry and embryological effects of Astatine-211 at Thomas Jefferson University in Philadelphia, PA, USA, as a Fulbright scholar. She has lectured in more than 300 seminars/courses/congresses, many organized by her; authored/contributed around 100 articles and six book chapters and edited two books. She is a Fellow of ACR, AAPM, IOMP, HPS, and IUPESM, and has received awards/recognitions from SEFM, AAPM, IOMP, ALFIM, ACCE, ACR, and ABR.

Michael G. Stabin is a Certified Health Physicist, President of the Radiation Dose Assessment Resource, Inc., living in Kennewick, WA, USA, where he worked for NV5 – Technical Engineering & Consulting Solutions and Hanford Mission Integration Solutions. He was an Associate Professor in the Radiology and Radiological Sciences Department at Vanderbilt University, in Nashville, TN, and a Scientist at the Radiation Internal Dose Information Center of Oak Ridge Institute for Science and Education. He received a Ph.D. in Nuclear Engineering (Health Physics emphasis) from the University of Tennessee, is a member of the HPS and the SNMMI, and is also a Fulbright scholar. He has over 225 publications in the open literature, most on internal dosimetry for nuclear medicine applications, including complete textbooks on health physics and internal dose assessment.

Series in Medical Physics and Biomedical Engineering

Series Editors: Kwan-Hoong Ng, E. Russell Ritenour, and Slavik Tabakov

Radiotheranostics – A Primer for Medical Physicists I

Physics, Chemistry, Biology and Clinical Applications

Edited by
Cari Borrás
Michael G. Stabin

CRC Press
Taylor & Francis Group
Boca Raton London New York

CRC Press is an imprint of the
Taylor & Francis Group, an **informa** business

Designed cover image: Aaron Kian-Ti Tong, Singapore General Hospital, Singapore

First edition published 2024
by CRC Press
2385 NW Executive Center Drive, Suite 320, Boca Raton FL 33431

and by CRC Press
4 Park Square, Milton Park, Abingdon, Oxon, OX14 4RN

CRC Press is an imprint of Taylor & Francis Group, LLC

© 2024 selection and editorial matter, Cari Borrás and Michael G. Stabin; individual chapters, the contributors

Library of Congress Cataloguing-in-Publication Data
Names: Borrás, Cari, editor. | Stabin, Michael G., editor.
Title: Radiotheranostics - a primer for medical physicists : physics, chemistry, biology and clinical applications / edited by Cari Borrás and Michael G. Stabin.
Other titles: Series in medical physics and biomedical engineering.
Description: First edition. | Boca Raton, FL : CRC Press, 2024. | Series: Series in medical physics and biomedical engineering | Includes bibliographical references and index. |
Summary: "The book provides a comprehensive introduction to the relevant theranostics aspects involving pairs of radiopharmaceuticals used in imaging and therapy for cancer treatments. Chapters explore the history of radiotheranostics, before discussing cancer biology and radiation biology models; clinical applications; radionuclide production and radiopharmaceutical preparation; source calibration and imaging instrumentation; biokinetic modelling and dosimetric formalisms; epidemiological studies and clinical trials. It also details radiation safety considerations; regulatory requirements; economic considerations, and discusses staff education, training and competences on radiotheranostics, and the future outlook for the field. It will serve as a valuable guide for academic and practicing clinical medical and health physicists with a basic knowledge of nuclear medicine, and although the book is not meant as a textbook, students and trainees in nuclear medicine physics may also find the book useful. This book will empower medical and health physicists with not only the necessary practical tools to estimate and document the individual dosimetry of patients undergoing radiotheranostic treatment, but it will enable them to convince the cancer community that such a dosimetry improves cancer control and results in longer survival times and also open conversations about organ dose estimates and calculations with policy makers to guide the future of the field"-- Provided by publisher.
Identifiers: LCCN 2023035615 | ISBN 9781032138978 (hardback) | ISBN 9781032169064 (paperback) | ISBN 9781003250913 (ebook)
Subjects: MESH: Neoplasms--radiotherapy | Radiopharmaceuticals--therapeutic use | Radioisotopes--therapeutic use | Theranostic Nanomedicine
Classification: LCC RC271.R27 | NLM QZ 269 | DDC 615.8/424--dc23/eng/20240102
LC record available at https://lccn.loc.gov/2023035615

ISBN: 978-1-032-13897-8 (hbk)
ISBN: 978-1-032-16906-4 (pbk)
ISBN: 978-1-003-25091-3 (ebk)

DOI: 10.1201/9781003250913

Typeset in Times
by MPS Limited, Dehradun

Contents

PART 1 Introduction

PART 2 Clinical Applications of Targeted Radionuclide Therapy in Cancer Control

PART 3   *Radiation Chemistry and Physics*

PART 4   *The Future*

About the Series

The *Series in Medical Physics and Biomedical Engineering* describes the ap- plications of physical sciences, engineering, and mathematics in medicine and clinical research.

The series seeks (but is not restricted to) publications in the following topics:

- Artificial organs
- Assistive technology
- Bioinformatics
- Bioinstrumentation
- Biomaterials
- Biomechanics
- Biomedical engineering
- Clinical engineering
- Imaging
- Implants
- Medical computing and mathematics
- Medical/surgical devices

- Patient monitoring
- Physiological measurement
- Prosthetics
- Radiation protection, health physics, and dosimetry
- Regulatory issues
- Rehabilitation engineering
- Sports medicine
- Systems physiology
- Telemedicine
- Tissue engineering
- Treatment

The *Series in Medical Physics and Biomedical Engineering* is an interna- tional series that meets the need for up-to-date texts in this rapidly developing field. Books in the series range in level from introductory graduate textbooks and practical handbooks to more advanced expositions of current research.

The *Series in Medical Physics and Biomedical Engineering* is the official book series of the International Organization for Medical Physics.

The International Organization for Medical Physics

The International Organization for Medical Physics (IOMP) represents over 18,000 medical physicists worldwide and has a membership of 80 national and 6 regional organizations, together with a number of corporate members. Individual medical physicists of all national member organisations are also automatically members.

The mission of IOMP is to advance medical physics practice worldwide by disseminating scientific and technical information, fostering the educational and professional development of medical physics and promoting the highest quality medical physics services for patients.

A World Congress on Medical Physics and Biomedical Engineering is held every three years in cooperation with International Federation for Medical and Biological Engineering (IFMBE) and International Union for Physics and En- gineering Sciences in Medicine (IUPESM). A regionally based international conference, the International Congress of Medical Physics (ICMP) is held be- tween world congresses. IOMP also sponsors international conferences, work- shops and courses.

The IOMP has several programmes to assist medical physicists in develop- ing countries. The joint IOMP Library Programme supports 75 active libraries in 43 developing countries, and the Used Equipment Programme coordinates equipment donations. The Travel Assistance Programme provides a limited number of grants to enable physicists to attend the world congresses.

IOMP co-sponsors the *Journal of Applied Clinical Medical Physics*. The IOMP publishes, twice a year, an electronic bulletin, *Medical Physics World*. IOMP also publishes e-Zine, an electronic news letter about six times a year. IOMP has an agreement with Taylor & Francis for the publication of the *Medical Physics and Biomedical Engineering* series of textbooks. IOMP members receive a discount.

IOMP collaborates with international organizations, such as the World Health Organisations (WHO), the International Atomic Energy Agency (IAEA) and other international professional bodies such as the International Radiation Protection Association (IRPA) and the International Commission on Radiological Protection (ICRP), to promote the development of medical physics and the safe use of radiation and medical devices.

Guidance on education, training and professional development of medical physicists is issued by IOMP, which is collaborating with other professional organizations in development of a professional certification system for medical physicists that can be implemented on a global basis.

The IOMP website (www.iomp.org) contains information on all the activi- ties of the IOMP, policy statements 1 and 2 and the 'IOMP: Review and Way Forward' which outlines all the activities of IOMP and plans for the future.

List of Common Acronyms

ABNM	American Board of Nuclear Medicine
AC	Atypical Carcinoids
ADME	Absorption, Distribution, Metabolism, And Excretion
ADT	Androgen Deprivation Therapy
AI	Artificial Intelligence
ALARA	As Low as is Reasonably Achievable
ALSYMPCA	Alpharadin In Symptomatic Prostate Cancer, An International Phase III Clinical Study
AML	Acute Myeloid Leukemia
ATA	American Thyroid Association
BCR	Biochemical Recurrence
BED	Biologically Effective Dose
BGO	Bismuth Germanate
BIPM	Bureau International des Poids et Mesures
BSOC	Best Standard Of Care
BSS	Basic Safety Standards
CAF	Cancer-Associated Fibroblast
CDC	Center for Disease Control
CERN	European Organization for Nuclear Research
CNR	Contrast-To-Noise Ratio
CQMP	Clinically Qualified Medical Physicist
CR	Complete Response
CRC	Colorectal Cancer
CSCS	Cancer Stem Cells
CT	Computed Tomography
CTCAE	Common Terminology Criteria for Adverse Events
CTDI	Computed Tomography Dose Index
CVOF	Central Field of View
CZT	Cadmium Zinc Telluride
DCR	Disease Control Rate
DDEP	Decay Data Evaluation Project
DEW	Dual-energy window method
DLT	Dose-Limiting Toxicity
DNA	Deoxyribonucleic Acid
DOTA	Dodecane Tetraacetic Acid
DOTANOC	DOTA-1-NaI3-octreotide
DOTATATE	DOTA-Tyr3-octreotate
DSMB	Data and Safety Monitoring Board
DTC	Differentiated Thyroid Cancer
DTPA	Diethylenetriamine Pentaacetate
EANM	European Association of Nuclear Medicine
EBNM	European Board of Nuclear Medicine
EBRT	External Beam Radiation Therapy
EC	Electron Capture
EDTMP	Ethylenediamine Tetra(Methylene Phosphonic Acid)
EGFR	Epidermal Growth Factor Receptor
eIND	Exploratory IND

EMA	European Medicines Agency
ERBB	Epidermal Growth Factor Receptors
EUS	Endoscopic Ultrasound
FAP	Fibroblast Activating Protein
FAPI	Fibroblast Activation Protein Inhibitor
FBP	Filtered back projection
FDA	Food And Drug Administration of The United States (also USFDA)
FOV	Field of View
FWHM	Full Width at Half Maximum
FWTM	Full Width at Tenth Maximum
GEP-NET	Gastroenteropancreatic-NET
GFR	Glomerular Filtration Rate
GLP/GMP	Good Laboratory/Manufacturing Practice
HCC	Hepatocellular Carcinoma
HEDP	Hydroxyethylidene Diphosphonic Acid
HEGF	Human Epidermal Growth Factor
HPV	Human Papillomavirus Cancer
HU	Hounsfield Unit
IAEA	International Atomic Energy Agency
ICH	International Conference on Harmonization
ICRP	International Commission on Radiological Protection
ICRU	International Commission of Radiation Units and Measurements
IMP	Investigational Medical Product
IMPCB	International Medical Physics Certification Board
IND	Investigational New Drug
IRB	Institutional Review Board
ISOL	Isotope-Separator-On-Line
IT	Isomeric Transition
JRCNMT	Joint Review Committee on Educational Programs in Nuclear Medicine Technology
LET	Linear Energy Transfer
LID	Low Iodine Diet
LOR	Line of Response
LQ	Linear Quadratic Model
mAb	Monoclonal Antibody
MCRPC	Metastatic Castration-Resistant Prostate Cancers
MDP	Methylene Diphosphate
MDS	Myelodysplastic Syndrome
MEN	Multiple Endocrine Neoplasia
MIBG	Meta-Iodobenzylguanidine
MIRD	Medical Internal Radiation Dose
ML-EM	Maximum-Likelihood Expectation Maximization
mPFS	Median Progression Free Survival
MRI	Magnetic Resonance Imaging
MTC	Medullary Thyroid Cancer
MTD	Maximum Tolerated Dose
MTF	Modulation Transfer Function
NaI	Sodium Iodide
NB	Neuroblastoma
NDA	New Drug Application
NEMA	National Electrical Manufacturers Association

NET	Neuroendocrine Tumors
NETTER 1	Neuroendocrine Tumors Therapy Clinical Trial
NF	Neurofibromatosis
NHL	Non-Hodgkin´s Lymphoma
NIS	Sodium Iodide Symporter
NIST	National Institute of Standards and Technology
NM	Nuclear Medicine
NMI	National Metrology Institute
NMT	Nuclear Medicine Technologist
NPs	Nanoparticles
NTCP	Normal Tissue Complication Probability
ORR	Overall Response Rate
OS	Overall Survival
OS-EM	Ordered-Subset Expectation-Maximization
PARP	Poly ADP-ribose polymerase
PC	Pheochromocytoma
PEG	Polyethylene Glycol
PET	Positron Emission Tomography
PFS	Progression Free Survival
PG	Paraganglioma
PK	Pharmacokinetic
PPGL	Pheochromocytoma and Paraganglioma
PR	Partial Response
PRRT	Peptide Receptor Radionuclide Therapy
PSA	Prostate-Specific Antigen
PSF	Point-Spread Function
PSMA	Prostate-Specific Membrane Antigen
PV	Polycythemia Vera
PVE	Partial Volume Effect
RADAR	Radiation Dose Assessment Resource
RAI	Radioactive Iodine
RAM	Radioactive Material
RCP	Radiochemical Purity
RCT	Randomized Controlled Trial
RFA	Radiofrequency Ablation
RHTSH	Recombinant Human Thyrotropin
RIB	Radioactive Ion Beam
RIT	Radioimmunotherapy
RNT	Radionuclide Therapy
RPO	Radiation Protection Officer
RPT	Radiopharmaceutical Therapy
RSO	Radiation Safety Officer
SA	Specific Activity
SBRT	Stereotactic body radiotherapy
SI	International System of Units
SIRT	Selective Internal Radiation Therapy
SNR	Signal to Noise Ratio
SOP	Standard Operating Procedures
SPECT	Single Photon Emission Computed Tomography
SPIONs	Superparamagnetic Iron Oxide Nanoparticles
SSAs	Somatostatin analogs

SST	Somatostatin
SSTR	Somatostatin Receptors
SUV	Standardized Uptake Value
TAC	Time-Activity Curve
TACE	Trans-Arterial Chemoembolization
TAE	Trans-Arterial Embolization
TC	Typical Carcinoids (TC)
TCP	Tumor Control Probability
TEI	Target Isotopic Enrichment
TEW	Triple-energy Window Method
THW	Thyroid Hormone Withdrawal
TMDD	Target-Mediated Drug Distribution
t-MN	Therapy-Related Myeloid Neoplasia
TOF	Time of Flight
TRIUMF	Canada's Particle Accelerator Centre
TRNT	Targeted Radionuclide Therapy (Also TRT)
TS	Tuberous Sclerosis
TSH	Thyroid Stimulating Hormone
TTFUS	Cooperative Thyrotoxicosis Therapy Follow-up Study
UFOV	Useful Field of View
VHL	Von-Hippel-Lindau Syndrome
VOI	Volume of Interest
WHO	World Health Organization

Contributors

Dale L. Bailey, PhD
Royal North Shore Hospital & The University
  of Sydney
Sydney, Australia

Maria Luisa Belli
IRST-IRCCS
Meldola, Italy

Eva Bezak, PhD
University of South Australia
Adelaide, Australia

John D. Boice, Jr., ScD
National Council on Radiation Protection and
  Measurements
Bethesda, Maryland, USA
And
Division of Epidemiology, Department of
  Medicine, Vanderbilt Epidemiology Center
  and Vanderbilt-Ingram Cancer Center,
  Vanderbilt University
Nashville, Tennessee, USA

Cari Borrás, DSc, FACR, FAAPM, FIOMP,
  FIUPESM, FHPS
Radiological Physics and Health Services
Washington DC, USA

Lawrence T. Dauer, PhD
Department of Medical Physics, Memorial
  Sloan Kettering Cancer Center
New York, New York, USA

Arianna Di Paolo, MD
IRST-IRCCS
Meldola, Italy

Gokce Engudar, PhD
TRIUMF Life Science Division
Vancouver, BC Canada

Frederic H. Fahey
Division of Nuclear Medicine and Molecular
  Imaging, Department of Radiology, Boston
  Children's Hospital, Harvard Medical School
Boston, MA, USA

Jake Forster, DSc
University of South Australia
Adelaide, Australia

Gopinath Gnanasegaran, MD
Royal Free London NHS Foundation Trust
London, United Kingdom

Frederick D. Grant, MD
Department of Radiology, Children's Hospital of
  Philadelphia, Perelman School of Medicine of
  the University of Pennsylvania
Philadelphia, PA, USA

Rodney J. Hicks, MD
Department of Medicine, St Vincent's Medical
  School, University of Melbourne, Melbourne
  Academic Centre for Health, University of
  Melbourne Centre for Cancer Research
Melbourne VIC, Australia
And
Victorian Comprehensive Cancer Centre, Central
  Clinical School, Alfred Hospital, Monash
  University, Melbourne VIC, Australia

Ashleigh Hull, PhD
University of South Australia
Adelaide, Australia

Angela Y. Jia, MD, PhD
Department of Radiation Oncology, Johns
  Hopkins University
Baltimore, USA
And
Department of Radiation Oncology, University
  Hospitals Seidman Cancer Center, Case
  Western Reserve University
Cleveland, OH, USA

Raghava Kashyap, MBBS, MD
Cancer Imaging, the Peter MacCallum Cancer
  Centre
Melbourne, Australia

Ana P. Kiess, MD, PhD
Department of Radiation Oncology, Johns
  Hopkins University
Baltimore, MD, USA

Ivan Kempson, PhD
Future Industries Institute, University of South
    Australia
Mawson Lakes, S.A., Australia

Grace Kong, MD
Cancer Imaging, the Peter MacCallum Cancer
    Centre
Melbourne, Australia
And
The Sir Peter MacCallum Department of
    Oncology, the University of Melbourne
Melbourne, Australia

Winnie Wing-Chuen Lam, MBBS, FRCR,
    FAMS
Singapore General Hospital
Singapore, Singapore

Nicole Lin, MD
Department of Radiation Oncology, Johns
    Hopkins University
Baltimore, MD, USA

Michael Ljungberg, PhD
Medical Radiation Physics, Lund University
Lund, Sweden

Kelvin Siu-Hoong Loke, MBBS, FRCR. FAMS
Singapore General Hospital
Singapore, Singapore

Irene Marini, MD
IRST-IRCCS
Meldola, Italy

Yiu Ming Khor, MBBS, MRCP
SingHealth – RADSC
Singapore, Singapore

Ali Nazarizadeh, DVM
Future Industries Institute, University of South
    Australia
Mawson Lakes, S.A., Australia

Diana Paez, MD, Med
Section of Nuclear Medicine and Diagnostic
    Imaging, International Atomic Energy
    Agency (IAEA), Vienna, Austria

Giovanni Paganelli, MD
IRST-IRCCS
Meldola, Italy

Thomas N.B. Pascual, MD, MSc MHPed
Department of Science and Technology,
    Philippines
And
College of Medical Imaging and Therapy, De
    La Salle Medical and Health Sciences
    Institute, Philippines

Kunthi Pathmaraj, MSc
Department of Molecular Imaging and Therapy,
    Austin Health
Melbourne, Australia

Valery Radchenko, PhD
TRIUMF Life Science Division
Vancouver, BC Canada

Andrew Robinson, PhD
National Physical Laboratory
Teddington, UK
And
The Christie Medical Physics and Engineering
    (CMPE), The Christie NHS Foundation
    Trust
Manchester, UK

Thomas J. Ruth, PhD, FRSC
TRIUMF Life Science Division
Vancouver, BC Canada

Anna Sarnelli, PhD
IRST-IRCCS
Meldola, Italy

Somanesan Satchi, MSc
Department of Nuclear Medicine and Molecular
    Imaging, Singapore General Hospital
Singapore

Michael G. Stabin, PhD
RADAR Inc
Kennewick WA, USA

Aaron Kian-Ti Tong, MBBS, MRCP, MMed,
    FAMS
Singapore General Hospital
Singapore, Singapore

Sue Ping Thang, MBChB, MRCP
Singapore General Hospital
Singapore, Singapore

Stephen Tronchin, MPhil
University of South Australia
Adelaide, Australia

Jarey H. Wang, MD, PhD
Department of Radiation Oncology,
    Johns Hopkins University
Baltimore, MD, USA

Chang-Tong Yang, PhD
Singapore General Hospital
Singapore, Singapore

Charles Xian-Yang Goh, MBBS, FRCR
SingHealth – RADSC
Singapore, Singapore

Sumbul Zaheer, MBBS, MRCP
SingHealth – RADSC
Singapore, Singapore

Acknowledgments

We are very grateful to all the authors for their cooperation in the delivery of their manuscripts despite the Covid pandemic. Special thanks go to Dale L. Bailey, Ph.D., from the University of Sydney, Australia, and to James Lamb, Ph.D., from CycloMedical, Knoxville, TN, USA, for their insightful advice on subjects and authors. One of the editors (CB) also acknowledges the help and support received during the editing process from M. Mahesh, Ph.D. of John Hopkins University, Baltimore, MD, USA, from William Roventine, MSc of Radiation Physics Services, Chepachet, RI, USA, and from Otto Martin, MD, MSc, Informatics in Healthcare, Miami, Fl, USA.

Part 1

Introduction

1 What Is Radiotheranostics?

Cari Borrás and Michael G. Stabin

1.1 DEFINITIONS

The term "theranostic" [thera(py) + (diag)nostic"] is attributed to the American John Funkhouser in a press release by the company Cardiovascular Diagnostics in August 1998 [1]. In 2020, Gomes Marin et al. defined theranostics as the pairing of diagnostic biomarkers with therapeutic agents that share a specific target in diseased cells or tissues; it is a medical procedure that uses the same or very similar biomolecules for both diagnosis and treatment of a disease [2]. It is important to understand that theranostics do not have to involve radionuclides, as a quick internet search can document [3–6]. However, when the diagnostic and therapeutic agents are either radionuclides or molecules labeled with radioactive materials, the term is called radiotheranostics. Some radionuclides, such as ^{131}I or ^{223}Ra, do not need to be conjugated to any biomolecule prior injection; they reach their target due to their biochemical properties. In other cases, it is necessary to produce "radiopharmaceuticals" by radiolabeling peptides, small molecules, antibodies, or nanoparticles that will bind to specific cells such as cancer cells. This type of treatment is called molecular or targeted radionuclide therapy (RNT), and it can be delivered using alpha, beta, Auger, and positron emitters (see Figure 1.1) [7].

In some parts of the world, like the United States, regardless of the mechanism the radionuclide is bound to cells, the therapy is designated as radiopharmaceutical therapy (RPT). In this book, our preferred term is RNT, but when referring to regulatory requirements or guidance publications of drug agencies, such as the Food and Drug Administration of the United States (FDA) [8], and international organizations, such as the International Commission on Radiological Protection (ICRP) [9] and the International Commission of Radiation Units and Measurements (ICRU) [10], RPT is used to retain consistency with the original documents.

1.2 SCOPE

This book addresses the most relevant aspects of radiotheranostic pairs used in imaging and therapy for cancer treatment. It is aimed at academic and practicing clinical medical and health physicists with basic knowledge of nuclear medicine. The text is rigorous, yet easily understandable to physics majors, and although the book is not meant as a textbook, medical physicists training in nuclear medicine physics may also find it useful.

Each chapter has been written as concisely as possible but offers extensive bibliographic references so that readers can delve deeper into whatever subjects they are interested in. We realize that the main interest of medical physicists will lie in dosimetry and radiation safety; however, it is our firm belief that it is essential for physicists to have a basic understanding of current clinical applications, including clinical trials and epidemiological studies; to understand that in addition to radiation effects, radiopharmaceuticals themselves are toxic; and to appreciate the need to work within a multidisciplinary team with specialized education, training, and experience.

To make it easier to read, the book is divided into two volumes. To set the framework, the first volume starts by explaining what radiotheranostics is and why this book is written (Chapter 1), the history of RNT and theranostics (Chapter 2), and the biology of cancer (Chapter 3). It then proceeds to

DOI: 10.1201/9781003250913-2

Beta-minus (β⁻)

- Most commonly used radionuclides for therapy
- Emitted as part of a radioactive decay
- Often have moderately long half-lives (10s to 100s of hours)
- Often accompanied by γ emissions which can be imaged
- Mid-range LET (linear energy transfer) – path lengths of ~mm
- Examples: ^{32}P, ^{67}Cu, ^{90}Y, ^{131}I, ^{177}Lu, ^{188}Re

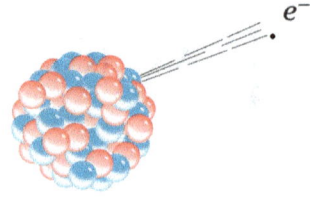

Alpha (α²⁺)

- Recently introduced for therapy
- Often emitted as part of a radioactive decay chain which may have daughters which also emit α-particles – can lead to radionuclide "escape"
- Usually given in small doses (MBqs) with low γ fluxes and hence are challenging to image
- High LET – path lengths of ~μm
- Examples: ^{149}Tb, ^{210}Pb, ^{211}At, ^{212}Pb, ^{213}Bi, ^{223}Ra, ^{225}Ac, ^{227}Th

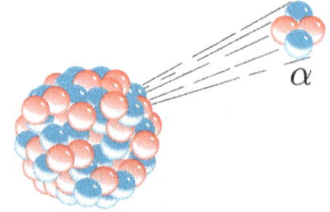

Auger e⁻

- Remains mostly experimental
- Emitted after an electron vacancy is created
- Vey high LET – path lengths are < μm; potentially most lethal particles if internalized by the cancer cell
- Examples: ^{111}In & ^{125}I have been used; ^{67}Ga, ^{99m}Tc ^{123}I potential candidates

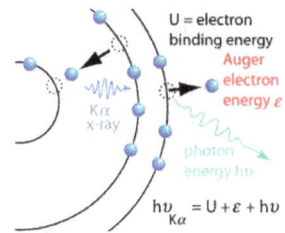

Positrons (β+)*

- Positively charged electrons emitted from nucleus – similar to β -
- Mid-range LET – path lengths of ~mm
- Candidates: $^{61/64}$Cu, ^{89}Zr, ^{124}I

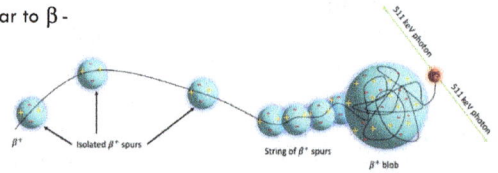

FIGURE 1.1 Particles for radiotheranostics (Courtesy of Dale L. Bailey [7]).

cover the clinical applications of unconjugated radionuclides, such as ^{131}I and ^{223}Ra (Chapter 4), and radionuclide-conjugated cancer-specific vectors – peptides (Chapter 5), small molecules and antibodies (Chapter 6), and nanoparticles (Chapter 7); provides an introduction to clinical trials and drug development (Chapter 8); discusses epidemiological studies (Chapter 9); and reviews the adverse effects of RNT – both from the radiation absorbed in organs and tissues and from the chemical toxicity of the radiopharmaceutical itself (Chapter 10). The next section focuses on the chemistry and physics of radionuclide production (Chapter 11), describes radioactivity measurements and traceability (Chapter 12), and addresses various aspects relative to instrumentation such as calibration, quantitative imaging, and quality control (Chapter 13). The first volume finishes with a section on the Future, which covers the education, training, and competence of the radiotheranostic multidisciplinary team – without them there is no future! – (Chapter 14), and has a final chapter (Chapter 15) that summarizes the most important physics characteristics of theranostics *today,* including many which will be expanded in the second volume, and it offers a glimpse into tomorrow.

   The second volume will start with a section on radiobiology to emphasize that radiobiology is the basis for dosimetry and radiation safety. The dosimetry chapters will cover mean absorbed dose formalisms and microdosimetric approaches; the safety section will include a review of current standards and regulations, both for radiopharmaceutical development and for radiological protection. After presenting an update on instrumentation and describing common economic constraints, the volume will end by exploring the role of artificial intelligence in radiotheranostics.

1.3 RADIOTHERANOSTIC PAIRS

A "theranostic pair" can be achieved in different ways: both the diagnostic component and the therapy component may be nuclides of the same element, for example $^{123/124}$I/^{131}I [11] or $^{61/64}$Cu/^{67}Cu [12,13]; the nuclides can be from the same chemical family, for example ^{18}F/^{211}At [14]; or they may be different radionuclide pairs, for example ^{99m}Tc-labeled albumin/^{90}Y microspheres [10]. Chapter 11 discusses the issues involved, and Chapter 15 adds more examples. It is important that the diagnostic component allows for imaging-based dosimetry so that it can be used to predict the absorbed dose delivered by the therapy administration. Although a direct imaging of the radionuclide used for therapy would be ideal, the therapy nuclide may not emit a positron or a gamma ray that is well suited for imaging with current radionuclide imagers. Tables 1.1–1.3, reproduced from ICRU 96 [10], list the selected alpha-, beta-, and Auger- emitting radionuclides used in RNT identifying the principal therapy radiations and the energy of their principal imaging radiations.

Should the therapy radionuclide not have an adequate imaging component, a chemically equivalent positron or gamma-emitting analog can be used for pretherapy imaging; the most important condition is that its half-life is sufficiently long to enable imaging over a few days to quantify time-varying biological distributions [10]. Figure 1.1 of Chapter 11 presents some examples. Tables 1.4 and 1.5 from reference [15] list selected radiotheranostic pairs in clinical use when both the imaging and the therapeutic agent are the same and when they are not. In addition to the clinical applications, the tables also list the targets and the pharmaceuticals involved.

In a 2022 review of theranostic pairs, Miller et al. [15] estimated the errors in theranostic absorbed dose when using imaging surrogates that may depend on differences in physical half-lives, radiopharmaceuticals' chemistry, radionuclide impurities, and biological effects between the pre-therapy and post-therapy imaging scans. They also recognize that "there is a large variability in radiation sensitivity and pharmacokinetics among patients". And although they "predict that most same-element isotope pairs are suitable for theranostic dosimetry", they conclude that: "if care is taken to consider differences in biological behavior and other aspects discussed in this work between radiopharmaceuticals labeled with different pairs of isotopes, theranostic dosimetry would be immensely beneficial for patient care".

1.4 THE NEED FOR PATIENT-INDIVIDUALIZED DOSIMETRY IN RADIONUCLIDE THERAPY

In radiotherapy with external sources of radiation (including brachytherapy), patient-individualized dose calculations are an established prerequisite to therapy. However, patient-individualized dose calculations are not routinely employed to optimize patients' therapy when radiopharmaceuticals are used for therapy. Physicians generally administer similar levels of activity to all patients, relying primarily on experience to determine the activity level desired to deliver a sufficient radiation dose to malignant tissues while avoiding adverse effects in other tissues. This works fairly well in the use of radioiodines for thyroid cancer, as the "therapeutic window" (difference in dose levels between what is experienced by the tumor and that experienced by the most important normal tissue) is large. However, patient-individualized dosimetry should be performed for patients with Graves' disease, and after decades of successful treatments with large numbers of patients, the use of a fixed activity approach has led to the fact that few investigators have characterized the radiation doses received by their subjects so that an understanding of normal and diseased tissue response to radiation dose could be well established. Traino and Di Martino showed how estimated thyroid dose varies considerably, with differences in target mass and patient biokinetics [16]. Kobe et al. [17] demonstrated dramatic differences in first treatment efficacy when individualized dosimetry was performed for Graves' disease. Jonsson and Mattsson [18] showed that not accouting for individual patient characteristics would result, on average, of 2.5 times *too much* activity prescribed; perhaps eight times too much in individual cases. In other forms of therapy, however, (e.g. the use of radiolabeled peptides for

TABLE 1.1

Selected Alpha-Particle-Emitting Radionuclides Suitable for Therapeutic Nuclear Medicine [10]

Radionuclide	Production	T_p	Principal Therapy Radiations	R_{CSDA} in Tissue[a]	Principal Imaging Radiations	References [From Original Publication]
^{211}At	Cyclotron ^{4}He-beam ^{209}Bi (α, 2n) ^{211}At	7.21 h	5.87 MeV α (^{211}At) 7.45 MeV α (^{211}Po)	48 μm 70 μm	^{211}At: 77 and 93 keV X-rays ^{211}Po: 570 and 898 keV γ-rays ^{207}Bi: 73 keV and 75 keV X-rays, and 590 keV γ-ray	(Sgouros et al., 2015)
^{212}Bi	Natural decay ^{232}Th ^{224}Ra/^{212}Bi generator ^{212}Pb/^{212}Bi generator	1.01 h	6.06 MeV α (^{212}Bi) 8.79 MeV α (^{212}Po)	50 μm 91 μm	^{212}Bi: 727 keV γ-ray ^{208}Tl: 583 keV and 860 keV γ-rays	(Sgouros et al., 2015)
^{213}Bi	^{225}Ac/^{213}Bi generator	45.6 m	5.87 MeV α (^{213}Bi) 8.38 MeV α (^{213}Po)	48 μm 85 μm	^{213}Bi: 440 keV γ-ray ^{209}Tl: 117 keV and 465 keV γ-rays	(Sgouros et al., 2015)
^{223}Ra	(n,γ) activation of ^{226}Ra to produce ^{227}Ac → ^{227}Th → ^{223}Ra	11.4 d	5.61 MeV α (^{223}Ra) 5.72 MeV α (^{223}Ra) 6.82 MeV α (^{219}Rn) 7.39 MeV α (^{215}Po) 6.62 MeV α (^{211}Bi) 7.45 MeV α (^{211}Po)	45 μm 46 μm 61 μm 69 μm 58 μm 70 μm	^{223}Ra: 144, 154, 269, 324 keV γ-rays ^{219}Rn: 271 keV and 402 keV γ-rays ^{211}Pb: 405 keV and 427 keV γ-rays ^{211}Bi: 351 keV γ-ray ^{211}Po: 570 keV and 898 keV γ-rays	(Sgouros et al., 2015)
^{225}Ac	Natural Decay of ^{233}U or Cyclotron p-beam ^{226}Ra (p,2n) ^{225}Ac	10.0 d	5.73 MeV α (^{225}Ac) 5.79 MeV α (^{225}Ac) 5.83 MeV α (^{225}Ac) 6.13 MeV α (^{221}Fr) 6.34 MeV α (^{221}Fr) 7.07 MeV α (^{217}At) 5.87 MeV α (^{213}Bi) 8.38 MeV α (^{213}Po)	46 μm 47 μm 48 μm 51 μm 54 μm 64 μm 48 μm 85 μm	^{225}Ac: 86 keV X-rays, 157 keV γ-ray ^{221}Fr: 218 keV γ-ray ^{213}Bi: 440 keV γ-ray ^{209}Tl: 117 keV and 465 keV γ-rays	(Sgouros et al., 2015)
^{227}Th	Natural Decay of ^{235}U or (n,γ) Activation of ^{226}Ra to ^{227}Ac → ^{227}Th	18.7 d	5.70 MeV α (^{227}Th) 5.71 MeV α (^{227}Th) 5.76 MeV α (^{227}Th) 5.98 MeV α (^{227}Th) 6.04 MeV α (^{227}Th) [plus ^{223}Ra α-particles]	46 μm 46 μm 47 μm 49 μm 50 μm	^{227}Th: 211, 236, 256, 286, 290, 300, 330 keV γ-rays (plus, ^{223}Ra series X-rays and γ-rays)	(Sgouros et al., 2015)

Note. CSDA = continuously slowing down approximation; R_{CSDA} = particle range using the continuously slowing down approximation; ICRU = International Commission on Radiation Units and Measurements.

[a] R_{CSDA} is given for E_{max} of the principal radiation based on the CSDA tabulated in ICRU Report 37 (ICRU, 1984).

TABLE 1.2

Selected Beta-Particle-Emitting Radionuclides Suitable for Therapeutic Nuclear Medicine [10]

Radionuclide	Production	T_p	Principal Therapy Radiations	R_{CSDA} in Tissue[a]	Principal Imaging Radiations Energy (Yield)	References [From Original Publication]
^{124}I	Cyclotron particles beams $^{127}Te\ (p,n)\ ^{124}I$ $^{127}Te\ (d,2n)\ ^{124}I$ $^{121}Sb\ (\alpha,n)\ ^{124}I$ $^{123}Sb\ (^3He,2n)\ ^{124}I$	4.18 d	β^+ (E_{max} = 0.61 MeV) ($\bar{E}_\beta$ = 0.188 MeV)	0.23 cm	511 keV (0.457) annihilation photons	(IAEA, 2011) $\bar{E}_\beta$ (Brown and Firestone, 1986)
^{131}I	Reactor production $^{130}Te\ (n,\gamma)\ ^{131}I$	8.02 d	β^- (E_{max} = 0.61 MeV) ($\bar{E}_\beta$ = 0.182 MeV)	0.23 cm	80 keV (0.026), 284 keV (0.06), 364 keV (0.82), 637 keV (0.07), 723 keV (0.018)	(IAEA,2011) $\bar{E}_\beta$ (Brown and Firestone, 1986
^{90}Y	Reactor production $^{89}Y\ (n,\gamma)\ ^{90}Y$ $^{235}U\ (n,f)\ ^{90}Sr \rightarrow {}^{90}Y$	2.67 d	β^- (E_{max} = 2.28 MeV) ($\bar{E}_\beta$ = 0.934 MeV)	1.1 cm	Bremsstrahlung, 511 keV (0.000032 annihilation photons	(IAEA,2011) $\bar{E}_\beta$ (Brown and Firestone, 1986)
^{89}Sr	Reactor production $^{88}Sr\ (n,\gamma)\ ^{89}Sr$	50.5 d	β^- (E_{max} = 1.49 MeV) ($\bar{E}_\beta$ = 0.583 MeV)	0.71 cm	Bremsstrahlung	(IAEA,2011) $\bar{E}_\beta$ (Brown and Firestone, 1986)
^{177}Lu	Reactor production $^{176}Lu\ (n,\gamma)\ ^{177}Lu$ $^{176}Yb\ (n,\gamma)\ ^{177}Yb \rightarrow {}^{177}Lu$	6.71 d	β^- (E_{max} = 0.50 MeV) ($\bar{E}_\beta$ = 0.133 MeV)	0.18 cm	113 keV (0.06), 208 keV (0.11)	(IAEA,2011) $\bar{E}_\beta$ (Brown and Firestone, 1986)
^{186}Re	Reactor production $^{185}Re\ (n,\gamma)\ ^{186}Re$	3.72 d	β^- (E_{max} = 1.07 MeV) ($\bar{E}_\beta$ = 0.323 MeV)	0.44 cm	137 keV (0.09)	(IAEA,2011) $\bar{E}_\beta$ (Brown and Firestone, 1986)
^{188}Re	Reactor production $^{187}Re\ (n,\gamma)\ ^{188}Re$	17.0 h	β^- (E_{max} = 2.12 MeV) ($\bar{E}_\beta$ = 0.765 MeV)	1 cm	155 keV (0.15), 478 keV (0.01) 633 keV (0.01)	(IAEA,2011) $\bar{E}_\beta$ (Brown and Firestone, 1986)
^{153}Sm	Reactor production $^{152}Sm\ (n,\gamma)\ ^{153}Sm$	46.3 h	β^- (E_{max} = 0.705 MeV) ($\bar{E}_\beta$ = 0.225 MeV)	0.28 cm	69 keV (0.0485),103 keV (0.298) 635 keV (0.322)	(IAEA,2011) $\bar{E}_\beta$ (Brown and Firestone, 1986)

Note. CSDA = continuously slowing down approximation: R_{CSDA} = particle range using the continuously slowing down approximation; IAEA = International Atomic Energy Agency, ICRU = International Commission on Radiation Units and Measurements.

[a] R_{CSDA} is given for E_{max} of the principal radiation based on the CSDA tabulated in ICRU Report 37 (ICRU, 1984).

TABLE 1.3

Selected Auger-Electron-Emitting Radionuclides Suitable for Therapeutic Nuclear Medicine [10]

Radionuclide	Production	T_p	Principal Therapy Radiations	R_{CSDA} in Tissue[a]	Principal Imaging Radiations Energy (Yield)	References [From Original Publication]
^{111}In	Cyclotron particles beams ^{111}Cd (p,n) ^{111}In ^{112}Cd (p,2n) ^{111}In	2.83 d	Conversion (145–219 keV, yield = 0.16) and Auger electrons (yield = 14.7)	0.05 cm	171.3 keV (0.906) 245.4 keV (0.941)	(IAEA, 2011) (Howell, 1992)
^{123}I	Cyclotron particles beams ^{124}Te (p,2n) ^{123}I ^{122}Xe (p,x) ^{123}I ^{127}I (p,5n) ^{123}Xe $\rightarrow$ ^{123}I ^{124}Xe (p,2n) ^{123}Cs $\rightarrow$ ^{123}Xe $\rightarrow$ ^{123}I	13.2 h	Conversion (127–154 keV, yield = 0.15) and Auger electrons (yield = 14.9)	0.02 cm	159 keV (0.833)	(IAEA, 2011) (Howell, 1992)
^{125}I	Reactor production ^{124}Xe (n,γ)^{125}Xe$\rightarrow$^{125}I	59.4 d	Conversion (30–35 keV, yield = 0.94) and Auger electrons (yield = 24.9)	0.0023 cm	35.49 keV (0.668)	(IAEA, 2011) (Howell, 1992)
^{193m}Pt	Cyclotron particle beams ^{192}Os (α,3n) ^{193m}Pt	4.33 d	Conversion (1–133 keV, yield = 3.0) and Auger electrons (yield = 26.4)	0.025 cm	135.5 keV (0.0011) 65–79 keV (0.143) Pt K X-rays	(Howell, 1992)
^{195m}Pt	Reactor production ^{194}Pt (n,γ) ^{195m}Pt	4.02 d	Conversion (17–117 keV, yield = 2.8), and Auger electrons (yield =32.8)	0.019 cm	30.89 keV (0.0228), 98.9 keV (0.114), 129.8 keV (0.0283),	(IAEA, 2011) (Howell, 1992)
^{117m}Sn	Reactor production ^{116}Sn (n,γ) ^{117m}Sn ^{117}Sn (n,n') ^{117m}Sn	13.6 d	Conversion (127–158 keV, yield = 1.14) and Auger electrons (yield = 2.9)	0.030 cm	156.2 (0.0211), 158.6 keV (0.864)	(IAEA, 2011) (Eckerman and Endo., 2008)
^{103}Pd	Reactor production ^{102}Pd (n,γ) ^{103}Pd	17.0 d	Auger electrons (yield = 7.4)	0.0009 cm	20–27 keV Rh X-rays (0.073)	(IAEA, 2011) (Eckerman and Endo., 2008)

Note. CSDA = continuously slowing down approximation; R_{CSDA} = particle range using the continuously slowing down approximation; IAEA = International Atomic Energy Agency, ICRU = International Commission on Radiation Units and Measurements,

[a] R_{CSDA} is given for E_{max} of the principal radiation based on the CSDA tabulated in ICRU Report 37 (ICRU, 1984).

TABLE 1.4

Popular Same-Element Pairs and Common Targets, Pharmaceuticals, and Treated Diseases [15]

Therapeutic Nuclides	Imaging	Targets	Pharmaceuticals	Applications	References [From Original Publication]
^{90}Y	^{86}Y (PET)	Somatostatin Receptors (SSTRs)	Somatostatin Analogs, e.g. DOTATOC	Neuro Endocrine Tumors (NETs)	[34]
		CD20 Antigens	mAbs, e.g. Ibritumomab Tiuxetan	Non-Hodgkin's Lymphoma (NHL)	[23]
		HER2/neu	Trastuzumab	Ovarian Cancer	[40]
		Prostate Specific Membrane Antigens (PSMA)	PSMA 4–6	Prostate Cancer	[41]
^{131}I	^{123}I	Thyroid-Stimulating Hormone (TSH)	Sodium Iodide (NaI)	Thyroid Diseases	[42]
	(SPECT)/	Norepinephrine Transporters	mIBG	Neuroblastomas, Pheochromocytomas, etc.	[35,43,44]
	^{124}I (PET)	PSMA	MIP-1095	Prostate Cancer	[45]
		The Extra Domain B of Fibronectin	L19-SIP	Multiple Cancers (Melanoma, Head/ Neck, etc.)	[46]
^{67}Cu	^{64}Cu (PET)	SSTRs	Octreotate, SarTATE	NETs Neuroblastomas	[47,48]
		CD20 Antigens	2IT-BAT-Lym-1	NHL	[49]
		PSMA	PSMA-617, RPS-085	Prostate Cancer	[50–52]
		Copper Transporter Protein 1	Cl_2	Multiple Cancers (Colorectal, Breast, Prostate, Melanoma, etc.)	[53,55]
^{47}Sc	$^{89}Sr*$ (PET)/	SSTRs	DOTANOC (A Somatostatin Analog)	NETs	[56]
	^{44}S (PET)	Folate Receptors	cm10 (a DOTA-Folate Conjugate)	Multiple Cancers (Breast, Ovarian, Lung, etc.)	[57]
^{89}Sr	$^{83}Sr*$ (PET)	Bone	Chloride (Cl)	Bone Metastases	[58]
$^{161}Tb/^{149}Tb$	$^{152}Tb(PET)/$	SSTRs	DOTANOC	NETs	[59]
	^{155}Tb	PSMA	PSMA-617	Prostate Cancer	[60]
	(SPECT)	Folate Receptors	cm09	Multiple Cancers (Breast, Ovarian, Lung, etc.)	[61]

* We list these pairs here for completeness, but they are not discussed further in this work.

TABLE 1.5
Popular Different-Element Pairs and the Common Targets, Pharmaceuticals, and Treated Diseases [15]

Therapeutic Nuclides	Imaging	Targets	Pharmaceuticals	Applications	References [From Original Publication]
^{177}Lu	^{68}Ga (PET)	SSTRs	DOTATATE, DOTATOC	NETs	[62,63]
		PSMA	PSMA-617/PSMA-11, PSMA-I&T	Prostate Cancer, Glioblastomas	[64,65]
		Gastrin-Releasing Peptide Receptor (GRPR)	NeoBOMB1, RM2, AMBA	Multiple Cancers (Prostate, Breast, etc.)	[66,68]
		Bone	DOTA^{ZOL}	Bone Metastases	[69,70]
	^{89}Zr (PET)	Epidermal Growth Factor Receptor (EGFR)	Cetuximab	Multiple Cancers (Colorectal, Head/Neck, Skin)	[71]
		CD38 Antigens	Daratumumab	Lymphoma	[72]
		Glypican-1	Miltuximab	Prostate Cancer	[73]
		PD-L1	αPD-L1, YO03	Colon Carcinoma	[74]
	^{64}Cu (PET)	SSTRs	DOTATOC DOTATATE	NETs	[37,75]
		PSMA	PSMA-617	Prostate Cancer	[76,77]
		Vascular EGFR	diZD	Breast Cancer	[78]
		L1-CAM	chCE7 fragments cA10-A3	Multiple Cancers (Neuroblastomas, Ovarian, Endometrial, etc.)	[79,80]
	^{18}F (PET)	EGFR	Cetuximab	Esophageal Squamous Cell Carcinoma	[81,82]
		PSMA	PSMA-617	Prostate Cancer	[77]
	^{44}Sc (PET)	PSMA	PSMA-617	Prostate Cancer	[83–85]
^{225}Ac	^{177}Lu (SPECT)	SSTRs	DOTATATE, DOTATOC	NETs	[86,87]
		PSMA	PSMA-617	Prostate Cancer	[88]
	^{89}Zr (PET)	CD20 Antigens	Ofatumumab	NHL	[89]
		EGRF	Nimotuzumab	Multiple Cancers (Squamous Cell Head/Neck, Breast, Cervical, etc.)	[90]
	^{111}In (SPECT)	Tumor-Associated-MUC1	TAB004	Breast Cancer	[25,91]
	^{177}Lu*(SPECT)	SSTRs	DOTATATE, DOTATOC	NETs	[92]
^{90}Y	^{111}In (SPECT)	PSMA	PSMA-617, J591	Prostate Cancer	[93,94]
		SSTRs	DOTATATE, DOTATOC	NETs	[95,96]
		CD20 Antigens	Ibritumomab Tiuxetan	NHL	[97]
		PSMA	J591	Prostate Cancer	[94,98]
		IL-2Rα	Anti-Tac	T-Cell Leukemia	[99]
		Lewis^Y Carbohydrate Antigen	mAbs, e.g. B3	Multiple Cancers (Colorectal, Breast, Esophageal, etc.)	[100]
	^{99m}Tc (SPECT)	–	[^{99m}Tc]Tc-MAA with ^{90}Y Microspheres	Hepatocellular Carcinoma, Metastatic Liver Cancers	[101,102]
	^{89}Zr* (PET)	CD20 Antigens	Ibritumomab Tiuxetan	NHL	[24]

* We list these pairs here for completeness, but they are not discussed further in this work.

radioimmunotherapy), the tumor-to-normal tissue absorbed dose ratio may be low, and without the use of a patient-specific treatment planning strategy based on radiation absorbed dose, patients are mostly given small amounts of the therapeutic agent, to cautiously avoid deleterious effects in normal tissues (most notably the kidneys or bone marrow). It is known that patients have significant variability in their tumor and normal tissue uptake concentrations as well as in the clearance rates at which activity leaves these tissues. Wahl [19] showed that activities administered to patients to treat non-Hodgkin's lymphoma (NHL) varied by factors of up to five in a large patient population. Thus, only a small fraction of the patient population receives optimal care, and patients may receive a lower than optimum administration of activity. This usually results in no deleterious effects in normal tissues, but suboptimal therapy generally being delivered to the malignant tissues with poorer response rates and higher rates of relapse.

The recommendation to perform patient-individualized dose calculations in RNT is not something new. For example, in 2002, Siegel et al. [20] stated: "If one were to approach the radiation oncologist or medical physicist in an external beam therapy program and suggest that all patients with a certain type of cancer should receive the exact same protocol (beam type, energy, beam exposure time, geometry, etc.), the idea would certainly be rejected as not being in the best interests of the patient. Instead, a patient-specific treatment plan would be implemented in which treatment times are varied to deliver the same radiation dose to all patients. Patient-specific calculations of doses delivered to tumors and normal tissues have been routine in external beam radiotherapy and brachytherapy for decades. The routine use of a fixed GBq/kg, GBq/m^2, or simply GBq, administration of radionuclides for therapy is equivalent to treating all patients in external beam radiotherapy with the same protocol. Varying the treatment time to result in equal absorbed dose for external beam radiotherapy is equivalent to accounting for the known variation in patients' uptake and retention half-time of activity of radionuclides to achieve equal tumor absorbed dose for internal-emitter radiotherapy. It has been suggested that fixed activity-administration protocol designs provide little useful information about the variability among patients relative to the normal organ dose than can be tolerated without dose-limiting toxicity compared to radiation dose-driven protocols".

In 2008, Stabin [21] addressed all of the main objections to performing patient-individualized dosimetry in RNT:

- Performing such calculations is difficult and expensive, requiring too much effort.
- There are no standardized methods for performing individualized dose calculations, and methods vary significantly among different institutions.
- Dose calculations to date have had poor success in predicting tissue response.
- With the level of difficulty involved, there must be some objective evidence that the use of radiation dose calculations provides positive benefit that justifies extra effort and cost.

In 2014, Strigari et al. published a study to determine a dose-effect relationship investigating 79 studies and found a correlation between absorbed dose and clinical effect in 48 of them [22].

Continued objections to the use of patient-specific dose calculations are not supported by recent clinical trials that have shown that patient-individualized dosimetry improves patient outcomes [23,24].

More recently, the ICRP and the ICRU have expressed strong views on the matter. The first "Main Point" of ICRP 140, published in 2019, states: "Individual absorbed dose estimates should be performed for treatment planning and for post administration verification of doses to tumours and normal tissues" [9]. And ICRU 96, published in 2021, affirms: "Radiopharmaceutical therapy has the advantage of delivering radiation, a treatment modality whose mechanism of action has been understood due to century-long experience in radiotherapy. These many years of experience have led to a rigorous treatment planning paradigm wherein the absorbed dose to tumor and normal tissues is calculated and used to optimally treat patients. Absorbed dose–driven implementation and treatment planning of RPT, as outlined in this report, will be adopted only if such treatment planning is shown to provide a long-term survival advantage over the more expedient approach of administered activity-based dosing paradigm. To date, studies demonstrating the advantages of dosimetry and treatment planning in RPT have not been conducted with the level of rigor and transparency required to change practice standards. The following are required before such studies can be conducted:

1. Standardized, well-validated quantitative imaging and dosimetry techniques.
2. Methods that reduce the logistical burden on patients and that are easy to implement while also preserving accuracy.
3. Reporting that includes an assessment of the uncertainty of the absorbed dose calculation (e.g., by providing the standard deviation of the reported absorbed dose result).
4. Development of organ models that are optimized to use activity distributions obtained from SPECT imaging" [10].

1.5   CONCLUSION

Although this volume only covers basic issues such as the physics, chemistry, clinical applications, and human resources involved in radiotheranostics, while dosimetry will be dealt in Volume 2; it was felt necessary to emphasize the need for individualized dosimetry here, since the goal of the book is to empower medical physicists with basic knowledge to lead the way towards achieving new treatment standards aimed at improving patient care.

We have to break the vicious cycle expressed in a 2022 JNM article: "Dosimetry is not performed because dose–response data are lacking, and dose–response data are lacking because dosimetry is not performed" [25]. The time has come for this reasonable paradigm shift in the practice of radiotheranostics, away from "one dose fits all" to patient-individualized dosimetry in RNT.

REFERENCES

1. PharmaNetics and Aventis Pharmaceuticals announce filing of 510K application for enoxaparin test [press release]. 1998. https://www.bizjournals.com/triangle/stories/2001/10/08/daily12.html. Accessed 31 October 2022.
2. Gomes Marin, JF, Nunes, RF, Coutinho, AM et al. Theranostics in nuclear medicine: emerging and re-emerging integrated imaging and therapies in the era of precision oncology. *Radiographics*. 2020; 40(6), 1715–1740.
3. Paradossi, G, Pellegretti, P, and Trucco, A (Editors). *Ultrasound Contrast Agents: Targeting and Processing Methods for Theranostics*. Springer, Milano, 2009.
4. Conde, J. *Handbook of Nanomaterials for Cancer Theranostics*. Elsevier, 2018.
5. Raju, GSR, and Bhaskar, LVKS (Editors). *Theranostics Approaches to Gastric and Colon Cancer*. Springer, Singapore, 2020.
6. Thorat, ND, and Kumar, N (Editors). *Nano-Pharmacokinetics and Theranostics: Advancing Cancer Therapy*. Academic Press, 2021.
7. Bailey, D. The Promise of Molecular Radionuclide Therapy. Special Symposium on "The Past, Present and Future of Targeted Radionuclide Therapy". IUPESM World Congress on Medical Physics and Biomedical Engineering, Singapore, 2022.
8. Food and Drug Administration. Radiopharmaceuticals. https://www.drugs.com/drug-class/radiopharmaceuticals.html Accessed 27 October 2022.
9. International Commission on Radiological Protection. Radiological Protection in Therapy with Radiopharmaceuticals. ICRP Publication 140. *Ann. ICRP* 48(1), September 2019. https://journals.sagepub.com/doi/full/10.1177/0146645319838665 Accessed 27 October 2022.
10. International Commission on Radiation Units and Measurements. Dosimetry-Guided Radiopharmaceutical Therapy. ICRU Report 96, *Journal of ICRU* 21(1)1–212, December 2021. https://www.icru.org/report/icru-report-96-dosimetry-guided-radiopharmaceutical-therapy/ Accessed 27 October 2022.
11. Iwano, S, Kato, K, Nihashi, T, Ito, S, Tachi, Y, and Naganawa, S. Comparisons of I-123 diagnostic and I-131 post-treatment scans for detecting residual thyroid tissue and metastases of differentiated thyroid cancer. *Ann Nucl Med*. 2009; 23(9), 777–782.

12. Mou, L, Martini, P, Pupillo, G, Cieszykowska, I, Cutler, CS, and Mikolajczak, R. (67)Cu production capabilities: a mini review. *Molecules*. 2022; 27(5), 1501.

13. Pupillo, G, Mou, L, Martini, P et al. Production of 67Cu by enriched 70Zn targets: first measurements of formation cross sections of 67Cu, 64Cu, 67Ga, 66Ga, 69mZn and 65Zn in interactions of 70Zn with protons above 45 MeV. *Radiochimica Acta*. 2020; 108(8), 593–602.

14. Zalutsky, MR, and Pruszynski, M. Astatine-211: production and availability. *Curr Radiopharm*. 2011; 4(3), 177–185.

15. Miller, C, Rousseau, J, Ramogida, CF et al. Implications of physics, chemistry and biology for dosimetry calculations using theranostic pairs. *Theranostics*. 2022; 12(1), 232–259.

16. Traino, A C, & Martino, F D. A dosimetric algorithm for patient-specific 131I therapy of thyroid cancer based on a prescribed target-mass reduction. *Physics in Medicine and Biology*. 2006; 51, 6449–6456.

17. Kobe, C, Weber, I, Eschner, W, Sudbrock, F, Schmidt, M, Dietlein, M, & Schicha, H. Graves' disease and radioiodine therapy. Is success of ablation dependent on the choice of thyreostatic medication? *Nuklearmedizin*. 2008; 47(4), 153–156.

18. Jönsson, H, & Mattsson , S. Excess radiation absorbed doses from non-optimised radioiodine treatment of hyperthyroidism. *Radiat Prot Dosimetry*. 2004; 108(2), 107–114.

19. Wahl , RL. Tositumomab and (131)I therapy in non-Hodgkin's lymphoma. *J Nucl Med*. 2005; 46, 128S–40S.

20. Siegel, JA, Stabin, MG, and Brill, AB. The importance of patient-specific radiation dose calculations for the administration of radionuclides in therapy. *Cell Mol Biol* (Noisy-le-Grand). 2002 Jul; 48(5), 451–459.

21. Stabin, MG. The case for patient-specific dosimetry in radionuclide therapy. *Cancer Biother Radiopharm* . 2008; 23(3), 273–284.

22. Strigari, L, Konijnenberg, M, Chiesa, C et al. The evidence base for the use of internal dosimetry in the clinical practice of molecular radiotherapy. *Eur J Nucl Med Mol Imaging*. 2014; 41, 1976–1988.

23. Garin, E, Tselikas, L, Guiu, B et al. Personalised versus standard dosimetry approach of selective internal radiation therapy in patients with locally advanced hepatocellular carcinoma (DOSISPHERE-01): a randomised, multicentre, open-label phase 2 trial. *Lancet Gastroenterol Hepatol*. 2021 Jan; 6(1), 17–29.

24. Lewandowski, RJ, and Salem, R. Radioembolisation with personalised dosimetry: improving outcomes for patients with advanced hepatocellular carcinoma. *Lancet Gastroenterol Hepatol*. 2021 Jan; 6(1), 2–3.

25. O'Donoghue, J, Zanzonico, P, Humm, J, and Kesner, A. Dosimetry in radiopharmaceutical therapy. *J Nucl Med*. 2022; 63, 1467–1474.

2 History of Radionuclide Therapy and Theranostics

Frederic H. Fahey, Frederick D. Grant, and Rodney J. Hicks

2.1 INTRODUCTION

The first targeted radionuclide therapy was performed by Saul Hertz and Arthur Roberts in March 1941. They administered a mixture of cyclotron produced iodine-130 and iodine-131 (^{130}I and ^{131}I) to a woman with hyperthyroidism. They subsequently reported their results in 29 patients in 1946 [1]. This advance in medical therapy did not occur spontaneously, but rather was developed on a background of many decades, and even centuries of prior scientific investigation and discovery, including important preclinical work by Hertz and Roberts themselves.

The development of a successful targeted radionuclide therapy would seem to depend on a small number of prerequisites. Some of these, like the discovery of radioactivity and ability to create artificial radionuclides, are common to all radionuclide therapy. Targeted radionuclide therapy requires an understanding of the physiology of the organ and disease of interest. For most therapies, a specific target must be chosen, and an appropriate targeting moiety identified. Radioiodine therapy for thyroid disease was very probably the first and is certainly the most successful targeted radionuclide therapy. An understanding of the physiological role of iodine in thyroid function allowed the radionuclide itself (radioiodine) to be chosen as the targeting moiety even before the specific characterization of the cellular target, the sodium-iodide transporter, or the genomic pathways that regulate its expression that underpins current diagnostic and therapeutic approaches [2]. Other radionuclide therapies such as bone-seeking agents were also introduced without a clear understanding of the target, but many emerging therapies are based on detailed molecular biology studies that characterize tractable targets. Finally, an appropriate therapeutic radioisotope must be chosen. The history of radioiodine therapy of thyroid disease demonstrates this, as targeted therapy of thyroid disease was not effective with short-lived radioisotopes of iodine and became feasible only after radioisotopes such as ^{131}I (half-life 8 days) could be produced. Thus, the development of targeted radionuclide therapy using radioiodine to treat benign and malignant thyroid disease can serve as a model for the development of subsequent targeted radionuclide therapies.

Here, we summarize the development of successful targeted radionuclide therapies over the past century or so, which have been increasingly based on an understanding of the underlying disease pathophysiology, identification of an appropriate biological target, development of an appropriate targeting moiety to carry the radionuclide to the target, and identification of an appropriate radionuclide for which production is feasible.

2.2 RÖNTGEN, BECQUEREL, AND THE CURIES

On November 8, 1895, Professor Röntgen was late for dinner. In his laboratory at the University of Würzberg, he had been investigating various aspects of the vacuum tubes being used to generate cathode rays, i.e. a stream of accelerated electrons. On that evening, he had encased the tube in a light-tight cardboard box to protect a thin aluminum window he had installed to allow the cathode rays to escape the tube. However, when he energized the tube, he noticed that a screen that was

DOI: 10.1201/9781003250913-3

coated with barium platinocyanide located nearby was fluorescing. After several experiments to confirm what he was seeing, he surmised that a new kind of invisible ray that he designated with the mathematical signal for the unknown, X, must be causing the fluorescence. Over the next several weeks, he ran additional experiments including taking a "shadowgram" photograph of his wife's hand using the new rays, the first radiograph. On December 28, 1895, less than 2 months since his initial discovery, Röntgen published his seminal paper entitled "A New Kind of Rays" [3]. Within just a few months, news of his "X-rays" had spread throughout the physics world and beyond as the medical implications were appreciated almost immediately. For his work, Professor Röntgen was awarded the very first Nobel Prize in Physics in 1901.

In the months following the publication of Röntgen's discovery, there was much excitement. In early 1896, Henri Becquerel was working at the École Polytechnique as well as succeeding his father as the chair of physics at the Muséum National d'Histoire Naturelle. His interest led him to wonder if phosphorescent materials such as uranium salts would emit rays similar to those observed by Röntgen after being exposed to sunlight. However, he found that not only did the salts exposed to sunlight emit such rays, but other salts kept in the dark did as well with essentially the same intensity. From this observation, he concluded that the salts themselves were emitting these rays. He also demonstrated that these rays differed from Röntgen's X-rays in that a component of the beam was affected by placement within an electric or magnetic field [4].

Marie Sklodowska Curie decided that further investigation of the rays emanating from uranium would be a possible area of research for her thesis at the University of Paris. The previous year, she had married Pierre Curie, a professor of physics at the university. Using a version of an electrometer devised by her husband, she found that the level of ionization in the air about the uranium samples was a reasonable measure of the intensity of the radiation. She found that the intensity of the radiation depended only on the quantity of uranium regardless of its chemical composition indicating that uranium itself was emitting the radiation. She found that the element, thorium, was also radioactive, a term she coined in 1898. About this same time, Pierre Curie decided to join his wife with her research on radioactivity.

They found that two materials containing uranium, pitchblende and torbenite, emitted substantially more radiation than uranium itself. From this observation, the Curies supposed that these materials must contain other elements that are much more radioactive than uranium. In 1898, the Curies announced their discovery of two new radioactive elements, polonium (named for Marie's homeland of Poland) and radium. For their work, they, along with Becquerel, were awarded the Nobel Prize in Physics in 1903 [5].

2.3 THE CURIE INSTITUTE AND OTHER EARLY USES OF RADIONUCLIDE THERAPY

How radium, now recognized to be ^{226}Ra, came to be used therapeutically has been elegantly described by Donald Blaufox, citing a *Comptes Rendue* report authored jointly by Henri Becquerel and Pierre Curie [6,7]. In early April 1901, having received a sample of radium contained in a glass tube from Madame Curie, Becquerel placed the small box in which it was contained in a pocket of his waistcoat, where it remained for several hours. Just over a week later, he noted a red mark on his skin in the shape of the tube, which began to desquamate towards the end of that month. In a compilation of various vignettes published previously by Mallinkrodt Nuclear, Marshall Brucer reported that Pierre Curie verified the effect of radium on skin by applying a sample to his own forearm [8]. This led Curie to postulate a potential medical use and providing a sample to a dermatologist by the name of Henri-Alexandre Danlos, of Ehlers-Danlos fame. Dr. Danlos began to use this small sample to successfully treat various skin conditions in his practice at the Saint Louis Hospital in Paris leading to the establishment of a laboratory to study the effects of radiation, which became the Curie Institute and was led by

Marie Curie herself. Madame Curie personally mentored small teams of researchers and students who independently investigated various aspects of radioactivity. She was known to sit with them on the stairs of the narrow entrance hall to discuss their findings, while also contributing her own research output [9].

Within a few short years and notwithstanding the extreme paucity of radium, given the difficulty in extracting it from various ores, radium therapy had reached the far corners of the Earth. In a book entitled *Radium: How and When to Use* authored by Dr. Herman Lawrence, a dermatologist at the Melbourne and St Vincent's Hospitals in Melbourne, Australia, which was published in 1911 by Stillwell and Co., patients were pictured applying radium to their own skin conditions at St Vincent's Hospital in 1905 (Figure 2.1) [10].

In a comprehensive description of the results that he had obtained in his own practice, Lawrence demonstrated significant efficacy in treating both squamous cell carcinoma, known at that time as epithelioma, and basal cell carcinoma, known then as rodent ulcer (Figure 2.2).

After inflammatory and desquamative phases, regression with minimal scarring but a tendency to hypopigmentation was noted. The use of radionuclides for the treatment of these non-melanomatous skin cancers has been recently revived with the use of rhenium-188 (^{188}Re) paste [11].

In the first half of the 20th century, radium therapy had grown into an accepted form of cancer treatment with both topical treatment by way of plaques applied to the skin and mucous membranes and radium needles inserted directly into tumor masses as a forerunner of seed brachytherapy. However, the risks of radium became increasingly recognized and there were many unethical practices that inevitably led to the demise of this treatment [12]. Interestingly, Henrietta Lacks, who was the donor of the first immortalized cancer cell line, the famous HeLa cells that have been an indispensable research tool, was treated with ^{226}Ra for her cervical cancer in 1951 at the Johns Hopkins Hospital in Baltimore [13].

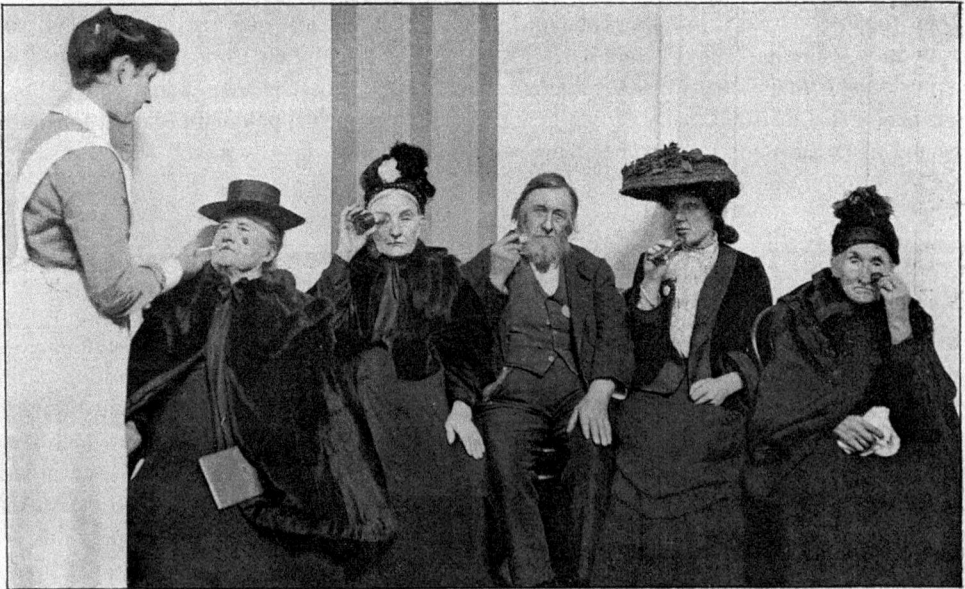

Radium being applied at the Skin Department, St. Vincent's Hospital, 1905.

FIGURE 2.1 Radium treatment in the Dermatology Clinic of St Vincent's Hospital, Melbourne, Australia, 1905 [As adapted from 10].

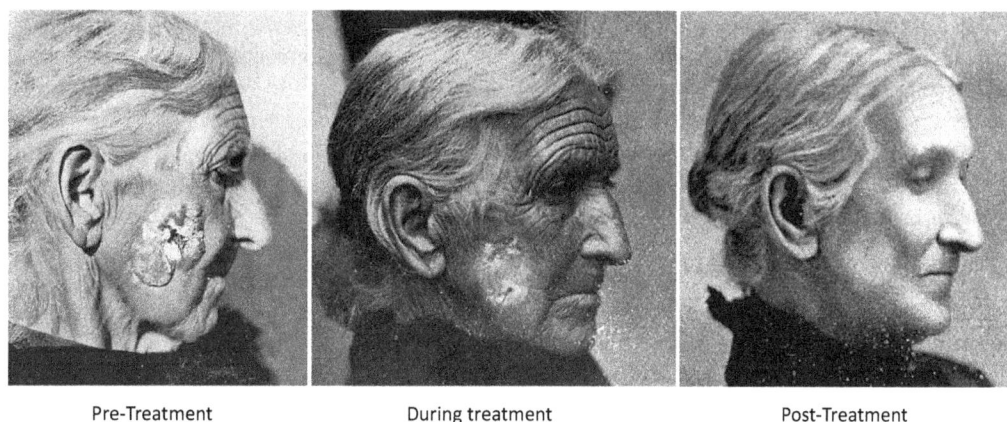

| Pre-Treatment | During treatment | Post-Treatment |

FIGURE 2.2 Patient before, during and after radium treatment, 1911 [As adapted from 10].

Nevertheless, polonium and other alpha-emitting radionuclides had an important part to play in establishing the ability to create artificial radiation with implications for the subsequent use of cyclotrons and reactors to make diagnostic and therapeutic radioisotopes as described below.

2.4 ADVANCES IN PHYSICS IN THE 1930S

Marie and Pierre Curie had two daughters, Irène, born in 1897, and Ève, born in 1904. Irène grew to follow in her parents' footsteps and pursued a career in physics at the University of Paris. In 1926, she married her colleague and co-investigator, Frédéric Joliot. In the following 10 years, Irène and Frédéric Joliot-Curie studied the effects of nuclear bombardment as were several other physicists of the time. These experiments could have possibly garnered them any one of three Nobel prizes.

In 1930, Bothe and Becker had demonstrated the emission of intense radiation when beryllium was bombarded by alpha particles. It was assumed at that time that this was high-energy gamma radiation. Early in 1932, the Joliot-Curies demonstrated that bombarding materials with this new radiation could lead to the emission of protons. However, later in that year, it was Sir James Chadwick who showed that this radiation consisted of neutrally charged particles, neutrons, for the discovery of which he was awarded the 1935 Nobel Prize in Physics [14].

In 1932, Carl Anderson, a postdoctoral fellow at the California Institute of Technology at the time, was obtaining photographs of cosmic-ray tracks inside a Wilson cloud chamber. During these experiments, he acquired several photographs of tracks resulting from a yet to be identified particle with the same positive charge as a proton but with a mass close to that of an electron. He referred to these particles as positive electrons, or "positrons" for short [15]. Although the initial photographs resulted from cosmic rays, he later used the bombardment of high-energy gamma rays from ^{208}Tl on a variety of materials to produce positrons via the process now known as pair production. For this work, Anderson, along with Victor Hess, was awarded the 1936 Nobel Prize in Physics.

In 1932, the Joliot-Curies were using the gamma rays from polonium to bombard a variety of materials, and in these experiments identified the production of both neutrons and positrons at about the same time as Chadwick and Anderson. Perhaps because they did not understand the importance of these discoveries, they did not report on these results in a timely fashion. However, they were the first to calculate an accurate estimate of the mass of the neutron.

In a similar experiment in January 1934, they bombarded aluminum with the alpha particles from polonium. They noted the prompt emission of neutrons. However, they also noticed that there was an emission of positrons over time with a half-life of about 2.5 minutes. They surmised that they had actually produced a new radioactive material that was now decaying via positron decay. The alpha irradiation of ^{27}Al had led to ^{30}P via an alpha-neutron (α,n) reaction which then decayed to ^{30}Si with the emission of the positron with the noted 2.5 min half-life. Whereas Irène's parents along with Becquerel had demonstrated the existence of naturally occurring radioactivity with the nuclides of uranium, thorium, polonium and radium, the Joliot-Curies had demonstrated the ability to artificially produce radioactivity leading to the potential use of many radionuclides for a variety of purposes including medicine. In their article published in 1934, they discussed the production of ^{13}N and ^{27}Si as well as ^{30}P [16]. For their work, the Joliot-Curies were awarded the 1935 Nobel Prize in Chemistry.

In 1928, Ernest Lawrence moved to the University of California at Berkeley after receiving his PhD from Yale in 1925 for his work on the photoelectric effect. While spending the summer in Schenectady, NY, he was introduced to engineers and physicists at General Electric who were investigating better approaches to accelerate electrons with high energy to produce X-rays. Like many physicists at the time, Lawrence was interested in generating charged particles such as protons with high energy. Since he was looking for a means to keep the acceleration as compact as possible, he was interested in the work of Rolf Widerøe who described a circular accelerator of charged particles [17]. Lawrence investigated the possibility of constraining the orbit of the charged particles by means of a uniform magnetic field while cycling the polarity of electrodes to provide nudges in energy in each half orbit. It turned out that the time for the charged particle to orbit was constant irrespective of its radius and thus its energy. Therefore, the switching frequency could be kept constant as the particle was being accelerated. This was basis of the particle accelerator that was to become known as the "cyclotron".

The first cyclotron designed in 1931 by Lawrence and his graduate student, Stanley Livingston, had a diameter of about 4.5 inches and accelerated hydrogen ions to an energy of about 80 eV [18]. A few years later, Lawrence and his team built a 27-inch version, and, by 1939, a 60-inch cyclotron had been constructed that could accelerate both hydrogen ions and deuterons to energies in excess of the nucleon binding energies. For his groundbreaking work, Lawrence was awarded the 1939 Nobel Prize in Physics. Early in Lawrence's experiments with the cyclotron, it had been observed that stray radiation was being produced. Only after the reports by the Joliot-Curies was it demonstrated that this was the result of the production of artificial radioactivity by the device. As a result, the cyclotron became a common method for the production of a number of artificially produced radionuclides. In 1939, Lawrence discussed the construction of a medical cyclotron at Crocker Radiation Laboratories [19].

2.5 SAUL HERTZ AND THE BIRTH OF RADIOIODINE THERAPY

In November 1936, Dr. Saul Hertz, the head of the Thyroid Unit at the Massachusetts General Hospital (MGH), attended a Harvard Medical School faculty luncheon with Dr. Howard Means, the chief of internal medicine at MGH. The invited speaker was Dr. Karl Compton, the president of the Massachusetts Institute of Technology (MIT). His lecture was entitled "What Physics Can Do for Biology and Medicine". It seems likely that Compton discussed the recent work of the Joliet-Curies and Enrico Fermi, as Dr. Hertz asked Compton if iodine could be made radioactive artificially [20].

Hertz's question was asked on the background of decades of prior scientific advances demonstrating a critical role of iodine in thyroid function. In the early 1800s, Robert Graves and others described cases of hypermetabolism, exophthalmos associated with diffuse enlargement of the thyroid gland (goiter), and the syndrome of toxic diffuse goiter became known as Graves' disease, although the underlying mechanism of disease was not understood [21]. Throughout most of the 19th century, the importance of iodine in thyroid function was unclear, and the role of iodine deficiency and the potential efficacy of iodine supplementation to treat or prevent endemic goiter remained controversial [22]. In 1896, Eugen Bauman reported that the thyroid gland contained high levels of iodinated protein, which he termed thyroiodine, and that oral administration of thyroiodine could reverse myxedema, the clinical symptoms of severe hypothyroidism [23]. In 1914, Edward Kendall crystallized and isolated thyroxine [24]. In subsequent years, O.P. Kimball and David Marine clearly demonstrated that iodine supplementation could treat and prevent endemic goiter in schoolgirls in Akron, OH [25]. Thus, a key role of iodine in thyroid function was confirmed.

In December 1936, a month after the faculty luncheon, Compton wrote to Hertz informing him that iodine indeed could be produced artificially radioactive and described what would now be recognized as the isotope ^{128}I, which decays primarily by beta decay with a half-life of 25 minutes. In his response to Compton's letter, Hertz wrote that he thought that radioactive iodine would be "a useful method of therapy in cases of over-activity of the thyroid gland", the first known expression of the concept of targeted radionuclide therapy. At MIT, ^{128}I was produced in the laboratory of Professor Robley Evans, using a radium-beryllium neutron source to irradiate "cold" ^{127}I, a technique first developed in the laboratory of Enrico Fermi [26]. A collaboration was established between the MIT and MGH groups, and Evans assigned Arthur Roberts to work with Hertz. Using tracer quantities of ^{128}I, Hertz and Roberts performed the first of a series of biokinetics studies of radioiodine in rabbits. These studies confirmed preferential uptake of iodine in the thyroid gland and demonstrated increased uptake of iodine in stimulated hyperplastic thyroid glands [27].

The work of Hertz and Roberts was limited by the small quantities and short half-life of ^{128}I. Further research and any attempt to use radioiodine as a therapeutic agent depended on advances in artificial radionuclide production made possible by the cyclotron developed by Lawrence and his group at Berkeley. In the mid-1930s, the Lawrence group, in collaboration with Enrico Fermi in Italy, recognized that the high-energy particles (in particular, protons) created by the cyclotron could be used to produce artificial radioactive elements in larger quantities than possible with small benchtop neutron sources. In addition, a different array of radioelements could be produced when targets were bombarded with high energy protons, rather than neutrons. Drs. Joseph Hamilton and Mayo Soley, collaborating with Lawrence, used a mixture of ^{130}I and ^{131}I produced in the cyclotron to perform tracer studies of iodine in humans, and demonstrated high uptake and retention of iodine in patients with Graves' disease, although they did not provide a quantitated assessment of uptake [28].

The Lawrence group already had administered therapeutic doses of a radionuclide to human patients, with the non-targeted intravenous administration of phosphorus-32 (^{32}P) to patients with leukemia. John Lawrence, brother of Ernest and a physician, had first given ^{32}P to a patient diagnosed with chronic myelogenous leukemia on November 28, 1938. This resulted in transient bone marrow suppression, and, after two additional doses of ^{32}P, the patient appeared to be in clinical remission. By mid-1940, John Lawrence had treated five patients with different forms of leukemia with ^{32}P. Early results were modest as ^{32}P was not curative for acute leukemia [29]. However, at the same time, cytotoxic chemotherapeutic agents were becoming available, with outcomes somewhat similar to ^{32}P therapy. Oncologists quickly came to favor the use of cytotoxic chemotherapy, as they could administer chemotherapy without training, licensure, or regulatory oversight, and the use of non-targeted ^{32}P fell into disfavor [30].

In 1940, the MGH and MIT collaborators received funding from the Markel Foundation to purchase and install a 42-inch cyclotron in Cambridge, MA to be used primarily for medical use. Using the mixture of ^{130}I and ^{131}I produced by the new cyclotron, Hertz and Roberts performed human studies and quantified high levels of radioiodine uptake (up to 80%) and retention in the thyroid glands of patients with Graves' disease [31]. Based on these results, on March 31, 1941, Hertz and Roberts administered the first therapeutic dose of radioactive iodine to a female patient with hyperthyroidism. A second dose of radioactive iodine was administered on April 16, 1941. After therapy, the patient's basal metabolic rate (the standard measure of the time for thyroid function) decreased, indicating a response to therapy. Over the next two years, Hertz and Roberts treated a total of 29 patients with hyperthyroidism, of which 20 were considered clinically to have been cured. Hertz and Roberts reported their early first in human radionuclide therapy at the annual meeting of the American Society for Clinical Investigation in May 1942. At the same meeting, Hamilton and Soley reported on their therapeutic administration of radioiodine for hyperthyroidism, starting in October 1941 [32]. In 1942, Hertz and Roberts also began investigating the uptake of radioiodine in patients with thyroid cancer.

In 1943, in the middle of World War II, Dr. Hertz was granted a military leave of absence from the MGH and joined the U.S. Navy at the rank of Commander. With his departure, Dr. Earl Chapman was appointed director of the Thyroid Unit at the MGH. At the end of the war, Hertz was not welcomed back to the MGH and instead joined the medical staff of the Beth Israel Hospital in Boston. He soon became aware that Chapman and Evans had submitted a manuscript describing their use of radioiodine to treat 22 patients with hyperthyroidism during Hertz's absence [33]. Hertz and Roberts quickly submitted a manuscript describing their earlier experience with the therapeutic use of radioactive iodine, with 22 of 29 patients becoming euthyroid. Both articles were published in May 1946 in the *Journal of the American Medical Association* [34,35]. That same year, Hertz facilitated the delivery of radioiodine from the MIT cyclotron to Montefiore Hospital in New York City, where Dr. Samuel Seidlin and his group performed the first therapeutic administration of radioiodine to patients with metastatic thyroid cancer. They reported their experience with 23 thyroid cancer patients in December 1946, also in the *Journal of the American Medical Association* [36].

With transfer of control of nuclear energy and radioisotope production in the United States from military to civilian control under the Atomic Energy Act of 1946, distribution of reactor-produced radionuclides for medical use, including ^{131}I, became feasible and widespread [37]. Hertz and others saw the potential for the therapeutic use of radionuclides, and in September 1947, Hertz was one of 19 physicians and scientists who presented at a symposium on the use of radioisotopes held at the University of Wisconsin [38]. Drs. Hertz and Seidlin co-founded the Radio Isotope Research Institute, based in Boston and New York, with the goal of using radioisotopes for the treatment of thyroid disease, including thyroid cancer, as well as other malignancies. Unfortunately, Hertz had little opportunity to advance the use of radioisotope therapy before dying of a heart attack in 1950 [20]. He also missed the chance of seeing the uptake of radiopharmaceuticals in the tissues being targeted, the second component of the theranostic paradigm.

2.6 RADIONUCLIDE THERAPY SINCE SAUL HERTZ, THERANOSTICS AND THE FUTURE

The therapeutic value of ^{131}I in treating thyroid disorders, particularly thyroid cancer, led William Beierwaltes of the University of Michigan to postulate that it might have efficacy in treating other endocrine disorders if appropriately complexed to targeting molecules [39]. This led to the development of ^{131}I meta-iodobenzylguanidine (MIBG), which had proven efficacy in these conditions [40–42]. This agent remains in use for the treatment of metastatic paraganglioma, pheochromocytoma, and neuroblastoma with high specific activity ^{131}I having been recently approved for use as an alternative to peptide receptor radionuclide therapy (PRRT), which will be further discussed below [43]. The University of Michigan group also radioiodinated a cholesterol precursor for the imaging of adrenocortical carcinoma but this was not used therapeutically [44]. An alternative agent, ^{131}I iodometomidate has been evaluated therapeutically for adrenocortical carcinoma and a newer agent with higher retention looks promising, but requires further evaluation in larger series [45,46].

The ease with which biomolecules can be radioiodinated has led to several other forms of radionuclide therapy. A logical extension of the development of monoclonal antibodies directed against antigenic targets expressed on various malignant blood cells and the high radiosensitivity of these cells was the development of ^{131}I anti-CD20 monoclonal antibodies [47]. The original iteration of this therapy was a murine antibody, tositumomab, but subsequent studies were performed with a chimeric antibody, ^{131}I rituximab [48]. This approach has also been applied using other radionuclides. Yttrium-90 (^{90}Y)-ibritumomab tiuxetan [49,50] and ^{177}Lu-DOTA-rituximab [51] are examples of this.

Also harking back to the historical development of radionuclides, ^{89}Sr, which had been investigated as a calcium analogue by Charles Pecher in the 1940s and found to provide significant relief of bone pain [52], was resurrected for treatment in the late 1980s [53] and was widely used in the treatment of metastatic prostate cancer through the 1990s, until largely being replaced as effective chemotherapeutic regimens and second-line androgen blocking drugs became available. Nevertheless, a randomized control trial did demonstrate a significant reduction in prostate-specific antigen (PSA) and prolonged event-free survival compared to hemi-body radiotherapy [54]. The success of this agent stimulated the investigation of other bone-seeking radiopharmaceuticals. [153]Sm EDTMP had the advantage of a shorter physical half-life and an imageable gamma emission that allowed dosimetry, which is useful in mitigating bone marrow toxicity [55,56]. [186]Re HEDP was also shown to be an effective palliative agent with possible antitumor efficacy [57]. [188]Re, which is a generator-produced radionuclide, has also been labeled to HEDP and shown to have dosimetric potential [58]. These beta-emitting radionuclides were used as a palliative therapy with a single cycle typically being administered. However, these agents were subsequently supplanted by alpha-emitting [223]Ra on the strength of the randomized control ALSYMPCA trial that demonstrated an overall survival advantage [59]. (See Chapter 8 for trial details.) It should be noted that this agent was administered over multiple cycles of treatment. Given the success of ^{177}Lu-based radionuclides, studies are ongoing using ^{177}Lu bisphosphonates [60].

The success of the theranostic paradigm in recent years has been driven by PRRT for neuroendocrine neoplasia and therapy based on prostate-specific membrane antigen (PSMA) for prostate cancer. PRRT grew out of the translation of ^{125}I autoradiography of somatostatin receptors to imaging with an ^{131}I somatostatin analogue [61]. Improved imaging characteristics of agents labeled with ^{111}In led to the Erasmus Medical Centre using a very high administered activity therapeutically in the case of a functioning metastatic pancreatic neuroendocrine tumor (NET) [62]. This demonstrated the stabilization of previously progressive disease and marked reduction in hormonal secretion. This stimulated larger studies [63] and combination of this Auger electron emitting radionuclide with chemotherapy [64]. However, objective responses were modest and led to the investigation of both ^{90}Y and ^{177}Lu agents with higher objective response rates, excellent disease control rates, and limited toxicity [65]. Most of these studies were retrospective and weren't widely accepted by the medical oncology community or regulatory authorities. This changed with the publication of the NETTER-1 randomized control trial of ^{177}Lu-DOTA-octreotate versus high-dose long-acting octreotide [66] which led to the approval of this agent in many countries. In addition to its efficacy in low-grade NET, studies have indicated effectiveness in higher grade NET [67], and in other tumor types including paraganglioma/pheochromocytoma [68] and neuroblastoma [69] (Chapter 8 also describes this trial).

PSMA is significantly overexpressed in metastatic castrate-resistant prostate cancer. The first agents to be developed were based on monoclonal antibodies developed in New York by the group of Neil Bander and Scott Tagawa [70,71]. This agent is now in multicenter trials as ^{177}Lu-J591 and a related radiopharmaceutical labeled with the alpha-emitter [225]Ac, J592, is also being evaluated. Pioneering studies were performed at the University of Heidelberg in developing both diagnostic and therapeutic small molecule ligands for this target with evidence of efficacy [72,73]. The first prospective trial of ^{177}Lu-PSMA-617 was performed at the Peter MacCallum Cancer Centre in Melbourne [74,75] and was followed by larger prospective multicenter trials including the randomized phase II TheraP and phase III VISION trials, which led to the regulatory approval of this agent [76,77].

The success of these theranostic paradigms with the diagnostic tracers becoming part of routine clinical evaluation and multiple trials evaluating whether the indications for use of the therapeutic agents can be brought earlier in the treatment pathway has led to very significant investment in the development of novel radiopharmaceuticals for both these and other targets. The topic of future theranostics is so vast that it is difficult to do it justice in the context of a historical review, but it would be remiss not to mention the emergence of exciting diagnostic/therapeutic pairs including ^{64}Cu/^{67}Cu and ^{203}Pb/^{212}Pb as PET/beta and SPECT/alpha agents, respectively, terbium-161 (^{161}Tb) as a combined beta and Auger emitter, and fibroblast activating protein as one of the most exciting pan-cancer targets identified in recent times.

^{64}Cu is a positron-emitting radionuclide with a 12.7 hour half-life that is sufficient to allow multiple timepoint imaging beyond 24 hours and, thereby, prospective dosimetry. It has been evaluated as the diagnostic pair of ^{67}Cu, a beta-emitting radionuclide, for NET [78,79] and PSMA theranostics [80,81]. These agents are now in phase II trials internationally.

^{203}Pb is suitable for SPECT imaging, while ^{212}Pb is a generator produced alpha-emitter with a half-life of 10.6 hours, making it potentially an ideal agent for radiopharmaceuticals with rapid, high, and specific uptake even if accompanied by relatively low retention. It is, however, only one of a palette of alpha-emitting radionuclides that are under investigation [82]. Interestingly, ^{212}Pb was one of the tracers that von Hevesy first applied in his development of the tracer dilution method, and the subject of another amusing historical vignette [83]. He was reported to have spiked his meal scraps with this radionuclide and proved that his boarding house was recycling leftovers.

The high linear energy transfer (LET) of alpha particles, imparting up to 400-fold DNA damage than beta-emitters, is attractive in controlling disease that is refractory to approved ^{177}Lu-based agents. However, there is concern regarding their greater toxicity to normal cells that might express the same target and their limited particle range may fail to deal with microscopic heterogeneity in target expression. ^{161}Tb has the advantages of beta-particle crossfire effect plus the presence of a high LET Auger electron that has theoretical advantages in controlling microscopic disease foci but lower toxicity than alphas due to lower tissue penetrance and offers a promising alternative to ^{177}Lu [84].

There is great excitement in the nuclear medicine community about fibroblast activating protein (FAP) as a pan-cancer target for theranostics given the very low uptake in most normal tissues [85]. A challenge for therapeutic applications of small molecule inhibitors (FAPI) has been their relatively low tissue residence time. However, various approaches are being applied to overcome these issues, including medicinal chemistry approaches and use of short half-life radionuclides. This might include the very same radionuclide, ^{212}Pb, that von Hevesy spiked his Sunday roast leftovers with more than a century ago.

2.7 CONCLUSION

The emergence of therapeutic nuclear medicine owes a great debt to its pioneers across many scientific domains. It has always benefited from, and leveraged, advances in physics, instrumentation, and chemistry, as well as medicine. Now, just over 125 years since the discovery of radioactivity, we remain dependent on advances in these fields, but the convergent science that is nuclear medicine is also being driven by advances in genomics, molecular biology, and computational sciences. The ability to not only treat what we can see, the essence of theranostics, but also combine multiple datapoints to select and prescribe an optimal treatment regimen for a given patient will respect and build on the legacy of the pioneers described above, and many others who we either knowingly or unwittingly have omitted. The advances will potentially see radionuclide therapy combined with other therapies to increase its efficacy and effect cures, just as radioiodine therapy still does.

REFERENCES

1. Hertz S, and Roberts A. Radioactive iodine in the study of thyroid physiology: VII. The use of radioactive iodine therapy in hyperthyroidism. *J Amer Med Assoc*, 1946. 131, 81–86.
2. Pattison DA, Solomon B, and Hicks RJ. A new theranostic paradigm for advanced thyroid cancer. *J Nucl Med*, 2016. 57, 1493–1494.

3. Röntgen WCF. On a new kind of rays. *Science*, 1896. 3(59), 227–231.
4. Becquerel H. Biographical. NobelPrize.org. Nobel Prize Outreach AB 2023. Wed. 25 Jan 2023. https://www.nobelprize.org/prizes/physics/1903/becquerel/biographical/ Retrieved 28-01-2023.
5. Curie P. Nobel Lecture. NobelPrize.org. Nobel Prize Outreach AB 2023. Wed. 25 Jan 2023. https://www.nobelprize.org/prizes/physics/1903/pierre-curie/lecture/ Retrieved 28-01-2023.
6. Blaufox, MD. Becquerel and the discovery of radioactivity: early concepts. *Semin Nucl Med*, 1999. 26(3), 145–154.
7. Becquerel H, and Curie P. Comptes Rendus Hebdomadaires des Seances de L'Academie des Sciences, 1901. 132, 1289.
8. Brucer, M. *A Chronology of Nuclear Medicine*, St. Louis, Robert R. Butaine, 1990, 101.
9. *Marie Curie and the Science of Radioactivity*. https://history.aip.org/exhibits/curie/radinst2.htm Retrieved 28-01-2023.
10. Lawrence H. *Radium: How and When to Use. Melbourne Stillwell and Co*, 1911.
11. Cipriani C, DeSantis M, Dahlhoff G et al. Personalized irradiation therapy for NMSC by rhenium-188 skin cancer therapy: a long-term retrospective study. *J Dermatolog Treat*, 2022, 33(2), 969–975.
12. Blaufox MD. Radioactive artifacts: historical sources of modern radium contamination. *Semin Nucl Med*, 1988. 18(1), 46–64.
13. Skloot R. *The Immortal Life of Henrietta Lacks*, New York, Crown Publisher, 2010.
14. Chadwick J. The Nobel Prize in Physics 1935. https://www.nobelprize.org/prizes/physics/1935/chadwick/facts/ Retrieved 28-01-2023.
15. Anderson CD. The positive electron. *Phys Rev*, 1933, 43(6), 491–494.
16. Joliot F, and Curie I. Artificial production of a new kind of radio-element. *Nature*, 1934, 133, 201–202.
17. Widerøe R (December 17, 1928). Ueber Ein Neues Prinzip Zur Herstellung Hoher Spannungen. *Arch Elektron Übertrag*, 1928. 21(4), 387–406 (in German).
18. Lawrence EO, and Cooksey D. On the apparatus for the multiple acceleration of light ions to high speeds. *Phys Rev*, 1936, 50, 1131.
19. Seaborg GTE. *EO Lawrence – Physicist, Engineer, Statesman of Science. Science*, 1958. 128, 1123–1124.
20. Fahey FH, and Grant FD. Celebrating eighty years of radionuclide therapy and the work of Saul Hertz. *J Appl Clin Medic Phys*, 2021. 22, 4–10.
21. Graves RJ. Clinical lectures delivered at the Meath Hospital during the session 1834–1835. Lecture XII: Dr. Graves's lectures: newly observed affection of the thyroid gland. *London Med Surg*, 1835. 7, 516–517.
22. Zimmerman MB. Research on iodine deficiency and goiter in the 19th and early 20th centuries. *J Nutrit*, 2008. 138, 2060–2063.
23. Bauman F. Ueber das normale vorkommen vod jod in thierkorper. *Z Physiol Chem*, 1896. 21, 319–330 (In German).
24. Kendall ED. The isolation in crystalline form of the compound containing iodin, which occurs in the thyroid. *J Am Med Assoc*, 1915. 64, 2042–2043.
25. Kimball OP, and Marine D. Prevention of simple goiter in man. 2nd paper. *J Lab Clin Med*, 1917. 3(1), 40–49.
26. Fermi E. Radioactivity induced by neutron bombardment. *Nature*, 1934. 133, 757.
27. Hertz S, Roberts A, and Evans RD. Radioactive iodine as an indicator in the study of thyroid physiology. *Proc Soc Exper Biol Med*, 1938. 38, 9915P.
28. Hamilton JG, and Soley MH. Studies in iodine metabolism of the thyroid gland in situ by the use of radio-iodine in normal subjects and in patients with various types of goiter. *Am J Physiol*, 1939. 127, 557.
29. Lawrence JH. Nuclear physics and therapy: preliminary report on a new method for the treatment of leukemia and polycythemia. *Radiology*, 194, 35, 51–60.
30. Brucer M. John Lawrence treats the first ^{32}P patient. In *A Chronology of Nuclear Medicine* Brucer M ed. Robert R. Butaine, St. Louis, 1990, pp. 225–226.
31. Hertz S, Roberts A, and Salter WT. Radioactive iodine as an indicator in thyroid physiology. IV. The metabolism of iodine in Graves disease. *J Clin Invest*, 1942. 21, 25–29.
32. Low-Beer BVA, Lawrence JH, and Stone RS. The therapeutic use of artificially produced radioactive substances. *Radiology*, 1942. 39, 573–597.
33. Fahey FH, Grant FD, and Thrall JH. Saul Hertz MD, and the birth of radionuclide therapy. *EJNMMI Phys*, 2017. 4, 15.

34. Hertz S, Roberts A. Radioactive iodine in the study of thyroid physiology. VII. The use of radioactive iodine therapy in Graves' disease. *J Am Med Assoc*. 1946, 131, 81–86.
35. Chapman EM, Evans RD. The treatment of hyperthyroidism with radioactive iodine. *J Am Med Assoc*, 1946. 131, 86–91.
36. Seidlin S, Marinelli L, and Oshry E. Radioactive iodine therapy: effect on functioning metastases of adenocarcinoma of the thyroid. *J Am Med Assoc*, 1946. 132, 838–847.
37. Availability of radioactive isotopes. *Science*, 1946. 103, 697–705.
38. Zirkle RE. A symposium on the use of isotopes in biology and medicine (book review). *Science*, 1949. 109, 70.
39. Haynie TP, Nofal MM, and Beierwaltes WH. Treatment of thyroid carcinoma with I-131. Results at fourteen years. *J Am Med Assoc*, 1963, 183, 303–306.
40. Shapiro B, Sisson JC, Eyre P et al. ^{131}I-MIBG – a new agent in diagnosis and treatment of pheochromocytoma. *Cardiology*. 1985. 72(1), 137–142.
41. Hutchinson RJ, Sisson JC, Miser JS et al. Long-term results of [131I]metaiodobenzylguanidine treatment of refractory advanced neuroblastoma. *J Nucl Biol Med*, 1991. 35(4), 237–240.
42. Shapiro B, Sisson JC, Wieland DM et al. Radiopharmaceutical therapy of malignant pheochromocytoma with [131I]metaiodobenzylguanidine: results from ten years of experience. *J Nucl Biol Med*, 1991. 35(4), 269–276.
43. Jha A, Taïeb D, Carrasquillo JA et al. High-specific-activity-131I-MIBG vs ^{177}Lu-DOTATATE based peptide receptor radionuclide therapy: an evolving conundrum in targeted radionuclide therapy of metastatic pheochromocytoma and paraganglioma. *Clin Cancer Res*, 2021. 27(11), 2989–2995.
44. Beierwaltes WH, Sisson JC, and Shapiro B. Diagnosis of adrenal tumors with radionuclide imaging. *Spec Top Endocrinol Metab*, 1984, 6, 1–54.
45. Hahner S, Kreissl MC, Fassnacht M et al. [131I]iodometomidate for targeted radionuclide therapy of advanced adrenocortical carcinoma. *J Clin Endocrinol Metab*, 2012. 97(3), 914–922.
46. Hahner S, Hartrampf PE, Mihatsch PW et al. Targeting 11-beta hydroxylase with [131I]IMAZA: a novel approach for the treatment of advanced adrenocortical carcinoma. *J Clin Endocrinol Metab*, 2022. 107(4), e1348–e1355.
47. Kaminski MS, Zasadny KR, Francis IR et al. Iodine-131-anti-B1 radioimmunotherapy for B-cell lymphoma. *J Clin Oncol*, 1996. 14(7), 1974–1981.
48. Leahy MF, Seymour JF, Hicks RJ, and Turner JH. Multicenter phase II clinical study of iodine-131-rituximab radioimmunotherapy in relapsed or refractory indolent non-Hodgkin's lymphoma. *J Clin Oncol*, 2006. 24(27), 4418–4425.
49. Wiseman GA, White CA, Witzig TE et al. Radioimmunotherapy of relapsed non-Hodgkin's lymphoma with zevalin, a ^{90}Y-labeled anti-CD20 monoclonal antibody. *Clin Cancer Res*, 1999. 5(10) Suppl:3281s–3286s.
50. Witzig TE, White CA, Wiseman GA et al. Phase I/II trial of IDEC-Y2B8 radioimmunotherapy for treatment of relapsed or refractory CD20(+) B-cell non-Hodgkin's lymphoma. *J Clin Oncol*, 1999. 17(12), 3793–3803.
51. Forrer F, Oechslin-Oberholzer C, Campana B et al. Radioimmunotherapy with ^{177}Lu-DOTA-rituximab: final results of a phase I/II Study in 31 patients with relapsing follicular, mantle cell, and other indolent B-cell lymphomas. *J Nucl Med*, 2013. 54(7), 1045–1052.
52. Pecher C. Biological investigations with radioactive calcium and strontium. Preliminary report on the use of radioactive strontium in the treatment of metastatic bone cancer. *Univ Calif Pub Pharmacol*, 1942. 11, 117–139.
53. Reddy EK, Robinson RG, and Mansfield CM. Strontium-89 for palliation of bone metastases. *J Natl Med Assoc*, 1986. 78(1), 27–32.
54. Porter AT, and McEwan AJ. Strontium-89 as an adjuvant to external beam radiation improves pain relief and delays disease progression in advanced prostate cancer: results of a randomized controlled trial. *Semin Oncol*, 1993. 20(3) Suppl 2:38–43.
55. Cameron PJ, Klemp PF, Martindale AA, and Turner JH. Prospective [153]Sm-EDTMP therapy dosimetry by whole-body scintigraphy. *Nucl Med Commun*, 1999. 20(7), 609–615.
56. Turner JH, Claringbold PG, Hetherington EL et al. A phase I study of samarium-153 ethylenediaminetetramethylene phosphonate therapy for disseminated skeletal metastases. *J Clin Oncol*, 1989. 7(12), 1926–1931.
57. Liepe K, Hliscs R, Kropp J et al. Rhenium-188-HEDP in the palliative treatment of bone metastases. *Cancer Biother Radiopharm*, 2000. 15(3), 261–265.

58. Liepe K, Hliscs R, Kropp J et al. Dosimetry of [188]Re-hydroxyethylidene diphosphonate in human prostate cancer skeletal metastases. *J Nucl Med*, 2003, 44(6), 953–960.

59. Parker C, Nilsson S, Heinrich D et al. Alpha emitter radium-223 and survival in metastatic prostate cancer. *N Engl J Med*, 2013. 369(3), 213–223.

60. Yadav MP, Ballal S, Meckel M et al. [177Lu] Lu-DOTA-ZOL bone pain palliation in patients with skeletal metastases from various cancers: efficacy and safety results. *EJNMMI Res*, 2020. 10(1), 130.

61. Lamberts SW, Reubi JC, Bakker WH, and Krenning EP. Somatostatin receptor imaging with ^{123}I-Tyr3-octreotide. *Z Gastroenterol*, 1990, 28 (2), 20–21.

62. Krenning EP, Kooij PP, Bakker WH et al. Radiotherapy with a radiolabeled somatostatin analogue, [111In-DTPA-D-Phe1]-octreotide. A case history. *Ann N Y Acad Sci*, 1994. 733, 496–506.

63. Krenning EP, Kooij PP, Pauwels S et al. Somatostatin receptor: scintigraphy and radionuclide therapy. *Digestion*, 1996. 57 (1), 57–61.

64. Kong G, Johnston V, Ramdave S et al. High-administered activity In-111 octreotide therapy with concomitant radiosensitizing 5FU chemotherapy for treatment of neuroendocrine tumors: preliminary experience. *Cancer Biother Radiopharm*, 2009. 24(5), 527–533.

65. Hicks RJ, Kwekkeboom DJ, Krenning E et al. ENETS consensus guidelines for the standards of care in neuroendocrine neoplasia: peptide receptor radionuclide therapy with radiolabeled somatostatin analogues. *Neuroendocrinology*, 2017. 105(3), 295–309.

66. Strosberg JR, Wolin EM, Chasen B et al. NETTER-1 phase III: Progression-free survival, radiographic response, and preliminary overall survival results in patients with midgut neuroendocrine tumors treated with 177-Lu-Dotatate. *J Clin Oncol*, 2016. 34 Suppl 4S:abstr.194.

67. Sorbye H, Kong G, and Grozinsky-Glasberg S. PRRT in high-grade gastroenteropancreatic neuroendocrine neoplasms (WHO G3). *Endocr Relat Cancer*, 2020. 27(3), R67–R77.

68. Kong G, Grozinsky-Glasberg S, Hofman M et al. Efficacy of peptide receptor radionuclide therapy (PRRT) for functional metastatic paraganglioma and phaeochromocytoma. *J Clin Endocrinol Metab*, 2017. 102(9), 3278–3287.

69. Kong G, Hofman MS, Murray WK et al. Initial experience with Gallium-68 DOTA-octreotate PET/CT and peptide receptor radionuclide therapy for pediatric patients with refractory metastatic neuroblastoma. *J Pediatr Hematol Oncol*, 2016. 38(2), 87–96.

70. Bander NH, Milowsky MI, Nanus DM et al. Phase I trial of [177]lutetium-labeled J591, a monoclonal antibody to prostate-specific membrane antigen, in patients with androgen-independent prostate cancer. *J Clin Oncol*, 2005. 23(21), 4591–4601.

71. Tagawa ST, Milowsky MI, Morris M et al. Phase II study of lutetium-177-labeled anti-prostate-specific membrane antigen monoclonal antibody J591 for metastatic castration-resistant prostate cancer. *Clin Cancer Res,* 2013. 19(18), 5182–5191.

72. Kratochwil C, Bruchertseifer F, Giesel FL et al. [225]Ac-PSMA-617 for PSMA-targeted α-radiation therapy of metastatic castration-resistant prostate cancer. *J Nucl Med*, 2016. 57(12), 1941–1944.

73. Kratochwil C, Giesel FL, Eder M et al. [177Lu]Lutetium-labelled PSMA ligand-induced remission in a patient with metastatic prostate cancer. *Eur J Nucl Med Mol Imaging*, 2015. 42(6), 987–988.

74. Hofman MS, Violet J, Hicks RJ et al. [177Lu]-PSMA-617 radionuclide treatment in patients with metastatic castration-resistant prostate cancer (LuPSMA trial): a single-centre, single-arm, phase 2 study. *Lancet Oncol*, 2018. 19(6), 825–833.

75. Violet J, Sandhu S, Iravani A et al. Long-term follow-up and outcomes of retreatment in an expanded 50-patient single-center phase II prospective trial of ^{177}Lu-PSMA-617 theranostics in metastatic castration-resistant prostate cancer. *J Nucl Med*, 2020. 61(6), 857–865.

76. Hofman MS, Emmett L, Sandhu S et al. [177Lu]Lu-PSMA-617 versus cabazitaxel in patients with metastatic castration-resistant prostate cancer (TheraP). a randomised, open-label, phase 2 trial. *Lancet*, 2021. 397, 797–804.

77. Sartor O, DeBono J, Chi KN et al. Lutetium-177-PSMA-617 for metastatic castration-resistant prostate cancer. *N Engl J Med*, 2021. 385(12), 1091–1103.

78. Cullinane C, Jeffery CM, Roselt PD et al. Peptide receptor radionuclide therapy with (67)Cu-CuSarTATE is highly efficacious against a somatostatin positive neuroendocrine tumor model. *J Nucl Med*, 2020. 61(12), 1800–1805.

79. Hicks RJ, Jackson P, Kong G et al. Cu-SARTATE PET imaging of patients with neuroendocrine tumors demonstrates high tumor uptake and retention, potentially allowing prospective dosimetry for peptide receptor radionuclide therapy. *J Nucl Med*, 2019. 60(6), 777–785.

80. McInnes LE, Cullinane C, Roselt PD et al. Therapeutic efficacy of a bivalent inhibitor of prostate-specific membrane antigen labeled with [67]Cu. *J Nucl Med*, 2021. 62(6), 829–832.

81. Zia NA, Cullinane C, Zuylekom V et al. A bivalent inhibitor of prostate specific membrane antigen radiolabeled with copper-64 with high tumor uptake and retention. *Angew Chem Int Ed Engl*, 2019. 58(42), 14991–14994.

82. Sgouros G. Dosimetry, radiobiology and synthetic lethality: radiopharmaceutical therapy (RPT) with alpha-particle-emitters. *Semin Nucl Med*, 2020. 50(2), 124–132.

83. Myers WG. Georg Charles de Hevesy: the father of nuclear medicine. *J Nucl Med*, 1979. 20(6), 590–594.

84. Baum RP, Singh A, Kulkarni HR et al. First-in-humans application of [161]Tb: a feasibility study using [161]Tb-DOTATOC. *J Nucl Med*, 2021. 62(10), 1391–1397.

85. Hicks RJ, Roselt PJ, Kallur KG et al. FAPI PET/CT: will it end the hegemony of ^{18}F-FDG in oncology? *J Nucl Med*, 2021. 62(3), 296–302.

3 Biological Principles behind Targeted Radionuclide Therapy for Cancer

Ashleigh Hull, Jake Forster, Stephen Tronchin, and Eva Bezak

3.1 A BRIEF INTRODUCTION TO BIOLOGY OF CANCER AND CANCER METASTASIS

According to the World Health Organization (WHO), "cancer is a leading cause of death worldwide, accounting for nearly 10 million deaths in 2020, or nearly one in six deaths"[1]. Cancer disease also represents a major economic burden. For example, "the estimated national expenditures for cancer care in the United States in 2018 were $150.8 billion" [2]. In future years, costs are likely to increase as the population ages and more people will be diagnosed with cancer and as new, more expensive treatments (such as particle therapy) become mainstream. Additionally, reported data show that cancer therapy responses exhibit large patient-to-patient variations irrespective of uniform treatment protocols, being a consequence of stochastic but primarily patient-specific factors. Hence, presently, considerable interest and effort in cancer therapy development are dedicated towards more personalised (or precision) and targeted approaches, including targeted radionuclide therapy (TRNT).

Cancer is a complex disease. The term actually covers a large group of diseases that have an abnormal and uncontrolled growth of cells in common [3]. Cancer can originate in any of the tissues and organs in a body and can also invade the surrounding tissues or spread (i.e., metastasise) to organs distant to its initial location.

If this uncontrolled cell growth occurs in a solid tissue (e.g., muscle, an organ), a tumor will be formed. Solid tumors can broadly be divided into three categories: **benign** (noncancerous and therefore non-invading and generally not life-threatening), **pre-malignant** (this tumor can in time turn malignant if not treated) and **malignant** (cancerous with the potential for tissue invasion). Based on the tissue of origin, tumors can also be categorized as, e.g., **carcinomas** (cancers of the epithelial tissue), sarcomas (bone and soft tissue cancers), **teratomas** (a germ cell origin), **gliomas** (cancers of the glial cells of the brain and nervous system), **melanomas** (cancer of the melanocytes, i.e., the skin cells that produce melanin) and others. Cancers of the blood system do not form solid tumors and are sometimes referred to as liquid cancers. They include **leukaemias** (most commonly, cancers of the white blood cells originating in the bone marrow), **lymphomas** (cancers of the lymphatic system) and **multiple myelomas** (cancers of the plasma cells in the bone marrow).

In general, tumors consist of multiple cell types and tumor stroma, i.e., the supportive framework of a tumor – just like in the case of a healthy organ's stroma. The stroma itself consists of (a) the extracellular matrix (ECM) – a non-cellular component of the stroma made of water, proteins, polysaccharides and others, and (b) stromal cells (fibroblasts and adipocytes), cells of the vascular system and cells of the immune system [4]. The tumor cells themselves vary in phenotype and degrees of differentiation. However, there also exists a subset of tumor cells that are analogous to stem cells in normal tissue. It is these **cancer stem cells** (CSCs), or **cancer clonogens**, that have the ability to self-renew indefinitely and differentiate to form the other cells of the tumor. CSCs are

DOI: 10.1201/9781003250913-4

also more treatment resistant and are responsible for tumor development, progression, metastasis and recurrence [5,6]. Additionally, a supportive microenvironment can provide conditions allowing CSCs to survive in a hypoxic state, rendering them, for example, more resistant to irradiation as the toxicity depends on cellular partial oxygen pressure [7,8].

Why does cancer happen? A simple answer is: cancer happens because of the changes in genes that control the functionality of cells, including their growth and division [9]. There can be numerous reasons for this genetic malfunction to happen, e.g., aging, exposure to harmful substances (including radiation), lifestyle (smoking, obesity), certain viral infections (e.g., human papillomavirus (HPV) positive cancers of cervix or head and neck), heredity and others. The relationship between family history and cancer has been confirmed for several cancers, including prostate and breast cancers [10,11].

And the picture is even more complex as various somatic genetic mutations in different tumors and the associated epigenetic changes (i.e., modifications to DNA that regulate whether certain genes are turned on or off) are highly varied between cancers and this may determine how the disease will evolve over time, including growth, invasiveness, response to therapy. Cancer is therefore also a very **heterogenous disease**.

Despite this high degree of heterogeneity, according to Hanahan and Weinberg [12–14], there are still some essential characteristics that are present in all cancers and are often called **the hallmarks of cancer**. These include [12,13]: (a) genome instability and mutation, (b) tumor promoting inflammation, (c) self-sufficiency in growth signals, (d) insensitivity to antigrowth signals, (e) evasion of apoptosis (the programmed cell death), (f) evasion of immune destruction, (g) sustained angiogenesis, (h) modification of cellular metabolism, (i) limitless replicative potential and (j) tissue invasion and metastasis. Cancer cells can also accelerate their own cell cycle, have increased mobility and have modified their cellular surface, thus changing their sensitivity to the regulating mechanisms of the host [15]. While the changes in the cell membrane (e.g., in proteins, enzymes, cell surface receptors) play an important role in the process of malignization, they also represent a point of differentiation between the normal and the malignant cells and therefore can offer solutions/targets for cancer cell identification and therapy. These changes can include structural changes of proteins and surface receptors, different (increased/decreased) receptor expressions, presence of new surface molecules, etc [15] – i.e., cancer specific surface characteristics that can be utilized in TRNT.

3.1.1 CANCER METASTASIS

The process of cancer metastasis is equally complex and consists of multiple steps, in which highly genetically mutated cancer cells detach from the tumor and its ECM and invade the surrounding tissue locally (i.e., **in situ**) [16]. In the next stage, these cells can infiltrate blood micro-vessels and the lymphatic system and thus be transported to other tissues and organs, a process known as **dissemination** [17]. The penetration of cancer cells inside the capillaries is a complex enzymatic process that depends on tissue vascularization and the enzymatic content of cancer cells. **Extravasation**, or leakage, into the appropriate secondary site, is then followed by the establishment of a new microenvironment to provide blood supply and nutrients. If the migrated cancer cells are able to settle in the new tissue and develop their own supportive microenvironment, they can eventually form a macroscopic metastasis, a process known as **colonization** [12,13]. It is apparent that for a "successful metastasis" the host tissues must have certain favorable characteristics to enable the metastatic process – this is sometimes called the "seed and soil hypothesis" [16–18]. There is evidence that certain cancers have metastases preferentially appearing in particular tissues or organs (e.g., in bones or lungs [19,20]). This is a consequence of the fact that different organs (or the "soils") have biologically unique microenvironments, with some being more pliant towards colonization by certain cancer cell phenotypes than others [16–18]. In addition, the metastasizing cells impact the normal tissue homeostasis (i.e., the self-regulating processes to maintain the tissue's normal functionality) and perturb the normal regulatory dynamics of the invaded tissues [21].

3.1.2 A NOTE ON CANCER THERAPIES

The most common therapies for cancer include surgery, chemotherapy, radiotherapy and immunotherapy, with many of these being used in combination. As a matter of fact, with modern treatment techniques, only a few primary cancers are fatal. It is the disseminated disease that is the primary cause of cancer death [22], requiring systemic treatment approaches to kill not only the metastases but also the circulating cancer cells and micro-metastases. The ability to kill subclinical cancer disease is one of the main challenges. Many current cancer therapies are unable to control metastatic disease and are often associated with insidious toxicities (such as chemotherapy). Additionally, micrometastases may be in the G0 phase (i.e., the resting, non-replicative phase of the cell cycle) and outside the cell cycle; as such these cells are insensitive to chemo and radiotherapy [22]. New targeted therapies are therefore needed that get around the current limitations of targeting and cancer cell toxicity.

Current targeted systemic therapies, among others, include immuno-, inhibitor and monoclonal antibody (mAb) therapies, based on selective targeting of function. However, mAbs are insufficiently toxic and the ongoing cancer mutations defy cure. Many targeting vectors are not toxic to cancer cells at all. At the same time, new advances in radiation oncology and nuclear medicine have led to the development of internal forms of radiation therapy, where the radiation is delivered directly to cells based on their molecular profile. This molecularly targeted radiation therapy, called targeted radionuclide therapy, is **systemic yet localized**, i.e., it can target primary, metastatic or circulating cancer cells relative to their expression of the target receptor. In 2019, the United States National Institute of Health predicted that TRNT will constitute up to 60% of all forms of radiation therapy by 2030, highlighting the high value of TRNT development in the oncology field.

The following sections of this chapter will talk on specific biological aspects of TRNT for treatment of cancer, from targeting mechanisms to specific receptors and delivery of therapy itself.

3.2 TARGETING MECHANISMS IN RADIONUCLIDE THERAPY

A rich variety of targeting mechanisms have been employed in TRNT (Figure 3.1). In the modern theranostics paradigm, the radiopharmaceutical used for TRNT consists of a radiometal that emits betas, alphas or Auger electrons labeled to a targeting vector via a chelator. Examples of chelators are tetraazacyclododecane tetraacetic acid (DOTA) and diethylenetriamine pentaacetate (DTPA). The targeting vector targets and binds to a cell surface receptor (a membrane or transmembrane receptor) overexpressed on target cells. The biodistribution and uptake of the radiopharmaceutical are intended to be dictated by the targeting vector alone, independent of the radionuclide. Consequently, the therapeutic radionuclide can be interchanged for a different radiometal suitable for diagnostic imaging for the purpose of patient screening.

TRNTs that use the radiometal-chelator-vector template can be classified according to the nature of the targeting vector.

3.2.1 RADIOLIGAND THERAPY

In radioligand therapy (RLT), a radiolabeled ligand targets a receptor overexpressed on cancer cells. Although RLT technically includes antibody ligands, these are discussed separately in the next section. The performance of the ligand is assessed in terms of its biokinetics (tumor and organ uptake, clearance rate, and clearance pathway), tissue penetration, receptor binding efficiency, persistence of the receptor–ligand complex, and whether the complex is internalized. When a ligand binds to a receptor, a possible outcome is that the receptor is agonized or antagonized, and molecular signalling effects result from activating or blocking the target receptor.

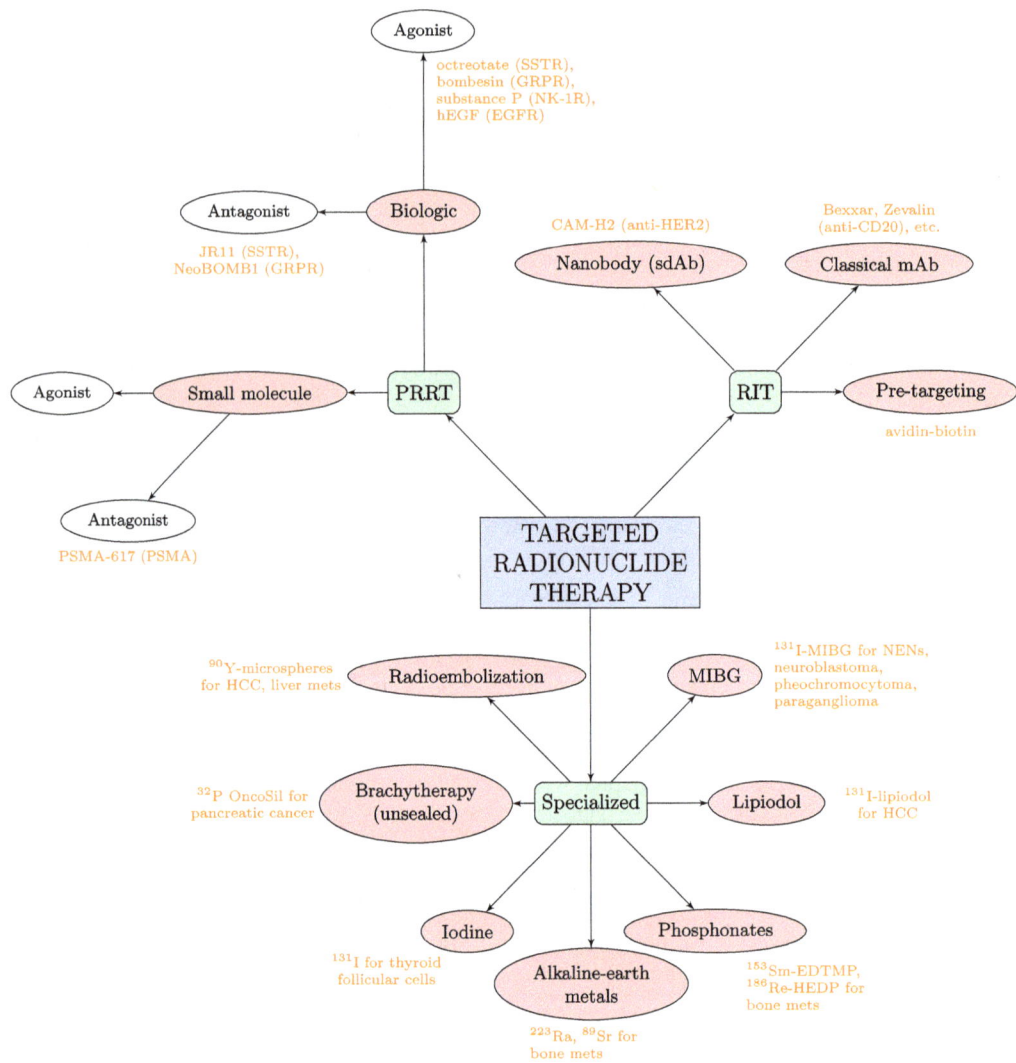

FIGURE 3.1   A flow diagram showing the various targeting mechanisms utilized in radionuclide therapy.

The ligand in RLT may be a protein, which is relatively large. For example, the epidermal growth factor receptor (EGFR) is overexpressed by a variety of cancers (lung, head and neck, colon, pancreas, breast, ovary, bladder and kidney) and can be targeted with human epidermal growth factor (hEGF). When hEGF binds to EGFR, EGFR is agonized, and the receptor–ligand complex is internalized. EGFR is recognized as an oncogene, with its activation associated with cell proliferation, so agonizing this receptor may not be desirable. In a phase I trial, hEGF was radiolabeled with the Auger-emitter ^{111}In (^{111}In-DTPA-hEGF) for the treatment of metastatic EGFR-positive breast cancer [23].

Peptide receptor radionuclide therapy (PRRT) is a kind of RLT in which the target receptor is a peptide receptor. Peptides are generally smaller than proteins and can be chemically synthesized. For example, neuorendocrine tumors (NETs) overexpress somatostatin receptors (SSTR), which provides a target for PRRT. Somatostatin (SST) is a peptide hormone and SSTR is a family of peptide receptors. There are SSTR subtypes 1–5, with SSTR2 the subtype most commonly over-expressed by NETs.

SSTR agonists are similar to SST; they bind to SSTR and activate the receptor. The receptor–agonist complex is internalized and retained in the cytoplasm. Activation of SSTR has an anti-proliferative effect, inducing cell cycle arrest and apoptosis. Low-grade metastatic NETs are treated with a long-acting-release SST agonist alone, which can reduce symptoms and halt tumor growth for some time. Octreotide and octreotate are examples of SSTR agonists that are used in NET PRRT, both of which mainly target SSTR2. PRRT with ^{177}Lu-DOTA-octreotate received the approval of the United States Food and Drug Administration (FDA) for SSTR-positive gastro-enteropancreatic NETs [24].

Peptides that are SSTR antagonists also bind to SSTR, but they block it rather than activate it, and there is limited or no internalization. SSTR antagonists may have greater binding efficiency than SSTR agonists [25]. This may be because antagonists bind to all SSTR states, whereas agonists only bind to states that represent a small proportion of the total receptor population [26]. JR11 is an example of an SSTR antagonist that has been used in NET PRRT [27]. Another example of PRRT is when the alpha-emitter ^{213}Bi was conjugated to substance P to target the NK-1 receptor overexpressed by glioblastoma multiforme [28].

The protein and peptide ligands mentioned above are classified as biologic. There are smaller ligands called small molecules. A small molecule is a ligand comprising 20–100 atoms and has a molecular mass less than 1000 g/mol (1 kDa). A small molecule can bind to an enzyme, or a receptor that has structural and functional homology with an enzyme, and activate or inhibit the enzyme activity. For example, small molecule inhibitors have been developed and radiolabeled to target the prostate-specific membrane antigen (PSMA).

PSMA is a transmembrane receptor expressed in normal prostate tissue but overexpressed 1000-fold on prostate cancer, and PSMA expression increases with disease progression. After a ligand binds to PSMA, there is internalization of the ligand–receptor complex. Small molecules that successfully bind end up in the late endosomes. The effects of PSMA's enzymatic activity are unclear, and inhibition of PSMA by small molecules is not believed to contribute to therapeutic effect. Examples of PSMA small molecule inhibitors are PSMA-I&T, PSMA-11, PSMA-617 and SAR-bisPSMA. ^{177}Lu-PSMA-617 received FDA approval for third-line treatment of metastatic castration-resistant prostate cancer (mCRPC) [29]. Peptides and small molecules have faster targeting and clearance than protein ligands, but may have shorter tumor retention times.

3.2.2 RADIOIMMUNOTHERAPY

In radioimmunotherapy (RIT), a radiolabeled antibody is used to target an antigen receptor over-expressed on cancer cells. If the antibody binds to the target antigen, an antigen–antibody complex forms. For example, PSMA is an antigen and thus can be targeted using an antibody called an anti-PSMA antibody. Antibodies are proteins, so technically RLT encompasses RIT, but there are additional considerations for antibody ligands discussed below, which makes the distinction worthwhile.

Conventional RIT uses a radiolabeled monoclonal antibody (mAb). Notable examples are ^{131}I-tositumomab (Bexxar) and ^{90}Y ibritumomab tiuxetan (Zevalin), both of which are anti-CD20 mAbs approved by the FDA for relapsed or refractory, low-grade or follicular B cell non-Hodgkin's lymphoma. CD20 is an antigen on the surface of B cells to which these mAbs are able to bind. Note that Bexxar and Zevalin are murine mAbs, which means they lose effectiveness in humans after the first administration.

For repeat administration of an antibody to be effective (i.e., for it to continue forming bonds to the target antigen), it must be nonimmunogenic, i.e., a patient must not develop immunity towards the antibody. Murine antibodies are immunogenic, while chimeric, humanized and fully human antibodies are less immunogenic. Cyclosporine may be administered to possibly prevent the development of human anti-mouse antibody.

If the mAb is humanized or fully human, there can be a cytotoxic immune effect following the formation of the antibody–antigen complex. This is desirable because it contributes to the inactivation of target cells, in addition to the ionizing radiation emitted by the conjugated therapeutic radionuclide. The latter mechanism is still dominant. An example of a humanized mAb used in RIT is huJ591 (rosopatamab), which is anti-PSMA and has been radiolabeled with ^{90}Y [30] and ^{177}Lu [31,32] for the treatment of mCRPC.

mAbs are generally much larger (about 100 times) than the biologic ligands in RLT. The larger size is necessary to elicit a cytotoxic immune response upon binding but may hinder tissue penetration and delivery. To address the size limitations of mAbs, another kind of antibody called a nanobody (a.k.a. single domain antibody; sdAb) can be used. Nanobodies are typically made from camelid heavy-chain-only antibodies. They are about a tenth of the size of mAbs, so they may have better access to tumors while still having the potential to generate a cytotoxic immune response. Importantly, nanobodies can also be radiolabeled and used for RIT. For example, ^{131}I was conjugated to the anti-HER2 sdAb 2Rs15d (CAM-H2) and administered for advanced HER2-positive breast cancer [33].

Another strategy that has been used to enhance the effectiveness of mAb-based RIT is pre-targeting. The mAb concentration in tumors reaches maximum after about 1 day, but the mAb concentration in the blood and normal tissue background decreases slowly, resulting in the tumor-to-normal tissue mAb concentration ratio reaching maximum 2–3 days after administration. In pre-targeted RIT, the mAb and the radionuclide are administered separately with a time delay to increase the ratio of tumor-to-normal tissue dose.

There have been two main approaches for pre-targeted RIT, each of which uses the avidin–biotin complex. In one approach, a streptavidin-conjugated mAb is administered and the mAb is given 48–72 h to bind to target antigens on tumor cells. A clearing agent is then administered, which binds to circulating streptavidin and mediates their hepatic clearance from circulation. Approximately 24 h later, radiolabeled biotin is administered, which binds to streptavidin presented on tumor cells. An example of this is a phase 1 trial for B cell NHL, wherein B9E9FP was administered, an anti-CD20-streptavidin murine mAb, followed by a synthetic clearing agent, followed by ^{90}Y/^{111}In-DOTA-biotin [34].

In another pre-targeting method, first a biotinylated mAb is administered, which binds to the target antigen and displays biotins at target cells. Then 24–36 h later, avidin and streptavidin are administered in turn. They bind to the biotins and display avidin at target cells. Finally, 16–24 h later, a radiolabeled biotin is administered, which binds to avidin on the target cells. There have been RIT trials using this pre-targeting method with the anti-tenascin mAb BC4 and ^{90}Y for glioma [35].

Note that antigens may be internalizing or not, and pre-targeting may not be effective if the target antigen is internalizing.

3.3 MOLECULAR TARGETS FOR TARGETED RADIONUCLIDE THERAPY

The effectiveness of TRNT is highly dependent on the expression profile of the target receptor. To ensure selective tumor targeting, the target receptor should be overexpressed on cancerous cells with minimal to no expression on healthy, normal cells. This expression profile optimizes the radiation dose to the tumor targets while reducing damage to normal tissues and limiting normal-tissue toxicities (i.e., treatment side effects). There are numerous targets being investigated for TRNT of cancer. This section will discuss some of the most promising molecular targets to date.

3.3.1 SODIUM IODIDE SYMPORTER

The sodium iodide symporter (NIS) is a cotransporter glycoprotein that facilitates the cellular uptake of iodide. NIS is normally located on the thyroid, salivary glands, breasts and stomach. It is the primary target of radioactive iodine treatment using iodine-131 for thyroid cancer. Using the physiological action of NIS, radioactive iodine is transported to both malignant and benign thyroid tissue where it is organified and trapped to decay. NIS expression can be both down- and upregulated in thyroid malignancies [36]. The expression of NIS is primarily regulated by the thyroid stimulating hormone (TSH). Given the variable expression pattern of NIS in thyroid malignancies, it is common for TSH levels to be artificially elevated to stimulate NIS expression prior to radioactive iodine therapy [37].

An example radiopharmaceutical is radioactive sodium iodide ($Na^{131}I$).

3.3.2 SOMATOSTATIN RECEPTOR

SSTRs are a family of five G-protein coupled receptors that provide inhibitory neuroendocrine functions. SSTRs are expressed across a range of tissue types including the brain, gastrointestinal tract, pancreas and lungs in differential patterns across the five subtypes. In normal cells, SSTRs bind with endogenous or synthetic SST to provide a range of intracellular signals such as decreasing cellular proliferation, inhibiting hormonal secretion and modulating neuronal activity [38]. Upregulation of SSTRs is prominent in neuroendocrine tumors including paraganglioma, pancreatic islet cell tumor, small cell lung carcinoma and medullary thyroid cancer. SSTR2 is the most prominently expressed SSTR in NETs [39,40]. Activation of SSTR2 in NETs stimulates tumor growth and is consequently a key therapeutic target [38].

An example radiopharmaceutical is ^{177}Lu-DOTATATE.

3.3.3 PROSTATE-SPECIFIC MEMBRANE ANTIGEN

PSMA is a type II transmembrane protein. It is normally expressed in the epithelium of secretory ducts of benign prostate tissue as well as in the lacrimal and salivary glands, kidneys and small intestine. In malignant prostate tissues, PSMA is translocated to the luminal surface of the ducts and aberrantly expressed at 100–1000 times the level of normal prostate cells [41]. PSMA provides enzymatic functions related to the prostate and acts as a glutamate-preferring carboxypeptidase [42–44]. The overexpression of PSMA suggests a role of PSMA in driving cancer progression via its enzymatic activity [45]. PSMA expression has been correlated with the Gleason score (grading system for prostate cancer) and the PSA level (biochemical indicator of high functioning prostate), suggesting its therapeutic targets may be most beneficial for advanced disease [46]. Interestingly, several other cancers, including glioblastoma, thyroid, gastric, breast, renal and colorectal, have shown PSMA expression which could be exploited in future therapeutic avenues [47,48]. An example radiopharmaceutical is ^{225}Ac-PSMA-617.

3.3.4 EPIDERMAL GROWTH FACTOR RECEPTOR

Epidermal growth factor receptors (ErbB) are a family of receptor tyrosine kinases consisting of ErbB-1 (EGFR or HER1), ErbB-2 (HER2), ErbB-3 (HER3) and ErbB-4 (HER4). ErbB functions to regulate cell proliferation, migration, growth and differentiation [49]. Almost all cell types express a member of the ErbB family. In normal cells, the density of ErbB expression is between 10^4 and 10^5 receptors per cell [50]. Upregulation of ErbB has been noted in several cancers, where receptor density increases to over 10^6 receptors per cell [51]. The amplification of ErbB expression is a primary driver of tumorigenesis in glioblastoma, breast and lung cancers, as well as renal, pancreatic, ovarian and head and neck cancers [49]. Mutations of the extracellular and kinase domains in ErbB promote oncogenic signals to increase cell proliferation and prevent apoptosis [52]. Given expression of ErbB can lead to metastases, advanced disease and poor survival, it is a favourable therapeutic target for a number of aggressive malignancies [53].

An example radiopharmaceutical is ^{131}I-trastuzumab.

3.3.5 Fibroblast Activation Protein

Fibroblast activation protein (FAP) is a membrane-bound serine protease found within cancer-associated fibroblasts (CAFs). CAFs are a key component of the tumor microenvironment and contribute to the development of the tumor stroma, a dense connection of fibrotic networks that support the tumor and provide a physical barrier to the infiltration of therapeutic agents [54,55]. Targeting of CAFs via FAP provides an opportunity to degrade the tumor stroma to improve the entry of other therapeutic substances. Expression of FAP is almost non-existent in normal tissue given the lack of CAFs and activated fibroblasts [56]. FAP expression increases exponentially in sites of inflammation, fibrosis and tumors. Overexpression of FAP is found in over 90% of epithelial tumors, including breast, ovarian, pancreatic, lung and colorectal cancers [54,57].

An example radiopharmaceutical is ^{90}Y-FAPI-46.

3.3.6 Mucins

Mucins are a family of heavily glycosylated proteins found on epithelial tissues. Currently, 22 mucins have been characterized as either secreted or transmembrane proteins. Both secreted and transmembrane mucins provide anti-adhesion properties by creating a physical barrier to protect the apical surface of epithelial cells [58]. Transmembrane mucins also regulate cell signals to promote cell growth and differentiation [58]. Of the 22 mucins, MUC1 is the primary mucin of interest involved in carcinogenesis, although MUC16 and others have also been assessed [59,60]. During carcinogenesis, epithelial cells lose polarization resulting in overexpression of mucins across the entire cell surface [59]. MUC1 also exhibits changes in the glycosylation pattern of the extra-cellular domain in malignant cells. These glycosylation changes reveal novel cancer-specific epitopes (MUC1-CE), the primary targets of mucin-based therapies. MUC1-CE have been shown to be expressed in over 90% of pancreatic and ovarian cancers [61,62]. Expression of MUC1-CE is also correlated with advanced disease, likely due to the dysregulated function of MUC1 in cancer which promotes metastases [63,64].

An example radiopharmaceutical is ^{225}Ac-DOTA-C595.

3.3.7 Integrins

Integrins are transmembrane proteins that facilitate adhesion and signalling of the ECM. The functions of integrins have been associated with tumor invasion, development and metastases [65]. Several integrins have been identified as cancer targets; however, most TRNT developments have centred around $\alpha_V \beta_3$. Integrin $\alpha_V \beta_3$ acts as a target for angiogenesis. Most normal tissues have low expression of $\alpha_V \beta_3$; yet areas of angiogenesis such as bone, endometrium and malignant tumors express high $\alpha_V \beta_3$ levels [66]. The close relationship of angiogenesis to tumor growth and invasion suggests $\alpha_V \beta_3$ is a valuable target for killing tumors during growth phases [67]. Integrin $\alpha_V \beta_3$ has been assessed as a therapeutic target in melanoma, colorectal and breast cancer [68–70].

An example radiopharmaceutical is ^{177}Lu-EB-RGD.

3.3.8 CD133

CD133 is a membrane bound glycoprotein expressed by CSCs. CSCs represent a population of cells within a tumor that have unlimited replicative potential. The ability of CSCs to self-renew can allow tumors to regenerate if CSCs remain after treatment. The presence of CSCs is also correlated with metastasis and treatment resistance [71]. CD133 is therefore a promising therapeutic target and has primarily been assessed for TRNT in colorectal cancer and leukaemia [72,73]. While the exact function of CD133 is unknown, it is believed to have a role in cell differentiation, apoptosis and organisation of the plasma membrane [74,75]. Aside from CSCs, CD133 is also expressed within stem cells associated with the central nervous system, hematopoietic system, renal and prostate tissues [76].

An example radiopharmaceutical is ^{211}At-CXCR4.

3.4 SPECIALIZED TARGETING MECHANISMS IN RADIONUCLIDE THERAPY – EXAMPLES

As discussed above, targeting the desired cancer cells can be achieved with specially designed molecules designed to bind to antigens or peptide receptors on the target cells. There are a number of other ways that targeting is achieved in TRNT. These other types of specialized targeting mechanisms (i.e., not targeting antigens or peptide receptors) are outlined in Figure 3.1 and are discussed below.

3.4.1 BRACHYTHERAPY

Brachytherapy is a form of internal TRNT in which radionuclides are placed into or near a tumor. The radionuclides (also called brachytherapy sources) may be left inside the patient or removed, depending on the treatment. Common radionuclides used for brachytherapy include cesium-131, iridium-192, iodine-125 and palladium-103. The sources are commonly "sealed" in small containers such as seeds, pellets and thin wires or tubes. The sources can be placed using catheters, needles or applicators.

Brachytherapy can also be performed with "unsealed" sources (liquid containing the radioactive material), which is injected into the desired location. In this sense, the targeting of the radionuclide is achieved through the direct injection at the desired site.

3.4.1.1 ^{32}P OncoSil for Pancreatic Cancer

^{32}P OncoSil^{TM} is an example of intratumoral brachytherapy. OncoSil consists of phosphorus-32 (^{32}P) microparticles suspended in a diluent. The ^{32}P microspheres are placed into a pancreatic tumor via injection under endoscopic ultrasound guidance.

^{32}P is a pure beta-emitter, decaying via beta-minus decay with a mean electron energy of 695 keV and a maximum electron energy of 1.71 MeV.

^{32}P OncoSil is indicated for patients with unresectable locally advanced pancreatic cancer (LAPC), used in combination with gemcitabine-based chemotherapy. A clinical study has shown that out of 42 patients with initially unresectable LAPC who received ^{32}P OncoSil in combination with standard of care chemotherapy (FOLFIRINOX or gemcitabine chemotherapy), 10 of them became resectable and 42 patients had a median overall survival of 15.5 months, compared to the median survival of approximately 13 months for LAPC patients treated with only chemotherapy [77].

3.4.1.2 ^{90}Y-Microspheres for Liver Cancer (Radioembolization)

Radioembolization, also called intra-arterial brachytherapy, is a type of TRNT used to treat liver cancer or cancers that have spread to the liver. Tiny glass or resin beads, called microspheres, are filled with the radioactive isotope yttrium-90 (^{90}Y). The ^{90}Y-microspheres are injected into the main blood vessel that supplies the tumor with blood. The microspheres lodge in the tumor where they deliver a dose of radiation directly to the cancer cells.

Radioembolization is commonly performed with the guidance of an angiogram, which uses a contrast material and X-ray imaging to visualize blood vessels, with at least two sessions required.

The first session involves a mapping angiogram, where a catheter is placed into the hepatic artery via the groin and angiography is used to map out the arteries involved in blood circulation in the liver. At this stage, any blood flow from the liver to healthy structures can be blocked off (embolized).

The radiation dose is delivered in the second session, where a catheter is placed into the artery supplying the tumor. Two major blood vessels supply blood to the liver, with normal liver tissue receiving about 75% of its blood supply from the portal vein and 25% from the hepatic artery. A tumor growing in the liver will receive the majority of its blood supply (80–100%) via the hepatic artery [78]. As such, the catheter is placed into the hepatic artery, with angiography used to confirm the correct placement of the catheter. The ^{90}Y-microspheres are then injected into the artery where they flow directly into and lodge in the tumor. ^{90}Y has a half-life of 2.7 days and undergoes beta-minus decay producing a mean electron energy of 932 keV and a maximum electron energy of 2.28 MeV. The ^{90}Y-microspheres deliver radiation directly to the tumor as the yttrium decays, with the radioactivity effectively disappearing after about 30 days.

Radioembolization is generally not considered a cure for liver cancer but can extend and improve quality of life for patients with inoperable tumors or help shrink liver tumors to make them operable. Further studies of radioembolization will help demonstrate the effect of this treatment.

3.4.2 Lipiodol

3.4.2.1 ^{131}I-Lipiodol for HCC

Lipiodol, also known as ethiodized oil, is a poppyseed oil. Lipiodol is used in diagnostic imaging as an iodinated contrast agent to enhance vascular structures and organs on plain X-ray and CT scans (lipiodol is naturally iodinated, with iodine naturally present in poppyseed oil).

Lipiodol can also be readily iodinated with ^{131}I to form a therapeutic agent (^{131}I-lipiodol). ^{131}I-lipiodol is used for patients with hepatocellular carcinoma (HCC), a type of primary liver cancer. The administration of ^{131}I-lipiodol is similar to the process used for radioembolization with ^{90}Y microspheres. The liver tumor receives the majority of its blood supply from the hepatic artery. ^{131}I-lipiodol is injected into the hepatic artery via a catheter, done under fluoroscopic guidance. The ^{131}I-lipiodol follows arterial flow towards the tumor and gets trapped in tumor micro-vessels, with the remainder distributing in the healthy liver tissue. Lipiodol is cleared from HCC cells at a slower rate compared to healthy liver cells, meaning ^{131}I-lipiodol is retained in the tumor for a longer period [79]. Twenty-four hours post administration, 75–90% of the administered activity is trapped in the liver, with tumor-to-normal tissue uptake ratios ranging from 2.3 to 12. There is also a 10–25% pulmonary uptake resulting from arteriovenous shunting [80]. The exact mechanism of lipiodol favouring deposition in hepatic tumors over healthy liver tissue is only partially understood and is briefly outlined here. Hepatic tumors have varying degrees of vascularization, with the tumors mostly vascularized with arterial supply mediated by the secretion of factors such as vascular endothelial growth factor [81]. Tumor arterial supply dominates over portal venous supply, and the progressive involution (reduction in size of the liver) results in a "siphon effect". The increased tumor neo-vasculature displays a high affinity for lipiodol [81].

Iodine-131 has a half-life of 8 days and undergoes beta minus decay to stable xenon-131. In 90% of decays, ^{131}I will produce an electron with a mean energy of 191.6 keV and maximum energy of 606.3 keV. A 364 keV gamma is then rapidly produced (with 82% abundance) as ^{131}Xe de-excites to the ground state. The therapeutic effect of ^{131}I-lipiodol is achieved primary from the beta radiation emitted by ^{131}I, which has a maximum penetration in human tissue of about 1 to 2 mm.

^{131}I-lipiodol has been demonstrated to be a useful therapy in the management of patients with advanced (unresectable) HCC [82], as well as an effective treatment of HCC with portal vein thrombosis and as an adjuvant to surgery after the resection of HCCs. ^{131}I-lipiodol has been found to be at least as effective as chemoembolization and is tolerated much better [83].

3.4.3 MIBG

3.4.3.1 ^{131}I-MIBG for Neuroendocrine Tumors

^{131}I-MIBG is a radiopharmaceutical used in the treatment of certain neuroendocrine tumors. MIBG is a molecule that is structurally very similar to norepinephrine (noradrenaline), a neurotransmitter that is taken up by certain neuroendocrine cells. MIBG therefore specifically targets neuro-endocrine cells including certain neuroendocrine tumors such as neuroblastoma (NB), pheochro-mocytoma (PC), paraganglioma (PG) and carcinoid tumors.

^{131}I-MIBG is injected into the bloodstream of the patient. The neuroendocrine tumor cells will selectively take up the ^{131}I-MIBG wherever they are located in the body. [131]I undergoes beta-minus decay, with 90% of decays producing an electron with a mean energy of 191.6 keV and a maximum energy of 606.3 keV. A 364 keV gamma is then rapidly produced (82% abundance) as the daughter [131]Xe de-excites. The gamma emission allows the biodistribution of ^{131}I-MIBG to be imaged, which provides information on the extend and spread of the neuroendocrine tumor being targeted.

The indications of ^{131}I-MIBG include treatment-resistant NB, unresectable or metastatic PC and PG, unresectable or metastatic carcinoid tumors, and unresectable or metastatic medullary thyroid cancer (MTC). ^{131}I-MIBG is considered an effective therapy for advanced NB, PC and PG. However, for advanced carcinoid tumors and MTC, ^{131}I-MIBG has largely been replaced by SSTR therapy [84].

3.4.4 ELEMENTAL ACCUMULATION AT DESIRED SITE

Certain radionuclides can be used to target specific types of cancers using the elemental behaviour of the radionuclide in the body.

3.4.4.1 ^{131}I for Thyroid Therapy

A well-known example of targeting achieved via a radionuclides natural behaviour in the body is iodine-131 for thyroid therapy. [131]I is used in the treatment of hyperthyroidism and well-differentiated thyroid cancer (papillary and follicular thyroid cancer).

Iodine is cleared from the body's circulation primarily via the thyroid and kidneys. The thyroid follicular cells (the structural and functional units of the thyroid gland) absorb iodine from the bloodstream via sodium-iodine symporters (proteins that transport two molecules across a mem-brane). The thyroid then uses the iodine in the synthesis of the body's thyroid hormones. The body of a healthy adult contains about 15–20 mg of iodine, with 70–80% of this being stored in the thyroid [85]. Certain malignant thyroid cells maintain the ability to take up iodine, allowing radioactive iodine (^{131}I) to be used to treat malignant thyroid cells.

[131]I therapy is employed in various scenarios. For hyperthyroidism, ^{131}I is used to destroy part of the thyroid gland to reduce the overactivity of the gland. For cancer therapy, ^{131}I is used to destroy any remaining thyroid cells after surgical removal of the thyroid; this use is referred to as remnant ablation. [131]I therapy is also used to treat the spread of thyroid cancer. Certain malignant cancer cells will take up ^{131}I regardless of where they are located in the body; this allows ^{131}I therapy to be used for thyroid cancers that have spread to any surrounding tissue, lymph nodes or any other parts of the body. The spread of the cancer from the thyroid is a strong indication for ^{131}I therapy. It is important to note that ^{131}I can only be used for thyroid cancer provided the malignant cells take up iodine. This is the case for well-differentiated thyroid cancers (papillary and follicular thyroid cancer); however, ^{131}I cannot be used for undifferentiated (anaplastic) and medullary thyroid cancer, since these cancers do not take up iodine.

Prior to therapy of thyroid cancer with ^{131}I, patients are often put on a low iodine diet for several weeks to starve the thyroid of iodine, and any anti-thyroid medication is stopped at least three days prior to therapy for hyperthyroidism. The patient swallows ^{131}I as sodium iodide in a liquid or capsule form. [131]I is absorbed into the bloodstream through the gastrointestinal tract and is circulated throughout the body via the bloodstream. Thyroid cells take up ^{131}I, with about 30% of the administered iodine trapped in the thyroid and 70% directly excreted in urine [86] when administered after thyroidectomy. The biological half-life of iodine in the thyroid gland is about 120 days [86], resulting in an effective half-life of iodine in the human body of about 7.6 days. [131]I decays via beta-minus decay (the principal electron has a mean energy of 191.6 keV and maximum energy 606.3 keV) delivering a local dose to the area it is concentrated. The principal gamma (364 keV) can be used to image the extent of the cancer.

3.4.4.2 ^{223}Ra, ^{89}Sr for Bone Metastases (Alkaline Earth Metals)

Bone-seeking radionuclides are isotopes that when administered systemically will naturally localize at the site of bone metastases, where they deliver a local dose of radiation. The bone matrix of mammals consists of about 30–40% organic matter (mostly type I collagen) and 60–70% inorganic minerals (mostly calcium and phosphate). The collagen provides a matrix that becomes filled with calcium phosphate crystals through bone mineralization, a process mediated by osteoblasts [87].

Bone-seeking radionuclides strontium-89 (^{89}Sr) and radium-223 (^{223}Ra) are calcium mimetics that accumulate in regions of high osteoblastic activity, such as bone metastases, where they are incorporated into the bone matrix through the bone mineralization process. ^{89}Sr and ^{223}Ra are used in the management of patients with bone metastases. They are injected intravenously in the form of ^{89}Sr chloride and ^{223}Ra chloride.

Bone-seeking radionuclides such as ^{89}Sr and ^{223}Ra (and also ^{153}Sm-EDTMP and ^{186}Re-HEDP, discussed in the phosphonates section) do not specifically target cancer cells. They are incorporated into the bone matrix and rely on regions of bone metastases having increased osteoblastic activity, so they are preferentially incorporated at these sites.

Bone metastases are grouped into three types: Osteolytic (e.g., multiple myeloma), Osteoblastic (e.g., prostate cancer) and Mixed (patients with both osteolytic and osteoblastic lesions, e.g., breast cancer) [88]. Since ^{89}Sr and ^{223}Ra are preferentially taken up at sites of bone formation, they are more likely to be effective for osteoblastic metastases [88].

^{89}Sr is a beta-emitter with 99.99% of decays producing an electron with mean energy 587 keV and maximum energy 1.5 MeV. A 909 keV gamma is produced with 0.01% abundance. The mean range of the electrons in soft tissue is 2.4 mm. The half-life of ^{89}Sr is 50.5 days. Ideally, the half-life should be long enough to allow time for accumulation in the bone matrix, but short enough to limit the risk of myelotoxicity. The longer half-life and higher energy emissions from ^{89}Sr, compared to other beta emitters like ^{153}Sm and ^{186}Re, increase the risk of myelotoxicity.

Radium-223 is an alpha-emitter that produces a mean alpha energy of 5.64 MeV. ^{223}Ra has a half-life of 11.4 days and undergoes a complex decay scheme, with six daughters, ending in stable lead. The total decay energy is 28.2 MeV with 95% from alpha emissions, 3.2% from beta emissions and less than 2% from gamma emissions [89]. The maximum tissue penetration of the alpha emissions is less than 0.1 mm [90]. Alpha emissions have an advantage over beta emissions due to the reduced marrow toxicity from the short range of alpha particles in tissue. Alpha particles are also more cytotoxic compared to beta particles, inducing mainly double-stranded DNA breaks.

Historically, bone-seeking radionuclides have been used in the palliation of patients with bone metastases to reduce pain and discomfort. However, ^{223}Ra has shown improved survival rates for patients with metastatic prostate cancer with a 30% reduction in risk of death compared to a placebo [90,91].

3.4.5   Phosphonates

3.4.5.1 ^{153}Sm-EDTMP, ^{186}Re-HEDP for Bone Metastases

Samarium-153 (^{153}Sm) and rhenium-186 (^{186}Re) are similar to strontium-89 in that they are bone-seeking beta-emitting radionuclides used in the palliative pain management of patients with bone metastases. ^{153}Sm and ^{186}Re have shorter half-lives, 1.9 days and 3.8 days, respectively, compared to the 50.5 day half-life of ^{89}Sr. The shorter half-life enables a faster radiation delivery and rapid clearance from the body, reducing the risk of myelotoxicity.

To increase their bone-seeking properties, ^{153}Sm is chelated with EDTMP (^{153}Sm-EDTMP) and ^{186}Re is chelated with HEDP (^{186}Re-HEDP). EDTMP and HEDP are bone-seeking phosphonates that increase the uptake of the radiopharmaceutical into the bone. During the mineral formation phase of bone, the material hydroxyapatite is formed, which consists primarily of calcium and phosphate. ^{153}Sm-EDTMP and ^{186}Re-HEDP localize into the bone by binding to the hydroxy-apatite crystals [92].

It has been observed that 24 hours post intravenous administration, the mean bone uptake for ^{153}Sm-EDTMP is about 50% of the initial total whole-body activity with about 40% cleared through urine, and for ^{186}Re-HEDP the mean bone uptake is about 22% of the initial whole-body activity with about 65% cleared through urine. Both radiopharmaceuticals also display an approximate 13% retention in soft-tissue 24 hours post administration [93].

Samarium-153 undergoes beta-minus decay producing electrons with a mean energy of 230 keV, a maximum energy of 810 keV, and a mean range in soft tissue of 0.6 mm. ^{153}Sm also produces a 104 keV gamma (28% abundance). ^{186}Re also undergoes beta-minus decay producing electrons with a mean energy of 349 keV, a maximum energy of 1071 keV, and a mean range in tissue of 1.1 mm [90]. ^{186}Re also produces a 137 keV gamma (9.5% abundance). The gamma emissions from these isotopes make it possible to image the extent of the bone metastases, making the isotopes useful for diagnostic and therapeutic purposes.

Bone-seeking beta-emitters such as ^{89}Sr, ^{153}Sm-EDTMP and ^{186}Re-HEDP have been shown to be useful options for managing pain and improving the quality of life for patients with metastatic bone cancer, especially for bone metastases from prostate and breast cancer [92,94]. As more attention is placed on the potential for alpha-emitting radionuclides, beta-emitters will continue to play a role in pain management for patients with bone metastases.

3.5   CONCLUSION

Cancer is a complex group of diseases characterized by an uncontrolled growth of cells that can form a tumor, infiltrate the surrounding healthy tissues, but can also invade (i.e., metastasize) organs distant to its primary location. The process of metastasis is precipitated by the presence of cancer cells in lymphatic and hemapoietic systems of the body. While surgery and external beam radiation therapy are excellent for the treatment of localized disease, targeted systemic therapies are required to eradicate the circulating cancer cells and micrometastases. Considering that one of the hallmarks of cancer is significant distinctive changes to the cancer cell membrane and its receptors, an opportunity is presented for TRNT that can "selectively" deliver cytotoxic radiation to cancer cells while minimizing the damage to healthy tissues. While this chapter provided an overall summary of various modalities and applications of TRNT, Chapters 4, 5, 6 and 7 describe in more detail the characteristics of the most common clinical applications in current use today.

REFERENCES

1. WHO, https://www.who.int/news-room/fact-sheets/detail/cancer#:~:text=Cancer%20is%20a%20leading%20cause,and%20rectum%20and%20prostate%20cancers. 2022 [cited 2022 5 July].
2. NIH National Cancer Institute, https://www.cancer.gov/about-cancer/understanding/statistics). 2022 [cited 2022 5 July].
3. Grizzi, F. and M. Chiriva-Internati, Cancer: looking for simplicity and finding complexity. *Cancer Cell Int*, 2006. 6: p. 4.
4. Egeblad, M., E. S. Nakasone, and Z. Werb, Tumors as organs: complex tissues that interface with the entire organism. *Dev Cell*, 2010. 18(6): pp. 884–901.

5. Reid, P. A., P. Wilson, Y. Li, L. G. Marcu, and E. Bezak, Current understanding of cancer stem cells: review of their radiobiology and role in head and neck cancers. *Head Neck*, 2017. 39(9): pp. 1920–1932.

6. Sayed, S. I., R. C. Dwivedi, R. Katna et al., Implications of understanding cancer stem cell (CSC) biology in head and neck squamous cell cancer. *Oral Oncol*, 2011. 47(4): pp. 237–243.

7. Cojoc, M., K. Mäbert, M. H. Muders, and A. Dubrovska, A role for cancer stem cells in therapy resistance: cellular and molecular mechanisms. *Semin Cancer Biol*, 2015. 31: pp. 16–27.

8. Borovski, T., E. M. Felipe De Sousa, L. Vermeulen, and J. P. Medema, Cancer stem cell niche: the place to be. *Cancer Res*, 2011. 71(3): pp. 634–639.

9. Weinberg, R. A., *The Biology of Cancer*, 2nd ed. 2014: Garland Science.

10. Brandao, A., P. Paulo, and M. R. Teixeira, Hereditary predisposition to prostate cancer: from genetics to clinical implications. *Int J Mol Sci*, 2020. 21(14).

11. Hu, C., S. N. Hart, R. Gnanaolivu et al., A population-based study of genes previously implicated in breast cancer. *N Engl J Med*, 2021. 384(5): pp. 440–451.

12. Hanahan, D. and R. A. Weinberg, The hallmarks of cancer. *Cell*, 2000. 100(1): pp. 57–70.

13. Hanahan, D. and R. A. Weinberg, Hallmarks of cancer: the next generation. *Cell*, 2011. 144(5): pp. 646–674.

14. Hanahan, D., Hallmarks of cancer: new dimensions. *Cancer Discov*, 2022. 12(1): pp. 31–46.

15. Baba, A. and C. Câtoi, *Chapter 3 Tumor cell morphology*, in *Comparative Oncology*. 2007, The Publishing House of the Romanian Academy.

16. Langley, R. R. and I. J. Fidler, Tumor cell-organ microenvironment interactions in the pathogenesis of cancer metastasis. *Endocr Rev*, 2007. 28(3): pp. 297–321.

17. Fidler, I. J., The pathogenesis of cancer metastasis: the 'seed and soil' hypothesis revisited. *Nat Rev Cancer*, 2003. 3(6): pp. 453–458.

18. Langley, R. R. and I. J. Fidler, The seed and soil hypothesis revisited – the role of tumor-stroma interactions in metastasis to different organs. *Int J Cancer*, 2011. 128(11): pp. 2527–2535.

19. Krishnan, K., C. Khanna, and L. J. Helman, The molecular biology of pulmonary metastasis. *Thorac Surg Clin*, 2006. 16(2): pp. 115–124.

20. Wong, S. K., N. V. Mohamad, T. R. Giaze et al., Prostate cancer and bone metastases: the underlying mechanisms. *Int J Mol Sci*, 2019. 20(10).

21. Basanta, D. and A. R. A. Anderson, Homeostasis back and forth: an ecoevolutionary perspective of cancer. *Cold Spring Harb Perspect Med*, 2017. 7(9): a028332.

22. Allen, B. J., E. Bezak, and L. G. Marcu, Quo vadis radiotherapy? Technological advances and the rising problems in cancer management. *Biomed Res Int*, 2013. 2013: p. 749203.

23. Vallis, K. A., R. M. Reilly, D. Scollard, P. Merante, A. Brade, S. Velauthapillai et al., Phase I trial to evaluate the tumor and normal tissue uptake, radiation dosimetry and safety of (111)In-DTPA-human epidermal growth factor in patients with metastatic EGFR-positive breast cancer. *Am J Nucl Med Mol Imaging*, 2014. 4(2): pp. 181–192.

24. Strosberg, J. R., M. E. Caplin, P. L. Kunz et al., 177Lu-Dotatate plus long-acting octreotide versus high-dose long-acting octreotide in patients with midgut neuroendocrine tumors (NETTER-1): final overall survival and long-term safety results from an open-label, randomised, controlled, phase 3 trial. *Lancet Oncol*, 2021. 22(12): pp. 1752–1763.

25. Nicolas, G. P., R. Mansi, L. McDougall et al., Biodistribution, pharmacokinetics, and dosimetry of (177)Lu-, (90)Y-, and (111)In-labeled somatostatin receptor antagonist OPS201 in comparison to the agonist (177)Lu-DOTATATE: the mass effect. *J Nucl Med*, 2017. 58(9): pp. 1435–1441.

26. Ginj, M., H. Zhang, B. Waser et al., Radiolabeled somatostatin receptor antagonists are preferable to agonists for in vivo peptide receptor targeting of tumors. *Proc Natl Acad Sci USA*, 2006. 103(44): pp. 16436–16441.

27. Reidy-Lagunes, D., N. Pandit-Taskar, J. A. O'Donoghue et al., Phase I trial of well-differentiated neuroendocrine tumors (NETs) with radiolabeled somatostatin antagonist (177)Lu-satoreotide tetra-xetan. *Clin Cancer Res*, 2019. 25(23): pp. 6939–6947.

28. Krolicki, L., F. Bruchertseifer, J. Kunikowska et al., Safety and efficacy of targeted alpha therapy with (213)Bi-DOTA-substance P in recurrent glioblastoma. *Eur J Nucl Med Mol Imaging*, 2019. 46(3): pp. 614–622.

29. Sartor, O., J. de Bono, K. N. Chi et al., Lutetium-177-PSMA-617 for metastatic castration-resistant prostate cancer. *N Engl J Med*, 2021. 385(12): pp. 1091–1103.

30. Milowsky, M. I., D. M. Nanus, L. Kostakoglu et al., Phase I trial of yttrium-90-labeled anti-prostate-specific membrane antigen monoclonal antibody J591 for androgen-independent prostate cancer. *J Clin Oncol*, 2004. 22(13): pp. 2522–2531.
31. Bander, N. H., M. I. Milowsky, D. M. Nanus et al., Phase I trial of 177lutetium-labeled J591, a monoclonal antibody to prostate-specific membrane antigen, in patients with androgen-independent prostate cancer. *J Clin Oncol*, 2005. 23(21): pp. 4591–4601.
32. Tagawa, S. T., M. I. Milowsky, M. Morris et al., Phase II study of Lutetium-177-labeled anti-prostate-specific membrane antigen monoclonal antibody J591 for metastatic castration-resistant prostate cancer. *Clin Cancer Res*, 2013. 19(18): pp. 5182–5191.
33. Keyaerts, M., J. De Vos, F. P. Duhoux et al., Phase I results of CAM-H2: safety profile and tumor targeting in patients. *J Clin Oncol*, 2018. 36(15): pp. e13017–e13017.
34. Forero, A., P. L. Weiden, J. M. Vose et al., Phase 1 trial of a novel anti-CD20 fusion protein in pretargeted radioimmunotherapy for B-cell non-Hodgkin lymphoma. *Blood*, 2004. 104(1): pp. 227–236.
35. Grana, C., M. Chinol, C. Robertson, C. Mazzetta, M. Bartolomei, C. De Cicco, et al., Pretargeted adjuvant radioimmunotherapy with yttrium-90-biotin in malignant glioma patients: a pilot study. *Br J Cancer*, 2002. 86(2): pp. 207–212.
36. Ringel, M. D., J. Anderson, S. L. Souza et al., Expression of the sodium iodide symporter and thyroglobulin genes are reduced in papillary thyroid cancer. *Mod Pathol*, 2001. 14(4): pp. 289–296.
37. Kogai, T. and G. A. Brent, The sodium iodide symporter (NIS): regulation and approaches to targeting for cancer therapeutics. *Pharmacol Ther*, 2012. 135(3): pp. 355–370.
38. Callison, J. C., Jr., R. C. Walker, and P. P. Massion, Somatostatin receptors in lung cancer: from function to molecular imaging and therapeutics. *J Lung Cancer*, 2011. 10(2): pp. 69–76.
39. Childs, A., C. Vesely, L. Ensell et al., Expression of somatostatin receptors 2 and 5 in circulating tumortumourstumour cells from patients with neuroendocrine. *Br J Cancer*, 2016. 115(12): pp. 1540–1547.
40. Guenter, R., T. Aweda, D. M. Carmona Matos et al., Overexpression of somatostatin receptor type 2 in neuroendocrine tumors for improved Ga68-DOTATATE imaging and treatment. *Surgery*, 2020. 167(1): pp. 189–196.
41. Lenzo, N. P., D. Meyrick, and J. H. Turner, Review of gallium-68 PSMA PET/CT imaging in the management of prostate cancer. *Diagnostics (Basel)*, 2018. 8(1): p. 16.
42. Halsted, C. H., Ling E. H., R. Luthi-Carter et al., Folylpoly-gamma-glutamate carboxypeptidase from pig jejunum. Molecular characterization and relation to glutamate carboxypeptidase II. *J Biol Chem*, 1998. 273(32): pp. 20417–20424.
43. Carter, R. E., A. R. Feldman, and J. T. Coyle, Prostate-specific membrane antigen is a hydrolase with substrate and pharmacologic characteristics of a neuropeptidase. *Proc Natl Acad Sci USA*, 1996. 93(2): pp. 749–753.
44. Pinto, J. T., B. P. Suffoletto, T. M. Berzin et al., Prostate-specific membrane antigen: a novel folate hydrolase in human prostatic carcinoma cells. *Clin Cancer Res*, 1996. 2(9): pp. 1445–1451.
45. Bařinka, C., C. Rojas, B. Slusher, M. Pomper, Glutamate carboxypeptidase II in diagnosis and treatment of neurologic disorders and prostate cancer. *Curr Med Chem*, 2012. 19(6): pp. 856–870.
46. Sanli, Y., S. Kuyumcu, O. Sanli et al., Relationships between serum PSA levels, Gleason scores and results of 68Ga-PSMAPET/CT in patients with recurrent prostate cancer. *Ann Nucl Med*, 2017. 31(9): pp. 709–717.
47. Gao, Y., H. Zheng, L. Li et al., Prostate-specific membrane antigen (PSMA) promotes angiogenesis of glioblastoma through interacting with ITGB4 and regulating NF-κB signaling pathway. *Front Cell Dev Biol*, 2021. 9: p. 598377.
48. Chang, S. S., Overview of prostate-specific membrane antigen. *Rev Urol*, 2004. 6(Suppl 10): pp. S13–S18.
49. Wieduwilt, M. J. and M. M. Moasser, The epidermal growth factor receptor family: biology driving targeted therapeutics. *Cell Mol Life Sci*, 2008. 65(10): pp. 1566–1584.
50. Carpenter, G. and S. Cohen, Epidermal growth factor. *Annu Rev Biochem*, 1979. 48: pp. 193–216.
51. Gullick, W. J., J. J. Marsden, N. Whittle et al., Expression of epidermal growth factor receptors on human cervical, ovarian, and vulval carcinomas. *Cancer Res*, 1986. 46(1): pp. 285–292.
52. Wee, P. and Z. Wang, Epidermal growth factor receptor cell proliferation signaling pathways. *Cancers (Basel)*, 2017. 9(5): 52.
53. Oliveira-Cunha, M., W. G. Newman, and A. K. Siriwardena, Epidermal growth factor receptor in pancreatic cancer. *Cancers*, 2011. 3(2): pp. 1513–1526.

54. Altmann, A., U. Haberkorn, and J. Siveke, The latest developments in imaging of fibroblast activation protein. *J Nucl Med*, 2021. 62(2): p. 160.

55. Dendl, K., S. A. Koerber, C. Kratochwil et al., FAP and FAPI-PET/CT in malignant and non-malignant diseases: a perfect symbiosis? *Cancers (Basel)*, 2021. 13(19).

56. Hamson, E. J., F. M. Keane, S. Tholen, O. Schilling, M. D. Gorrell, Understanding fibroblast activation protein (FAP): substrates, activities, expression and targeting for cancer therapy. *Proteomics Clin Appl*, 2014. 8(5–6): pp. 454–463.

57. Huang, R., Y. Pu, S. Huang et al., FAPI-PET/CT in cancer imaging: a potential novel molecule of the century. *Front Oncol*, 2022. 12.

58. Kufe, D. W., Mucins in cancer: function, prognosis and therapy. *Nat Rev Cancer*, 2009. 9(12): pp. 874–885.

59. Nath, S. and P. Mukherjee, MUC1: a multifaceted oncoprotein with a key role in cancer progression. *Trends Mol Med*, 2014. 20(6): pp. 332–342.

60. Aithal, A., S. Rauth, P. Kshirsagar et al., MUC16 as a novel target for cancer therapy. *Expert Opin Ther Targets*, 2018. 22(8): pp. 675–686.

61. Wang, L., J. Ma, F. Liu et al., Expression of MUC1 in primary and metastatic human epithelial ovarian cancer and its therapeutic significance. *Gynecol Oncol*, 2007. 105(3): pp. 695–702.

62. Qu, C., Y. Li, Y. Song et al., MUC1 expression in primary and metastatic pancreatic cancer cells for in vitro treatment by 213Bi-C595 radioimmunoconjugate. *Br J Cancer*, 2004. 91(12): pp. 2086–2093.

63. Suh, H., K. Pillai, and D. L. Morris, Mucins in pancreatic cancer: biological role, implications in carcinogenesis and applications in diagnosis and therapy. *Am J Cancer Res*, 2017. 7(6): pp. 1372–1383.

64. Tinder, T. L., D. B. Subramani, G. D. Basu et al., MUC1 enhances tumor progression and contributes toward immunosuppression in a mouse model of spontaneous pancreatic adenocarcinoma. *J Immunol (Baltimore, MD.: 1950)*, 2008. 181(5): pp. 3116–3125.

65. Desgrosellier, J. S. and D. A. Cheresh, Integrins in cancer: biological implications and therapeutic opportunities. *Nat Rev Cancer*, 2010. 10(1): pp. 9–22.

66. Wilder, R. L., Integrin alpha V beta 3 as a target for treatment of rheumatoid arthritis and related rheumatic diseases. *Ann Rheum Dis*, 2002. 61 (Suppl 2): pp. ii96–ii99.

67. Yoshimoto, M., K. Ogawa, K. Washiyama et al., alpha(v)beta(3) Integrin-targeting radionuclide therapy and imaging with monomeric RGD peptide. *Int J Cancer*, 2008. 123(3): pp. 709–715.

68. Felding-Habermann, B., T. E. O'Toole, J. W. Smith et al., Integrin activation controls metastasis in human breast cancer. *Proc Natl Acad Sci USA*, 2001. 98(4): pp. 1853–1858.

69. Reinmuth, N., W. Liu, S. A. Ahmad et al., Alphavbeta3 integrin antagonist S247 decreases colon cancer metastasis and angiogenesis and improves survival in mice. *Cancer Res*, 2003. 63(9): pp. 2079–2087.

70. Nip, J., H. Shibata, D. J. Loskutoff, D. A. Cheresh, P. Brodt, Human melanoma cells derived from lymphatic metastases use integrin alpha v beta 3 to adhere to lymph node vitronectin. *J Clin Investig*, 1992. 90(4): pp. 1406–1413.

71. Yang, L., P. Shi, G. Zhao et al. Targeting cancer stem cell pathways for cancer therapy. *Signal Transduct Target Ther*, 2020. 5(1): p. 8.

72. Oriuchi, N., M. Aoki, N. Ukon et al., Possibility of cancer-stem-cell-targeted radioimmunotherapy for acute myelogenous leukemia using 211At-CXCR4 monoclonal antibody. *Sci Rep*, 2020. 10(1): p. 6810.

73. Lang, J., X. Lan, Y. Liu et al. Targeting cancer stem cells with an 131I-labeled anti-AC133 monoclonal antibody in human colorectal cancer xenografts. *Nucl Med Biol*, 2015. 42(5): pp. 505–512.

74. Irollo, E. and G. Pirozzi, CD133: to be or not to be, is this the real question? *Am J Transl Res*, 2013. 5(6): pp. 563–581.

75. Barzegar Behrooz, A., A. Syahir, and S. Ahmad, CD133: beyond a cancer stem cell biomarker. *J Drug Target*, 2019. 27(3): pp. 257–269.

76. Fan, X., L. G. Salford, and B. Widegren, Glioma stem cells: evidence and limitation. *Semin Cancer Biol*, 2007. 17(3): pp. 214–218.

77. Ross, P. J., H. S. Wasan, D. Croagh et al. Results of a single-arm pilot study of (32)P microparticles in unresectable locally advanced pancreatic adenocarcinoma with gemcitabine/nab-paclitaxel or FOLFIRINOX chemotherapy. *ESMO Open*, 2022. 7(1): p. 100356.

78. Lien W. M. A. N., The blood supply of experimental liver metastases. II. A microcirculatory study of the normal and tumor vessels of the liver with the use of perfused silicone rubber. *Surgery*, 1970. 68(2): p. 334:40.

79. Raoul, J. L., P. Bourguet, J. F. Bretagne et al. Hepatic artery injection of I-131-labeled lipiodol. Part I. Biodistribution study results in patients with hepatocellular carcinoma and liver metastases. *Radiology*, 1988. 168(2): pp. 541–545.
80. Guidelines for 131I-ethiodised oil (lipiodol) therapy. *Eur J Nucl Med Mol Imaging*, 2003. 30(3): pp. BP20–BP22.
81. Nezami, N., J. M. M. VAN Breugel, M. Konstantinidis et al. Lipiodol deposition and washout in primary and metastatic liver tumors after chemoembolization. *In Vivo*, 2021. 35(6): pp. 3261–3270.
82. Kallur, K. G., B. Aditi, G. R. Prashanth et al. I-131-lipiodol therapy in local disease control and survival in patients with advanced hepatocellular carcinoma: an observational study. *J Clin Oncol*, 2012. 30(15): p. e14721.
83. Ahmadzadehfar, H., A. Sabet, K. Wilhelm et al. Iodine-131-lipiodol therapy in hepatic tumours. *Methods*, 2011. 55(3): pp. 246–252.
84. Kayano, D. and S. Kinuya, Current consensus on I-131 MIBG therapy. *Nucl Med Mol Imaging*, 2018. 52(4): pp. 254–265.
85. Chung, H. R., Iodine and thyroid function. *Ann Pediatr Endocrinol Metab*, 2014. 19(1): pp. 8–12.
86. Wyszomirska, A., Iodine-131 for therapy of thyroid diseases. Physical and biological basis. *Nucl Med Rev Cent East Eur*, 2012. 15(2): pp. 120–123.
87. Kuhn, L. T., Bone mineralization, in *Encyclopedia of Materials: Science and Technology*, R. W. C. K. H. Jürgen Buschow, M. C. Flemings, B. Ilschner, E. J. Kramer, S. Mahajan, and P. Veyssière, Editors. 2001, Elsevier. pp. 787–794.
88. Macedo, F., K. Ladeira, F. Pinho et al. Bone metastases: an overview. *Oncol Rev*, 2017. 11(1): p. 321.
89. Flux, Glenn D., Imaging and dosimetry for radium-223: the potential for personalized treatment. *The British Journal of Radiology*, 2017. 90(1077), 20160748. https://doi.org/10.1259/bjr.20160748.
90. Goyal, J. and E. S. Antonarakis, Bone-targeting radiopharmaceuticals for the treatment of prostate cancer with bone metastases. *Cancer Lett*, 2012. 323(2): pp. 135–146.
91. Parker, C., S. Nilsson, D. Heinrich et al. Alpha emitter radium-223 and survival in metastatic prostate cancer. *N Engl J Med*, 2013. 369(3): pp. 213–223.
92. Frantellizzi, V., M. Montebello, F. Corica, and G. De Vincentis, Therapy of bone metastases with beta emitters, in *Nuclear Medicine and Molecular Imaging*. 2022, Elsevier. pp. 233–240.
93. Brenner, W., W.U. Kampen, A.M. Kampen, and E. Henze, Skeletal uptake and soft-tissue retention of 186Re-HEDP and 153Sm-EDTMP in patients with metastatic bone disease. *J Nucl Med*, 2001. 42(2): pp. 230–236.
94. Usuki, K. Y., M. T. Milano, M. David, and P. Okunieff, Metastatic disease, in *Clinical Radiation Oncology*, J. E. T. Leonard, and L. Gunderson, Editors. 2016, Elsevier. pp. 432–448.e4.

Part 2

Clinical Applications of Targeted Radionuclide Therapy in Cancer Control

4 Unconjugated Radionuclides

Aaron Kian-Ti Tong, Sue Ping Thang,
Winnie Wing-Chuen Lam, and Kelvin Siu-Hoong Loke

4.1 RADIOIODINE THERAPY (^{131}I) FOR DIFFERENTIATED THYROID CANCER

4.1.1 INTRODUCTION

Thyroid cancer is the most common endocrine tumor, and differentiated thyroid cancer comprises more than 90% of the cases [1]. Standard-of-care management of differentiated thyroid cancer typically involves surgery, radioiodine therapy with ^{131}I and thyroid hormone therapy. Radioiodine therapy can be deemed to have several fairly distinct clinical functions.

(1) Ablative – to ablate small normal thyroid remnants or residues in the thyroid bed after near-total or total thyroidectomy.
(2) Adjuvant – to reduce the risk of recurrence post-operatively and disease-specific mortality by presumably destroying low-volume disease.
(3) Treatment – to treat known local disease or distant metastases.
(4) Diagnostic – for detection of iodine-avid disease in a surveillance setting.

The American Thyroid Association (ATA) guidelines (2015) have stratified thyroid cancer patients into low-, intermediate- and high-risk categories [2]. The current evidence appears to support that there is no need for radioiodine ablation for low risk thyroid cancer (unifocal intra-thyroidal papillary microcarcinoma without adverse features). However, it is reasonable to consider radioiodine remnant ablation and adjuvant treatment for intermediate to high risk thyroid cancer. There is some evidence that overall survival may see benefit in such patients [3].

4.1.2 RADIOACTIVE DOSING

There are classically two major methodologies for deciding radioiodine dosing. Most centers use the empirical method which has standardized ranges of prescribed activity for different categories of patients. A few centers use lesion and body dosimetry to estimate the maximum tolerated absorbed dose to the bone marrow or whole body and calculate the radioiodine activity to be given for individual patients.

Current empirical dosing depends to a large extent on the risk-stratification of patients. Specifically, for low-risk thyroid cancer, two major clinical trials showed that as far as ablation success is concerned, 1.11 GBq is not statistically inferior to 3.7 GBq [4,5]. For intermediate-risk thyroid cancer, the ATA guidelines consider it reasonable to consider dosing activity in between 1.11 and 5.55 GBq. For high-risk thyroid cancer patients, there is more consensus opinion for a range of dose activity to be administered, particularly for those with iodine-avid distant metastases. For iodine-avid bone metastases, typical dose activities range from 3.7 to 7.4 GBq or more, or as determined by dosimetry. For lung metastases, it is recommended that the activity should be limited to a whole-body retention of below 2.96 GBq at 48 hours or 2 Gy to the bone marrow. It is also well known that in renal failure, the retention time of radioiodine in the body can be significantly increased and the dosing should be correspondingly adjusted lower. For pediatric subjects, the ATA guidelines do not specify recommended therapeutic radioiodine activities. Radioiodine activity adjusted for body weight based on a 70 kg adult weight has been proposed [6,7].

4.1.3 PROCEDURE

4.1.3.1 Patient Preparation

The effectiveness of radioiodine therapy depends on the patient's serum with thyroid stimulating hormone (TSH) level being adequately elevated. A TSH level of at least 30 mU/L is believed to increase sodium-iodide symporter (NIS) expression, thereby optimizing radioiodine uptake [8].

The TSH elevation can be achieved via two main ways:

1. Thyroid hormone withdrawal (THW): TSH is stimulated through thyroid hormone deprivation. For those on hormone replacement therapy, withdrawal of levothyroxine should be at least 3–4 weeks prior to radioiodine administration. For those post thyroidectomy and not on hormone replacement therapy, waiting for at least 3 weeks after surgery is recommended.
2. Recombinant human thyrotropin (rhTSH, trade name Thyrogen) administration: TSH stimulation is elevated through administration of rhTSH. Radioiodine is typically given 1 day after two consecutive daily intramuscular injections of 0.9 mg rhTSH. Patient can continue with hormone replacement therapy.

The ATA guidelines (2015) suggest that the use of rhTSH is an acceptable alternative to THW in patients with low-to-intermediate risk in the absence of distant metastasis. However, in patients with high-risk DTC and higher risks of disease-related mortality and morbidity, more randomized controlled trial data from long-term outcome studies are needed before rhTSH preparation can be recommended.

Iodine excess may result in competitive handling by NIS of non-radioactive iodine rather than radioiodine, and potentially resulting in reduced efficacy of radioiodine therapy. Patients should be advised to avoid iodine-containing medications prior to radioiodine therapy [9]. The use of low iodine diet (LID) is also recommended. Systematic review of observational studies showed that LIDs (≤50 μg/d of iodine) for 1–2 weeks appeared to be associated with reduction in urinary iodine excretion as well as increase in radioiodine uptake [10]. Food intake may alter the absorption of orally administered radioiodine. The patient should not take any food or water by mouth for approximately 2 hours before and 1–2 hours after the oral administration of radioiodine.

4.1.3.2 Radiation Safety Aspects

Depending on the dose of radioiodine administered, the patient may require hospitalization during radioiodine therapy to avoid unnecessary radiation exposure to others. Inpatient stay can be required when the administered activity is more than 1.22 GBq [9]. The patient can be discharged when the radiation exposure is less than 0.07 mSv/h at 1 m.

Written instructions on how to reduce radiation exposure should be given to patients and these typically last up to a week after therapy. Prolonged use of public transportation is discouraged for the first 24 hours after radioiodine therapy. Patients should sleep alone and should abstain from intercourse for approximately 1 week after therapy. Alternative care arrangements for up to a week may be necessary for patients with infants and small children. Close contact of approximately 10 minutes daily is allowed but patients should otherwise maintain a distance of about 0.9–1.8 m from pregnant women and children. Exposure of family members from items contaminated by patient's saliva or urine must be prevented (e.g. dishes and utensils should not be shared before washing, toilet should be flushed twice after use followed by hand washing for 20 seconds).

Pregnancy must be excluded within a few days before each radioiodine therapy. As radioiodine can accumulate in the breasts, radioiodine therapy should be deferred until lactating women have stopped breastfeeding for at least 3 months. Most experts recommend that both men and women use effective contraception for 6–12 months after radioiodine therapy before trying to conceive.

4.1.3.3 Post-Therapy Scintigraphy

Patients who received radioiodine therapy should undergo whole-body scintigraphy (WBS) approximately 3–7 days after treatment. This is to document the iodine uptake of any structural disease as well as to stage the disease. In some cases, hybrid SPECT/CT scan (if available) may often have incremental value when there is a diagnostic uncertainty, or when disease was advanced and 2-dimensional WBS was inconclusive.

4.1.3.4 Avoidance of "Stunning"

Stunning is defined as diminution of radioiodine uptake and efficacy following recent diagnostic radioiodine administration. In cases where radioiodine therapy is clearly necessary, a pre-therapeutic ^{131}I diagnostic scan should be avoided. To reduce the possibility of stunning when it is not yet known whether radioiodine therapy is indicated, an ^{131}I diagnostic WBS or thyroid uptake quantification of low activity should be performed. Recommended quantities are approximately 10–185 MBq for WBS and 3–10 MBq for uptake quantification. Alternatively, the use of 40–200 MBq of ^{123}I for diagnostic imaging can minimize the risk of stunning. ^{124}I PET/CT is emerging as an attractive modality for pre-radioiodine therapy imaging and dosimetry [11–13]. The extent of stunning effects with ^{124}I is still unknown, but as a precaution, activities of this radioisotope should be kept to a minimum.

4.1.4 SIDE EFFECTS

In general, radioiodine is a reasonably safe therapy, associated with low-risk cumulative dose-related early and late onset complications. Some early onset side effects may include sialadenitis (with possible alteration of taste and dental caries in long term; this side effect can be reduced by giving sweet candies or sour foods), nasolacrimal duct obstruction, nausea and occasional vomiting. Transient decrease in white blood cell and platelet counts may occur up to 6–10 weeks following ^{131}I activity of more than 5.55–7.4 GBq or with multiple therapies. Rarely, there can be late onset side effects such as secondary malignancies and male infertility.

4.2 UNCONJUGATED RADIONUCLIDES FOR BONE THERAPY

4.2.1 INTRODUCTION

Bone pain is the most frequent clinical manifestation of bone metastases, especially in patients with breast, prostate, lung, colon, stomach, bladder, uterus, rectum, thyroid and kidney cancers. Thirty percent of patients in the course of malignant disease development report bone pain with 60–90% of patients experiencing pain in the advanced stages of their disease. Majority of bone metastases are found in the axial skeleton [14]. Bone metastases and pain can be debilitating, affecting patients' quality of life, increasing morbidity with pathological fractures as well as reducing life expectancy. A direct correlation has been identified between the burden of bone metastases and overall survival of patients [15]. Bone pain and metastases thus pose a significant healthcare management burden internationally.

4.2.2 CLINICAL ASPECTS

Bone-seeking radiopharmaceutical therapy is an underutilised form of targeted radionuclide therapy which has had a history of more than 6 decades of use. It can be easily administered through intravenous injections/infusions with minimal side effects [16,17]. They can be used for bone pain palliation and the treatment of primary and metastatic bone tumors (osteoblastic or mixed osteoblastic). Other advantages include their ability to simultaneously treat multiple metastatic foci, the repeatability of procedure and possibility of combination therapy. Scanning with ^{99m}Tc-Methylene Diphosphate (MDP) or Oxidronate (HDP) bone scans or ^{18}F-sodium fluoride (^{18}F-NaF) PET scans can be used as the diagnostic determinant of tumor burden and uptake prior to this theranostic procedure.

Radiopharmaceuticals developed for these purposes are predominantly beta and alpha radiation emitting radionuclides: [89]Sr, [117m]Sn, [153]Sm, [166]Ho, ^{177}Lu, [186]Re, [188]Re, and [223]Ra [18]. The disease extent, tumor size, renal function, bone marrow reserve, local availability, multi-disciplinary team discussions and life expectancy of the patient determine the choice of appropriate radiopharmaceutical. The time to symptom relief, degree of pain palliation, adverse effects, duration of response (2–6 months) and retreatment timing vary with the physical properties, retention within the site of action, physical half-life and dose rate of the different radionuclides used. Radiopharmaceuticals with a longer biological half-life have a more delayed onset of response, possibly greater complication rate and longer retreatment period but also a longer duration of pain analgesia.

Overall, survival benefits from radionuclide therapies are limited and these treatments are mainly palliative – offering the potential of pain relief, reducing the need for oral analgesics and delaying/preventing skeletal related events. A noteworthy exception is the landmark study reported in the *New England Journal of Medicine* [19]. In this phase-III randomized control trial, 6 injections of radium-223 were compared with best standard of care in 921 metastatic castration-resistant prostate cancer patients with at least 2 symptomatic bone metastases who had received, were not eligible to receive, or declined docetaxel chemotherapy. Interim and final study analysis confirmed that radium-223 treatment was associated with statistically significant prolonged overall survival compared with placebo (median 14.9 vs 11.3 months) and this benefit was consistent across all patient subgroups.

All main secondary efficacy endpoints supported the benefit of radium-223 therapy (including a 30% reduction in death risk, significantly prolonged time to first symptomatic skeletal event, time to increase in total alkaline phosphatase level and time to increase in prostate-specific antigen (PSA) level). More patients in the radium-223 recipient group had meaningful improvement in quality of life during treatment.

Despite the physical and chemical differences, published data have shown rather similar efficacy of pain reduction between the different radiopharmaceuticals and similar clinical outcomes regardless of the type of the primary tumor from which bone metastases originated. α emitters are more toxic for tumoral cells, dispensing higher linear energy in a shorter range, which induces permanent DNA double-strand breaks and lesser radiation for surrounding normal tissues as compared to β^- emitters [20]. The response rate has been reported to be 70% using β^- emitters in a systematic review including 57 studies [21]. However, the majority of the published literature includes patients with bone metastases from lung, prostate and breast cancer. Slightly higher response rates have been reported in patients in whom lesions are osteoblastic, the skeletal involvement is limited and where the performance status of the patient is higher [22].

More commonly used radiopharmaceuticals in clinical practice are strontium-89 ([89]SrCl, Metastron), samarium-153 ([153]Sm-EDTMP, Quadramet) and radium-223 ([223]RaCl$_2$, Xofigo) with emerging use of lutetium-177 (^{177}Lu-EDTMP). The sources of radiation within the bone differ with the radiopharmaceutical chosen: metallic-chelated radiotracers tend to chemically absorb to the trabecular surface, whereas ^{32}P, ^{89}Sr and [223]Ra distribute more widely throughout bone. Bone uptake is proportional to the bone regenerative activity so that uptake is highest in the most osteogenic sites. Their mechanisms of action include acting at the peripheral nerve ends where inflammatory cells, tumor cells and cells with immune modulatory activity and chemical substances modulating pain accumulate, reducing cytokines and growth factors secreted by tumor and inflammatory cells and radiation-induced mechanical factors such as reduced periosteal swelling [23].

4.2.2.1 Post-Therapy Scintigraphy and Side Effects

Post radionuclide therapy scintigraphy can be performed with most agents using gamma photon emissions to assess tumor extent, evaluation of treatment response, ensure radiopharmaceutical distribution and perform dosimetry calculations. Due to the heterogeneity of radiopharmaceutical uptake, specula thickening, tumor and marrow distribution, there is large variation in dosimetry as a result [16]. Unsurprisingly, the most common adverse effect from radionuclide bone pain palliation therapy is mild and reversible hematological toxicity, allowing retreatment of patients who respond to this therapeutic modality.

4.3 UNCONJUGATED RADIONUCLIDES FOR SELECTIVE INTERNAL RADIATION THERAPY IN LIVER TUMORS

4.3.1 Introduction

Primary and secondary hepatic malignancies are a leading cause of cancer death worldwide. Hepatocellular carcinoma (HCC) is the fifth most prevalent human cancer with nearly 1 million deaths worldwide each year. Moreover, the worldwide incidence of HCC is increasing by 4.6% per annum [24]. The liver is also a common site for metastases from various cancers, especially colorectal cancer (CRC). As the third most common malignancy and the second deadliest cancer, CRC induces estimated 1.9 million incidence cases and 0.9 million deaths worldwide in 2020. The liver is the most common site for CRC metastases (approximately 70% of cases). The scale of the problem warrants more treatment options and locoregional therapies, especially with SIRT, have seen incremental use in the past decade. Due to the dual blood supply of the liver, SIRT can be safely administered intra-arterially to target liver tumors that preferentially derive their blood supply from the hepatic arteries while sparing the portal venous supply to the liver parenchyma.

4.3.1.1 Types of Unconjugated Radionuclides and Microspheres

Iodine-131 is a mixed beta and gamma emitting radionuclide with a physical half-life of 8.04 days. The maximum and mean beta particle energies are 0.61 MeV and 0.192 MeV, respectively, while the principal gamma photon emission is of 364 keV (81% abundance). While it has never been fixed onto microspheres, ^{131}I can be chemically bound to lipiodol (a naturally iodinated fatty acid ethyl ester of poppy seed oil) and has been used since the 1990s for palliation in HCC.

The most utilized radionuclide for SIRT is yttrium-90. It is a stronger beta emitter than ^{131}I with a mean energy of 0.9367 MeV and physical half-life of 64.1 hours (2.67 days). ^{90}Y microspheres entrapped within the liver parenchyma have a mean tissue penetration of 2.5 mm and maximum range of 11 mm in tissues. More than 90% of the ^{90}Y microspheres' radiation dose is delivered in the first 11 days post treatment. According to the Medical Internal Radiation Dose (MIRD) schema, an absorbed dose of approximately 50 Gy is provided by 1 GBq of ^{90}Y distributed homogenously throughout 1 kilogram of tissue [25]. It also has minimal internal pair production (32 ppm), which allows for diagnostic PET imaging. ^{90}Y has been fixed onto two types of microspheres for commercial use: resin and glass. The average size of resin microspheres is about 30% larger than glass microspheres, while glass microspheres have a higher specific activity than resin microspheres. Glass microspheres contain 2,500 Bq per microsphere and about 1–2 million microspheres are infused for a typical patient. Resin microspheres contain about 50 Bq per microsphere and a typical treatment contains 40–60 million microspheres.

Holmium-166 microspheres have recently become available for commercial use in Europe for SIRT in unresectable hepatic tumors. As ^{166}Ho microspheres emit both gamma (81 keV) and beta radiation, this new treatment modality has unique imaging as well as dosing possibilities as compared to treatments using ^{90}Y microspheres. Additionally, ^{166}Ho microspheres can be used in lower quantities (and activity) as a "scout scan" and theoretically should have superior performance for a radiation simulation scan as compared to using ^{99m}Tc macro aggregated albumin (MAA).

4.3.2 Treatment Strategies and Considerations

4.3.2.1 Intent of Treatment

Broadly, the intent of SIRT may be classified into three categories, namely curative, neoadjuvant and palliative treatments. The details of each treatment intents are as follows.

1. Curative – If the tumor is relatively confined to a limited area of the liver, it is theoretically possible for SIRT to achieve cure. Curative treatment typically involves the administration of a high radiation activity to a small region of the liver (usually 1 or 2 segments) in a technique known as radiation segmentectomy, which is defined as complete ablation of segmental tissue. This has been shown to be an effective treatment with clinically meaningful response rates and prolonged duration of response in unresectable solitary HCC $\leq$ 8 cm [26]. To a lesser degree, a similar concept can be applied to a technique called radiation lobectomy to achieve the ablation of hepatic lobar tissue (or at least marked tumor response) and at the same time simultaneously promoting contralateral lobe hypertrophy. This is especially so in patients with inadequate future liver remnant volumes and unable to proceed for surgical resection [27].

2. Neo-adjuvant – SIRT using ^{90}Y microspheres is able to downstage large and unresectable tumors and hence function as a bridge to surgical resection for patients that might otherwise only be directed to non-curative options. In addition, the increased progression free survival seen from SIRT has allowed for this treatment to also act as a bridge to liver transplant by halting tumor progression for many patients and prevent dropout while still on an orthotopic liver transplant waiting list [28].

3. Adjuvant/palliative – For locally advanced liver HCC, locoregional therapy with SIRT can play a part in both adjuvant therapy and palliative setting. Recent phase III trials evaluating ^{90}Y SIRT against standard of care sorafenib showed no significant difference in overall survival between the two treatment modalities. The SIRveNIB trial in Asia Pacific patients, however, found that fewer patients experienced grade $\geq$ 3 adverse events such as ascites, abdominal pain or anemia in the SIRT group compared to sorafenib [29]. In patients with portal vein tumor thrombosis, limited treatment options exist and SIRT has been found to provide benefits. Combination therapies with systemic treatment as well as external beam radiotherapy are the subject of ongoing research.

4.3.2.2 Radiation Simulation Study and Personalized Predictive Dosimetry

A routine practice is to perform a liver–lung shunt study using technetium-99m MAA prior to the actual delivery of radionuclide microspheres in order to determine the safety of SIRT. Figure 4.1 shows an example of a planar scintigram depicting the liver–lung shunt by administration of ^{99m}Tc-MAA during the exploratory hepatic angiogram. The scan is also useful to assess for other sites of extrahepatic MAA uptake such as the stomach and bowels that may require the attending interventional radiologist to manage via various techniques so as to proceed with a safe radio-embolization procedure.

In the past decade, there has been increasing use of personalized predictive dosimetry to obtain better patient outcomes. Currently, the ^{90}Y resin manufacturer still utilizes a semi-empirical (e.g. body surface area) method for activity prescription in their instructions for use, while the ^{90}Y glass manufacturer prescribes radiation activity based on a single compartment model. The pivotal randomized prospective trial DOSISPHERE-01 provided the first level I evidence that personalized dosimetry provided a strong response rate following ^{90}Y SIRT. A statistically significant increase in median overall survival (26.7 months versus 10.7 months, $p = 0.012$) was also observed in the personalized dosimetry arm [30]. Together with concerns over the manufacturers' prescription methods after several negative multicentre trials, such evidence on personalized

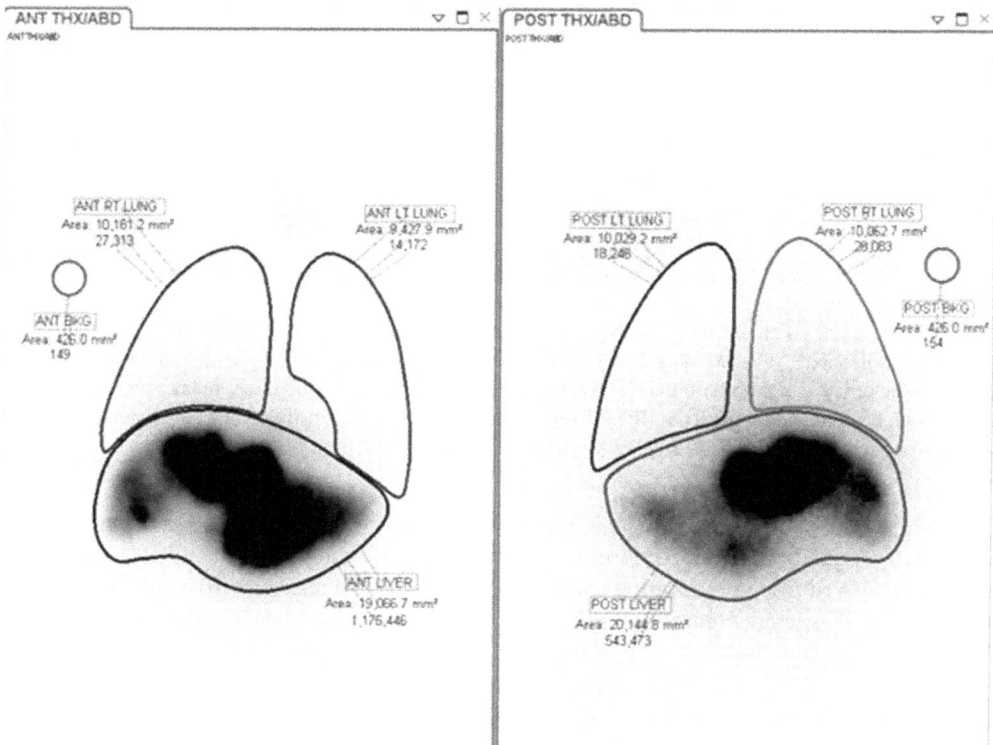

FIGURE 4.1   Anterior and posterior views of the thorax/abdomen following ^{99m}Tc-MAA planar imaging. Regions-of-interest (ROIs) are drawn to outline the lung and liver. The counts obtained and corrected for background will then be used to calculate the liver–lung shunt expressed as a percentage.

dosimetry helped lead to published recommendations of a multidisciplinary expert panel to advocate use of more personalized predictive dosimetry methods for activity prescription [31].

There are two main methods recognized for personalized predictive dosimetry: the more widely used partition (tri-compartmental) modeling and voxel-based dosimetry which has seen growing interest. It is in this situation that the ^{99m}Tc-MAA study has found itself additionally placed in the role of a radiation simulation scan for either methodologies. Similarly, ^{166}Ho microspheres can likewise play the role of a radiation simulation scan as mentioned earlier.

Usually, the partition model divides the target distribution for the ^{90}Y microspheres into three separate compartments, namely the hepatic tumor, non-tumoral hepatic tissue and the lung parenchyma. A radiation simulation scan using hybrid SPECT/CT, with appropriate regions-of-interest (ROIs) drawn either manually or automated using commercial dosimetric programs, allows for volumetric assessment on the CT as well as tracer count assessment based on the SPECT of various compartments. An example of this liver volumetry and count statistic generation is depicted in Figure 4.2. A tumor-to-normal liver ratio can be obtained by a ratio of the count density in the hepatic tumor to the normal liver parenchyma and this will be the basis for an activity prescription using the MIRD formula. The predicted absorbed dose can also be calculated for the normal liver and lung parenchyma to avoid the complications of radiation hepatitis/radioembolization-induced liver disease and radiation pneumonitis. Current state-of-the-art catheter-directed CT-angiography can allow for several hepatic arterial territories to be individually targeted in the same treatment setting and this may lead to "multi-partition" modeling with potentially better clinical outcomes [32].

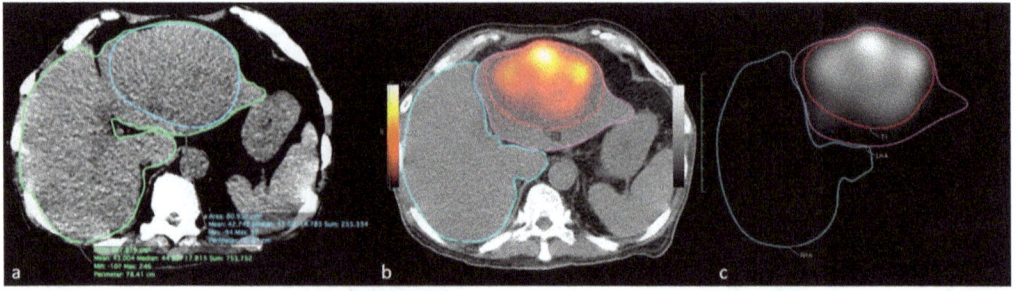

FIGURE 4.2   Axial CT image in (a) shows how to generate the liver and tumor volumes by drawing regions-of-interest (ROIs). The ^{99m}Tc-MAA axial SPECT/CT image in (b) outlines the right and left hepatic lobes and delineates the tumor based on both the CT component and with the aid of the tracer uptake on SPECT. Count statistics can be obtained on the axial SPECT image in (c) and a count density can be calculated based on the amount of counts within the ROI divided by the volume of the ROI.

Quantitative SPECT/CT has seen improvements over the years and voxel-based dosimetry promises the visualized absorbed dose at a voxel level for radionuclide therapies. Dose volume histograms derived from the radiation simulation SPECT/CT are also attractive tools for treatment planning as well as tumor control probability and normal tissue complication probability, similar to external beam radiotherapy. Currently, issues of noise and partial-volume errors from a nuclear medicine image still result in some uncertainty but it is hoped that this will gradually be overcome. An increasing number of commercial software solutions for dosimetry analyses are readily becoming available.

4.3.2.3   Tumor and Normal Organ Absorbed Dose Thresholds

There is growing data on tri-compartmental dosimetry indicating a dose–response relationship, although much variation exists. Absorbed dose recommendations and their respective level of evidence can be referenced in the recently published guidelines for both ^{90}Y glass and resin microspheres from The European Association of Nuclear Medicine [31].

Of importance, curative radiation segmentectomy has seen strong interest and efforts into finding a relationship between absorbed dose and complete response are ongoing with a recent study involving ^{90}Y glass microspheres for HCC showing complete pathological necrosis on histopathological correlation in all patients receiving >400 Gy [33].

4.3.2.4   Post-Therapy Imaging

Bremsstrahlung SPECT/CT can be used as a post-treatment scan to ascertain the successful treatment of ^{90}Y SIRT as per the radiation simulation scan using ^{99m}Tc-MAA. Unfortunately, it suffers from the problem of poor spatial resolution and at best might serve as an adjunct to this therapy. On the other hand, although more expensive and limited by poor count emission with longer scan times, ^{90}Y PET/CT imaging is gaining traction to replace bremsstrahlung due to its multifold uses in post SIRT analysis. In clinical practice, ^{90}Y PET/CT imaging allows for better assessment of the microspheres localization to ascertain if targeting was appropriate and also in predicting response to treatment. Figure 4.3 shows an example of a case that demonstrates the usefulness of ^{90}Y PET/CT in evaluating tumor response. The quantification of counts in ^{90}Y PET/CT imaging can be utilized for post-treatment dosimetry and identify tumor heterogeneity as well as provide intra-tumoral dose-histograms [34]. Occasionally, post-treatment imaging has led to further treatment such as repeat SIRT or external beam radiotherapy as a radiation boost to areas that were deemed under-treated.

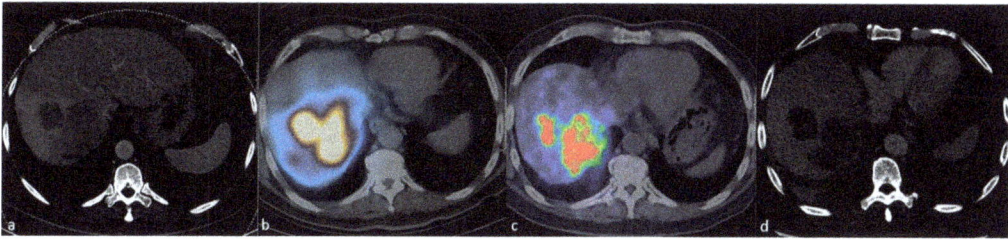

FIGURE 4.3 Axial contrast CT image in (a) shows the large right hepatic lobe tumors before ^{90}Y SIRT. The ^{99m}Tc-MAA axial SPECT/CT image in (b) shows good tracer uptake in the right hepatic tumors predicting good tumor targeting. After treatment, the ^{90}Y axial PET/CT image in (c) confirms excellent microsphere deposition in the right hepatic tumors. The axial CT image in (d) shows the right hepatic tumors two weeks post ^{90}Y SIRT with mild reduction in size indicating some initial treatment response.

4.3.3 SIDE EFFECTS

SIRT is a safe and efficacious procedure and the most common side effect of ^{90}Y SIRT will be the post-embolization syndrome (fever, abdominal pain and fatigue) which is usually mild. Other more serious complications usually arise from unintended deposition of ^{90}Y microspheres into non-target tissue in adjacent organs such as non-tumoral liver, lungs, biliary system, stomach and bowels. Depending on the site and absorbed dose, this may cause severe radiation-induced inflammation and subsequent damage along with potential organ failure. Treatment is usually symptomatic or with steroids and rarely requiring surgical intervention.

REFERENCES

1. Avram A. M., Zukotynski K., Nadel H. R., Giovanella L. Management of differentiated thyroid cancer: the standard of care. *J Nucl Med*. 2022 Feb;63(2):189–195.
2. Haugen Bryan R., Alexander Erik K., Bible Keith C., Doherty Gerard M., Mandel Susan J., Nikiforov Yuri E., et al. 2015 American Thyroid Association Management Guidelines for adult patients with thyroid nodules and differentiated thyroid cancer: The American Thyroid Association Guidelines Task Force on thyroid nodules and differentiated thyroid cancer. *Thyroid*. 2016; 26: 1–133.
3. Ruel E., Thomas S., Dinan M., Perkins J. M., Roman S. A., Sosa J. A. Adjuvant radioactive iodine therapy is associated with improved survival for patients with intermediate-risk papillary thyroid cancer. *J Clin Endocrinol Metab*. 2015 Apr; 100(4): 1529–1536. doi: 10.1210/jc.2014-4332. Epub 2015 Feb 2. PMID: 25642591; PMCID: PMC4399282.
4. Mal Mallick U., Harmer C., Yap B., Wadsley J., Clarke S., Moss L., et al. Ablation with low-dose radioiodine and thyrotropin alfa in thyroid cancer. *N Engl J Med*. 2012; 366: 1674–1685.
5. Schlumberger M., Catargi B., Borget I., Deandreis D., Zerdoud S., Bridji B., et al. Strategies of radioiodine ablation in patients with low-risk thyroid cancer. *N Engl J Med*. 2012; 366: 1663–1673.
6. Parisi M. T., Eslamy H., Mankoff D. Management of differentiated thyroid cancer in children: focus on the American Thyroid Association pediatric guidelines. *Semin Nucl Med*. 2016; 46: 147–164. 36.
7. Machac J. Thyroid cancer in pediatrics. *Endocrinol Metab Clin North Am*. 2016; 45: 359–404.
8. Edmonds C. J., Hayes S., Kermode J. C., Thompson B. D. Measurement of serum TSH and thyroid hormones in the management of treatment of thyroid carcinoma with radioiodine. *Br J Radiol*. 1977; 50: 799–807.
9. Silberstein E. B., Alavi A., Balon H. R., Clarke S. E., Divgi C., Gelfand M. J., et al. The SNMMI practice guideline for therapy of thyroid disease with 131I 3.0. *J Nucl Med*. 2012; 53: 1633–1651.
10. Sawka A. M., Ibrahim-Zada I., Galacgac P., Tsang R. W., Brierley J. D., Ezzat S., et al. Dietary iodine restriction in preparation for radioactive iodine treatment or scanning in well-differentiated thyroid cancer: a systematic review. *Thyroid*. 2010; 20: 1129–1138.
11. Freudenberg L. S., Jentzen W., Görges R., Petrich T., Marlowe R. J., Knust J., et al. 124I-PET dosimetry in advanced differentiated thyroid cancer: therapeutic impact. *Nuklearmedizin*. 2007; 46(4): 121–128.

12. Pentlow K. S., Graham M. C., Lambrecht R. M., Daghighian F., Bacharach S. L., Bendriem B., et al. Quantitative imaging of iodine-124 with PET. *J Nucl Med.* 1996 Sep; 37(9): 1557–1562.

13. Sgouros G., Kolbert K. S., Sheikh A., Pentlow K. S., Mun E. F., Barth A., et al. Patient-specific dosimetry for 131I thyroid cancer therapy using 124I PET and 3-dimensional-internal dosimetry (3D-ID) software. *J Nucl Med.* 2004 Aug; 45(8): 1366–1372.

14. Nielsen O. S., Munro A. J., Tannock I. F. Bone metastases: pathophysiology and management policy. *J Clin Oncol.* 1991; 9: 509–524.

15. Soloway M. S., Hardeman S. W., Hickey D., Raymond J., Todd B., Soloway S., et al. Stratification of patients with metastatic prostate cancer based on extent of disease on initial bone scan. *Cancer.* 1988 Jan 1; 61(1): 195–202.

16. Hamdy N. A., Papapoulos S. E. The palliative management of skeletal metastases in prostate cancer: use of bone-seeking radionuclides and bisphosphonates. *Semin Nucl Med.* 2001; 31: 62–68.

17. Silberstein E. B. Dosage and response in radiopharmaceutical therapy of painful osseous metastases. *J Nucl Med.* 1996; 37: 249–252.

18. Loke K. S. H., Padhy A. K., Ng D. C. E., Goh A. S. W., Divgi C. Dosimetric considerations in radioimmunotherapy and systemic radionuclide therapies: a review. *World J Nucl Med.* 2011 Jul-Dec; 10(2): 122–138.

19. Parker C., Nilsson S., Heinrich D., Helle S. I., O'Sullivan J. M., Fosså S. D. et al. Alpha emitter radium-223 and survival in metastatic prostate cancer. *N Engl J Med.* 2013; 369: 213–223.

20. Bruland, Ø.S., Nilsson, S., Fisher, D. R., Larsen, R. H. High-linear energy transfer irradiation targeted to skeletal metastases by the α-emitter 223Ra: Adjuvant or alternative to conventional modalities? *Clin Cancer Res.* 2006; 12: 6250s–6257s.

21. D'Angelo, G., Sciuto, R., Salvatori, M., Sperduti, I., Mantini, G., Maini, C. L., et al. Targeted "bone-seeking" radiopharmaceuticals for palliative treatment of bone metastases: A systematic review and meta-analysis. *Q J Nucl Med Mol Imaging.* 2012; 56: 538–543.

22. Dafermou A., Colamussi P., Giganti M., Cittanti C., Bestagno M. A Piffanelli. A multicentre observational study of radionuclide therapy in patients with painful bone metastases of prostate cancer. *Eur J Nucl Med.* 2001 Jul; 28(7): 788–798.

23. Juan C. V. Metastasic bone pain management with radioactive isotopes. *Braz Arch Biol Technol.* October 2005; 48, Special: 127–135.

24. Kew M. C. Epidemiology of hepatocellular carcinoma. *Toxicology.* 2002 Dec 27; 181–182: 35–38.

25. Kennedy A., Nag S., Salem R., Murthy R., McEwan A. J., Nutting C. W., et al. Recommendations for radioembolization of hepatic malignancies using yttrium-90 microsphere brachytherapy: a consensus panel report from the radioembolization brachytherapy oncology consortium. *Int J Radiat Oncol Biol Phys.* 2007; 68: 13–23.

26. Salem R., Johnson G. E., Kim E., Riaz A., Bishay V., Boucher E., et al. Yttrium-90 radioembolization for the treatment of solitary, unresectable HCC: the LEGACY study. *Hepatology.* 2021 Nov; 74(5): 2342–2352.

27. Entezari P., Gabr A., Kennedy K., Salem R., Lewandowski R. J. Radiation lobectomy: An overview of concept and applications, technical considerations, outcomes. *Semin Intervent Radiol.* 2021 Oct; 38(4): 419–424.

28. Gabr A., Kulik L., Mouli S., Riaz A., Ali R., Desai K., et al. Liver transplantation following yttrium-90 radioembolization: 15-year experience in 207-patient cohort. *Hepatology.* 2021 Mar; 73(3): 998–1010.

29. Chow P. K. H., Gandhi M., Tan S. B., Khin M. W., Khasbazar A., Ong J., et al. Asia-Pacific Hepatocellular Carcinoma Trials Group. SIRveNIB: selective internal radiation therapy versus sorafenib in Asia-Pacific patients with hepatocellular carcinoma. *J Clin Oncol.* 2018 Jul 1; 36(19): 1913–1921.

30. Garin E., Tselikas L., Guiu B., Chalaye J., Edeline J., de Baere T., et al. DOSISPHERE-01 Study Group. Personalised versus standard dosimetry approach of selective internal radiation therapy in patients with locally advanced hepatocellular carcinoma (DOSISPHERE-01): a randomised, multi-centre, open-label phase 2 trial. *Lancet Gastroenterol Hepatol.* 2021 Jan; 6(1): 17–29.

31. Weber M., Lam M., Chiesa C., Konijnenberg M., Cremonesi M., Flamen P., et al. EANM procedure guideline for the treatment of liver cancer and liver metastases with intra-arterial radioactive compounds. *Eur J Nucl Med Mol Imaging.* 2022 Apr; 49(5): 1682–1699.

32. Zhuang K. D., Tong A. K., Ng D. C. E., Tay K. H.. The role of catheter-directed CT-angiography in radioembolisation. *Cardiovasc Intervent Radiol.* 2022 May 20; 45: 1651–1658. doi: 10.1007/s00270-022-03157-4. Epub ahead of print. PMID: 35595985.

33. Gabr A., Riaz A., Johnson G. E., Kim E., Padia S., Lewandowski R. J., et al. Correlation of Y90-absorbed radiation dose to pathological necrosis in hepatocellular carcinoma: confirmatory multicenter analysis in 45 explants. *Eur J Nucl Med Mol Imaging*. 2021 Feb; 48(2): 580–583.
34. Kao Y. H., Steinberg J. D., Tay Y. S., Lim G. K., Yan J., Townsend D. W., et al. Post-radioembolization yttrium-90 PET/CT - part 2: dose-response and tumor predictive dosimetry for resin microspheres. *EJNMMI Res*. 2013 Jul 25; 3(1): 57.

5 Radionuclide-Conjugated Cancer-Specific Vectors
Peptides

*Arianna Di Paolo, Irene Marini, Anna Sarnelli,
Maria Luisa Belli, and Giovanni Paganelli*

5.1 INTRODUCTION

As introduced in Chapter 3, the biologic basis for receptor radionuclide diagnosis and therapy is the overexpression of specific receptors and the subsequent receptor-mediated retention of a radionuclide or a radiolabeled molecule at tumor site. The term targeted radionuclide therapy (TRNT) stands for the systemic administration of radionuclides or radiolabeled drugs directed against tumor-associated targets. This approach allows the selective irradiation of tumor cells, sparing, to some extent, the surrounding normal tissues [1].

The molecules studied as a vehicle for TRNT are antibodies, peptides, small molecules (e.g. enzyme substrate), and nanoparticles. Peptides, small molecules, and antibodies are the most clinically investigated agents, while liposomal or nanoconstruct-based techniques are currently being studied mostly in preclinical settings. Glass and resin microspheres are another way to perform TRNT. This approach is relatively well established in the treatment of hepatocellular carcinoma or hepatic metastases from other cancers.

5.2 PEPTIDES

Natural or synthetic peptides are chains of a certain number of amino acids linked by peptide bonds. The amino acid sequence along the chain, the spatial configuration of amino acid residues, their local and overall conformation, together with the intra and intermolecular interactions are all important factors in determining the biological activity of each peptide.

Human cancers overexpress receptors for a variety of peptides such as somatostatin (SST), bombesin, vasoactive intestinal peptide, cholecystokinin, and substance P. These peptides could be used as a "trojan horse" to vehicle radioisotopes within cancer cells. In principle, any over-expressed cancer cell receptor could be suitable for radiopeptide therapy. Peptide receptor radionuclide therapy (PRRT) based on somatostatin receptor (SSTR) overexpression in neuro-endocrine tumors (NETs) is the most studied system in clinical practice.

5.3 SOMATOSTATIN, SOMATOSTATIN RECEPTORS, SOMATOSTATIN ANALOGS, AND SOMATOSTATIN ANTAGONISTS

SST is a polypeptide hormone, first discovered in hypothalamic samples and identified as an inhibitor of growth hormone. There are two biologically active forms of this hormone: SS-14 (primary form in the brain) and SS-28 (primary form in the gut), with a 14 or 28 amino acids chain, respectively. They are both produced by proteolytic cleavage of precursors called prepro-somatostatin and pro-somatostatin. In the amino acid sequence of somatostatin, the essential

DOI: 10.1201/9781003250913-7

region for receptor binding is the tetrapeptide Phe-Trp-Lys-Thr (corresponding to the amino acid residues 7–10 in SS-14).

SST acts through both endocrine and paracrine pathways by binding to its receptor (SSTR), with a large variety of effects on multiple targets such as the inhibition of growth hormone secretion from the pituitary gland, paracrine inhibition of both insulin and glucagon secretion in the pancreas, inhibition of gastrin, cholecystokinin, secretin, and vasoactive intestinal peptide secretion in the gastrointestinal (GI) tract. Initially identified in pituitary adenomas, **SSTRs** have a wide expression in both normal tissues and solid tumors. They belong to the family of 7-transmembrane-domain G-protein-coupled molecules, with a weight of approximately 80 kDa. There are five different subtypes of SSTRs, showing 50% amino acids homology, most pronounced in the transmembrane regions. They are divided into two subgroups according to their structural homology and pharmacological profile: SSTR1 and 4 versus SSTR2A and B, 3, and 5. In the group of tumors that overexpress SSTR2, gastroenteropancreatic and bronchial NET, meningiomas, neuroblastomas, medulloblastomas and paragangliomas, renal cell and hepatocellular carcinomas, lymphomas, breast, and small-cell lung cancers can be mentioned. SSTR1 is often found in sarcomas and prostate cancers; less frequently they express SSTR5. SSTR1 is also found in gastroenteropancreatic tumors, gastric carcinomas, phaeochromocytomas, and ependymomas, often alternating with SSTR2 or SSTR5. Pituitary adenomas often express SSTR3, while SSTR4 is generally less represented.

Considering the distinct signaling cascades regulated by SSTRs, multiple signaling-targeted agents and receptor-targeted SST analogs/antagonists have been developed as antitumoral drugs. The ability of SSTR to be internalized constitutes the rationale both for the therapeutic use of "non-radioactive" **SST analogs** (SSAs) in NETs and for the use of radiolabeled SST analogs for diagnostic and therapeutic purposes.

In humans, the short plasma half-life (1–3 min) of native SST limits its clinical usefulness. Therefore, long-acting SSAs have been developed, such as octreotide and lanreotide, which differ from native SST-14 in terms of receptor affinity (they preferentially bind SSTR2 with high affinity) and in terms of longer half-life. Among octreotide analogs, Tyr3-octreotide (TOC) shows high affinity to SST2 and moderate affinity to SST5, while 1-Nal3-octreotide (NOC) and BzThi3-octreotide (BOC) show affinity also to SST3. [Tyr3, Thr8]-octreotide ([Tyr3]-octreotate or TATE), instead, shows almost selective affinity to SST2, while [1-Nal3, Thr8]-octreotide (NOC-ATE) and [BzThi3, Thr8]-octreotide (BOC-ATE) also bind to SST5 and SST3 [2].

Among **radiolabeled SSAs**, the first synthesized radioactive compound useful to imaging NET in 1989 was ^{123}I-labeled TOC [3]. Its clinical use was hampered by a difficult labeling process; moreover, the relatively high hepatic and intestinal uptake makes the interpretation of scintigraphic images suboptimal. The introduction of chelators for labeling with radiometals revolutionized the field. The first conjugated compound was ^{111}In-DTPA (Indium-111 diethylenetriaminepentaacetic acid)-octreotide or ^{111}In-pentreotide, also known as Octreoscan®, which remained for many years the gold standard for NET imaging. Nevertheless, gamma camera imaging was burdened by limited spatial resolution and by the interference of physiological uptake (e.g. spleen and kidneys). Following the development of PET imaging, new tracers have been investigated for NET, obtaining higher spatial resolution and better image quality. The use of the macrocyclic chelator DOTA (1,4,7,10-tetraazacyclododecane-1,4,7,10-tetraacetic acid) paved the way for a new era in NET imaging. It forms stable complexes with Gallium-68 (^{68}Ga) and with SSAs (known as [68]GaDOTA-peptides). Gallium-68 (^{68}Ga) is a positron-emitting isotope that can be obtained "on-site" from a [68]Ge/^{68}Ga generator. Its half-life of 67.6 minutes and its hydrophilic nature guarantee a rapid renal clearance and reduce the radiation dose for patients. Among [68]GaDOTA-peptides, ^{68}Ga-DOTA-Tyr3-octreotide (^{68}Ga-DOTATOC) was the first synthesized radiopharmaceutical, followed soon after by ^{68}Ga-DOTA-Tyr3-octreotate (^{68}Ga-DOTATATE) and ^{68}Ga-DOTA-1-NaI3-octreotide (^{68}Ga-DOTANOC). The introduction of ^{68}Ga-DOTA-peptides improved the detection of smaller or low-grade SSTR expression lesions and they allowed faster image acquisition, with a lower radiation exposure.

In the field of NET imaging, **SSTR antagonists** are emerging agents. Antagonists differ from octreotide agonists for the inversion of chirality at positions 1 and 2. The first SST2 antagonist ^{111}In-DOTA-BASS showed higher tumor uptake compared to the agonist ^{111}In-DTPA-TATE, despite its lower affinity, and it also showed to bind to a higher number of sites on the cell membrane. Antagonists are still under study; up to date, the most promising antagonists seem to be JR11 and LM3, which can be coupled to different chelators, DOTA and NODAGA, and radiolabeled with various radiometals.

5.4 RADIONUCLIDES FOR PRRT

Apart from the established diagnostic radionuclides gallium-68 and indium-111, several other radiometals have been proposed to label DOTA-peptides for therapeutic purposes. Among them, β^- emitters such as yttrium-90 and lutetium-177 are the two most commonly used isotopes for PRRT, with ^{177}Lu-DOTATATE (^{177}Lu-oxodotreotide or Lutathera®) being the only agent approved in most countries that use TRNT to date.

Yttrium-90 is a pure β^- emitting isotope, with a half-life of 64 hours, E_{max} of 2.28 MeV, and max tissue penetration of 11.3 mm. Lutetium-177 has a longer half-life (6.7 days), E_{max} 0.5 MeV, a lower tissue penetration (R_{max} 1.8–2 mm), and it emits both photons (two main γ emissions: 113 keV and 208 keV) and β^- particles, making it suitable both for imaging (γ emission) and for therapy (β^- emission) (Table 5.1).

A newly explored area in PPRT is the delivery of α emitter radiopharmaceuticals. Alpha particles have a very short range of penetration in tissues (20–100 μm) and a much higher linear energy transfer (LET) compared to β^- particles (50–230 versus 0.2 keV/μm). These features make α emitters more cytotoxic for tumor cells and more able to spare the surrounding normal cells. Among the α emitters, [213]Bi in combination with DOTATOC, [212]Pb-DOTAMTATE (AlphaMedix™), and [225]Ac-DOTATOC are currently under investigation.

5.5 NEUROENDOCRINE TUMORS

5.5.1 Epidemiology, Clinic, Classification, and Prognostic Factors

NETs constitute a heterogeneous group of predominantly slow-growing neoplasms, arising from the diffuse neuroendocrine cell system; they share the distinctive trait of overexpressing SSTRs on the cell membrane.

The incidence rates and the prevalence of NETs, generally considered relatively rare tumors, have been constantly increasing over the last 30 years, particularly those originating from the pancreas and small intestine.

TABLE 5.1
Physical Properties of ^{90}Y and [177]Lu

	[90]Y	[177]Lu
Physical Half-Life (days)	2.7	6.7
Emission Spectrum	β^-	β^- and γ
Particle Penetration (mm)	11.3	1.8–2
Maximum Beta Energy (MeV)	2.28	0.5
Imaging	Bremsstrahlung	γ emission

About 72% of NETs primarily arise from the GI system and about 25% from the bronchopulmonary system. Rarely, NETs can also originate from other sites where neuroendocrine cells are present (e.g. adrenal glands, thyroid, prostate, and ovary).

Generally sporadic, in some cases NETs can be associated with hereditary conditions such as type 1 multiple endocrine neoplasia (MEN 1), Von Hippel–Lindau Syndrome (VHL), neurofibromatosis (NF), and tuberous sclerosis (TS). In these scenarios, NETs can show a more precocious onset and are frequently multifocal.

NETs can be either non-functional (asymptomatic) or functional (symptomatic), due to NETs property of secreting hormones (e.g. glucagon, insulin, and gastrin) and/or amines (e.g. serotonin). In case of hypersecretion of serotonin, patients could present the so-called carcinoid syndrome (including diarrhea, flushing, and right heart failure). Other functioning tumors include insulinomas (hypoglycemia), gastrinomas (Zollinger–Ellison syndrome), and VIP-omas (watery diarrhoea, hypokalaemia, and achlorhydria).

The 2019 World Health Organization (WHO) classification [4] uses the term neuroendocrine neoplasms (NENs) to globally indicate tumors arising from the diffuse neuroendocrine cell system and categorizes the gastroenteropancreatic ones in three grades on the basis of cell proliferation, nuclear-antigen Ki-67 expression, and number of mitosis per high-power fields (HPF). Grade 1 (G1) refers to a Ki-67 <3% (and <2 mitoses per 10HPF), Grade 2 (G2) to Ki-67 of 3–20% (or 2–20 mitoses per 10 HPF), and Grade 3 (G3) to Ki-67 >20% (or >20 mitoses per 10 HPF). The WHO classification also divides gastroenteropancreatic neuroendocrine neoplasms (GEP-NENs) into well-differentiated gastroenteropancreatic neuroendocrine tumors (GEP-NETs – G1-G3) and poorly differentiated neuroendocrine carcinomas (NECs – always G3), reflecting their molecular differences (Figure 5.1).

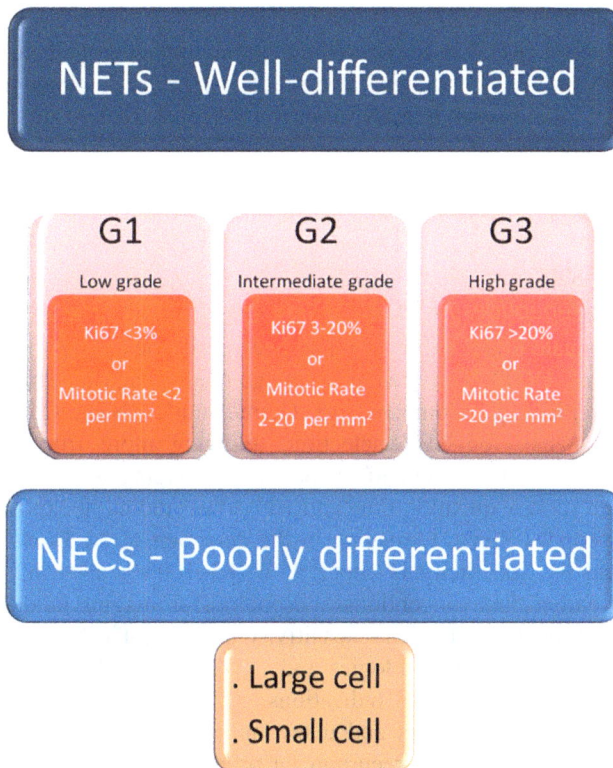

FIGURE 5.1   GEP-NETs: 2019 World Health Organization (WHO) classification.

The proliferation index relates to prognosis, biological behavior, and clinical evolution of the disease. High-grade tumors often demonstrate a reduced SSTR expression, limiting imaging sensibility and PRRT efficacy. Another relevant prognostic factor is the site of primary tumor: NETs arising from the small intestine and rectum generally show a better prognosis compared with those originating in pancreas or right colon. The presence of a functioning tumor is a negative prognostic factor, as well as the presence of a high tumor burden and FDG PET/CT-positive lesions. Instead, highly positive somatostatin receptor imaging (SRI) is a favorable prognostic factor and has an important predictive value for response to PRRT. However, FDG PET/CT-positive lesions have the worse prognostic factor for NETs undergoing PRRT [5].

5.5.2 DIAGNOSIS

Anatomic location of the primary tumor, grade, stage, local invasion, functionality, and SSTR expression are of pivotal importance in order to choose the best suitable therapeutic strategy in metastatic patients.

5.5.2.1 Conventional Imaging

Computed tomography (CT) is considered the basic radiological imaging modality for NET staging (because of wide availability, good standardization, and reproducibility). The sensitivity of CT to detect NETs is 61–93% and the specificity is 71–100%. CT is the method of choice for lung imaging but its sensitivity for bone metastases is poor, and small pathological lymph nodes or peritoneal metastases could be difficult to identify.

Magnetic resonance imaging (MRI) has been demonstrated superior to CT for the evaluation of liver metastases, for the pancreas, and in the imaging of bone and brain metastases.

Endoscopic ultrasound (EUS) is considered the optimal imaging method for the diagnosis of small pancreatic NETs (p-NETs), allowing also needle aspiration cytology or biopsy.

Contrast-enhanced ultrasound is a useful tool for the characterization of equivocal liver lesions at MR or CT imaging.

Intra-operative ultrasound facilitates localization, biopsy, and eventually removal of pancreatic and hepatic lesions.

5.5.2.2 PET/CT Imaging

5.5.2.2.1 ^{68}Ga-DOTA-peptides PET/CT

The first studies to evaluate SSTR expression had been performed using the tracer ^{111}In-DTPA-octreotide (OctreoScan®, OCT). Time required, image quality, and detection accuracy favored ^{68}Ga-DOTA-peptides PET/CT. Compared to OctreoScan®, ^{68}Ga-DOTA-peptides PET/CT showed better performance for NET detection, allowing more true positive tumor foci identification; it was also better tolerated by patients providing a non-invasive, whole-body 3D evaluation in quite short acquisition time and with lower radiation exposure. The sensitivity of the ^{68}Ga-DOTA-peptides PET/CT imaging in the detection of NETs is approximately 92% (range 64–100%) and the specificity is about 95% (83–100%), allowing the recognition of disease localizations earlier than conventional morphological imaging modalities. An important issue to take into account is that the sensitivity of ^{68}Ga-DOTA-peptides PET/CT can significantly vary among different histologies and tumor grades, depending on the density of SSTR expression on the cell membrane. Indications to ^{68}Ga-DOTA-peptides PET/CT currently include localization of primary tumors and detection of eventual sites of metastatic disease (staging); follow-up to detect residual, recurrent, or progressive disease (restaging); determination of SSTR status (assessed both visually and with semiquantitative methods) to select patients suitable for SSA therapy and PRRT. The evaluation of the response to therapy has been proposed as an indication, but standardization is still under debate because a reduction in receptor expression does not necessarily reflect a response to therapy (due to possible de-differentiation of the neoplasms).

Based on a qualitative evaluation of the tracer uptake in lesions, a "modified" Krenning score (on the basis of the Octreoscan Krenning score) has been proposed to select patients suitable for PRRT. It's a 5 points scale: 0 = no uptake; 1= very low uptake; 2 = uptake ≤ liver; 3 = uptake > liver; 4 = uptake > spleen. A score ≥3 sets the indication for PRRT. According to Kratochwil and co-workers [6], the semiquantitative parameter maximum standardized uptake value (SUV_{max}) at baseline ^{68}Ga-DOTA-peptides imaging in liver metastases can be considered predictive of response to PRRT; they propose a SUV_{max} cut-off > 16.4 to select patients suitable for PRRT. Moreover, the assessment of SSTR status allows the estimation of the absorbed dose for dosimetric purposes.

5.5.2.2.2 ^{18}F-FDG PET/CT

The routinary use of ^{18}F-FDG PET for the diagnosis of both primary tumor and metastases is limited by the high number of false negative scans in NET of every grade. Nevertheless, some evidence in literature has shown that patients with positive FDG imaging have a worst prognosis, paving the way to the use of this metabolic tracer for prognostic purpose. The concomitant use of ^{18}F-FDG PET/CT can be considered as complementary predictive option and its utilization in clinical protocols is becoming more common (Figures 5.2 and 5.3).

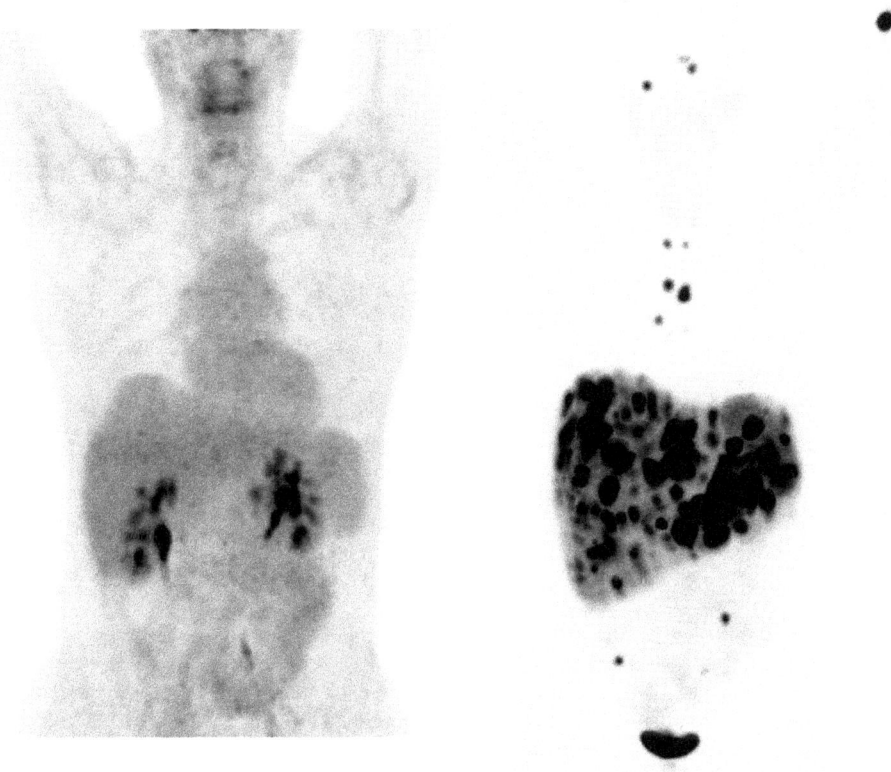

FIGURE 5.2 Patient with negative ^{18}F-FDG PET/CT (left) and positive ^{68}Ga-DOTA-peptides PET/CT (right). Images from Nuclear Medicine Unit – IRCCS Istituto Romagnolo per lo Studio dei Tumori (IRST) "Dino Amadori", Meldola, Italy.

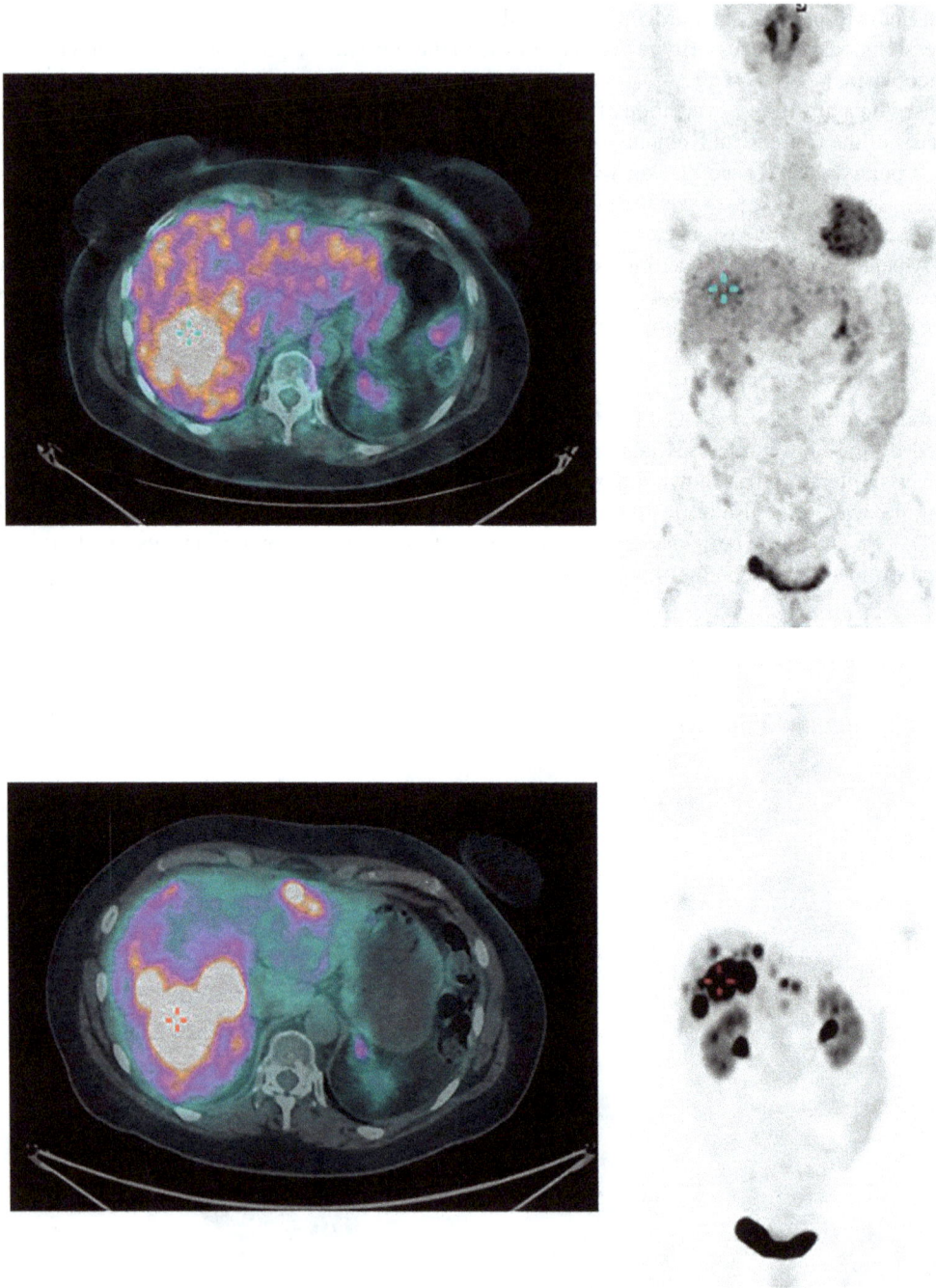

FIGURE 5.3 Patient with positive ^{18}F-FDG PET/CT (above) and positive ^{68}Ga-DOTA-peptides PET/CT (below). Even if in maximum intensity projection image the hepatic lesion is not so evident, in the transaxial image the same lesion clearly shows an elevated FDG metabolism. Images from Nuclear Medicine Unit – IRCCS Istituto Romagnolo per lo Studio dei Tumori (IRST) "Dino Amadori", Meldola, Italy.

5.5.3 Conventional Therapeutic Strategies

Nowadays, multiple treatment options are available for NET patients and the management should be tailored on the basis of tumor site, histology, extent, grade, stage, symptoms, and patient performance status.

5.5.3.1 Surgery

For local and loco-regional disease control, surgery is the treatment of choice. Whenever feasible, removal of the primary tumor should be attempted in order to reduce loco-regional invasion, the likelihood of metastatic spread, symptoms (in functional NETs), risk of recurrences, potential local events (e.g. obstruction, ischemia, perforation, or bleeding), and for palliative purpose.

Other options also include *radiofrequency ablation* (RFA)*, trans-arterial embolization* (TAE)*, trans-arterial chemoembolization* (TACE)*, and selective internal radiation therapy* (SIRT). Combined approaches could also be considered.

5.5.3.2 Long-Acting Somatostatin Analogs (SSAs)

SSAs are the standard first-line therapeutic strategy in NET patients. Usually well tolerated, SSAs can achieve an improvement of symptoms in 70–80% of the patients and, in selected cases, can obtain some inhibitory effect on primary and metastatic lesions growth. Subcutaneous injections of short-acting octreotide can be considered in cases of intermittingly increasing symptoms.

5.5.3.3 Interferon-Alpha (INF-α) and Other Treatments

INF-α is approved for the control of symptoms, usually as second-line treatment in refractory syndromic patients. In functioning tumors (e.g. insulinomas or gastrinomas), also other pharmacological treatments for the management of the symptoms, like *anti-hypoglycemic agents or proton pump inhibitors*, are usually effective.

5.5.3.4 Chemo-Biotherapy

Generally, traditional chemotherapeutic agents have little space for the control of well-differentiated NETs because of the indolent behavior of most of them. However, in some specific settings (e.g. advanced p-NET and in G3 NETs and NECs), the administration of systemic chemotherapy (e.g. *capecitabine* alone or in combination with *temozolomide* or the combined use of *carboplatin/etoposide* or *cisplatin/etoposide*) could be considered.

In recent years, some novel agents like *Everolimus, Sunitinib, and Bevacizumab* with different molecular targets (e.g. mTOR, TKI, and VEGF) have been introduced for the management of NET patients.

5.6 PEPTIDE RECEPTOR RADIONUCLIDE THERAPY

The majority of GEP-NETs express SSTRs on the cell membrane and can therefore be treated with radiolabeled SST analogues (PRRT). It involves the systemic administration of a radiopharmaceutical composed of a radionuclide (usually a β^- emitter) chelated to a specific SST analogue. The radiopharmaceutical binds to the SSTR over-expressed on the cell surface; it is internalized and concentrated in the tumor cells, where the targets (e.g. DNA) are attained. Afterward, the receptor is either recycled on the cell membrane or trapped in lysosomes for degradation.

In the 1990s, the first therapeutic experiences in NETs were performed using the Auger electron-emitting ^{111}In-pentetreotide, often producing clinical benefits on symptoms, even if the objective radiological response was rare. Afterward, the high-energy β^- emitter yttrium-90 linked to octreotide, constituting ^{90}Y-DOTA-Tyr3-octreotide (^{90}Y-DOTATOC) was evaluated. This radiopharmaceutical that showed a good affinity for SSTR2 has reported in clinical trials objective response rates (ORR) in 6–37% of patients and has shown a positive impact on overall survival (OS). In the mid-2000s, ^{177}Lu-DOTA-Tyr3-octreotate (^{177}Lu-DOTATATE) was synthesized. Compared to ^{90}Y, this new radiopharmaceutical shows a lower tissue penetration, a longer half-life, and a higher peptide receptor affinity (ninefold higher) for SSTR2s. Lutetium-177 also shows another relevant advantage due to its significant γ emission (113 and 208 keV). This allows us to obtain a good quality post-treatment whole-body imaging, providing an accurate representation of its distribution in neoplastic lesions and favoring disease monitoring after each treatment cycle.

PRRT has been used for over two decades as an effective systemic treatment option in metastatic and/or inoperable patients with SSTR positive GEPs, bronchopulmonary, and other NETs within the framework of specific research protocols because an approved radiopharmaceutical was lacking until the registration of ^{177}Lu-oxodotreotide (Lutathera®). The two most used radionuclides are yttrium-90 and lutetium-177. The more favorable combinations of radionuclide/DOTA-peptide are ^{90}Y-DOTATOC and ^{177}Lu-DOTATATE, while other different combinations resulted in either causing more toxicity or being less effective.

Over the years, the safety aspects and the effectiveness of PRRT have been evaluated in multiple protocols differing for administered activity (total or per cycle), number of cycles, and administration intervals. At present, for ^{90}Y-DOTATOC the recommended administered activities for each cycle range from 1.8 to 2.5 GBq (interval between cycles: 8–10 weeks) with a median of 4 cycles; for ^{177}Lu-DOTATATE the recommended administered activities range from 3.7 to 7.4 GBq (interval between cycles: 6–12 weeks) for 4 or 5 cycles. ^{90}Y-DOTATOC takes advantage of the higher β⁻ particle emission and is generally preferred for the treatment of larger neoplastic lesions because of its high β⁻ emission range (maximum tissue penetration of 11 mm, with a median of 5–7 mm). ^{177}Lu-DOTATATE avails of higher SSTR2 affinity, a longer residence time in the tumor, and a lower kidney exposure. ^{177}Lu-DOTATATE β⁻ rays have a smaller range (2 mm) and are consequently preferred for smaller lesions. The above-mentioned preferable properties favored ^{177}Lu-DOTATATE that, for its effectiveness and good tolerability, became the more widely used radiopharmaceutical (Figures 5.4 and 5.5).

After the pivotal NETTER-1 trial, ^{177}Lu-oxodotreotide (Lutathera®) was finally approved as a therapeutic option for patients with progressive, advanced, SSTR-positive, well-differentiated (G1/2) GEP-NETs. The preliminary results of the NETTER-1 trial showed the superiority of ^{177}Lu-DOTATATE over high-dose SSAs in midgut NETs, paving the way to the radiopharmaceutical trade registration in 2019. (See Chapter 8 for details of this trial).

5.6.1 INDICATIONS AND SAFETY ASPECTS

According to the current guidelines of the International Atomic Energy Agency, the European Association of Nuclear Medicine, and the Society of Nuclear Medicine and Molecular Imaging, PRRT is indicated as second-line treatment in patients with metastatic or inoperable (and possibly well to moderately differentiated, G1/G2) gastrointestinal NETs and positive SSRT status. As part of specific trials, PRRT may also be applied to patients with NETs of the bronchial tract, or with pheochromocytomas, paragangliomas, neuroblastomas, and medullary thyroid carcinomas.

It requires a baseline, in vivo, assessment of the SSTR density status of the tumor, generally obtained with a ^{68}Ga-DOTA-peptides PET/CT. The indication for the treatment can be assessed with a qualitative evaluation (the above-mentioned modified Krenning score >3) or with a semi-quantitative evaluation ($SUV_{max} > 16.4$) of the SSTR density. PRRT is contraindicated in case of pregnancy, severe concomitant illness or severe psychiatric disorder, breastfeeding, and severely compromised renal or bone marrow functions.

It is generally well tolerated, with in most cases no or only minimal toxicity to the target organs, especially kidney and bone marrow. The total scheduled activity is divided into multiple

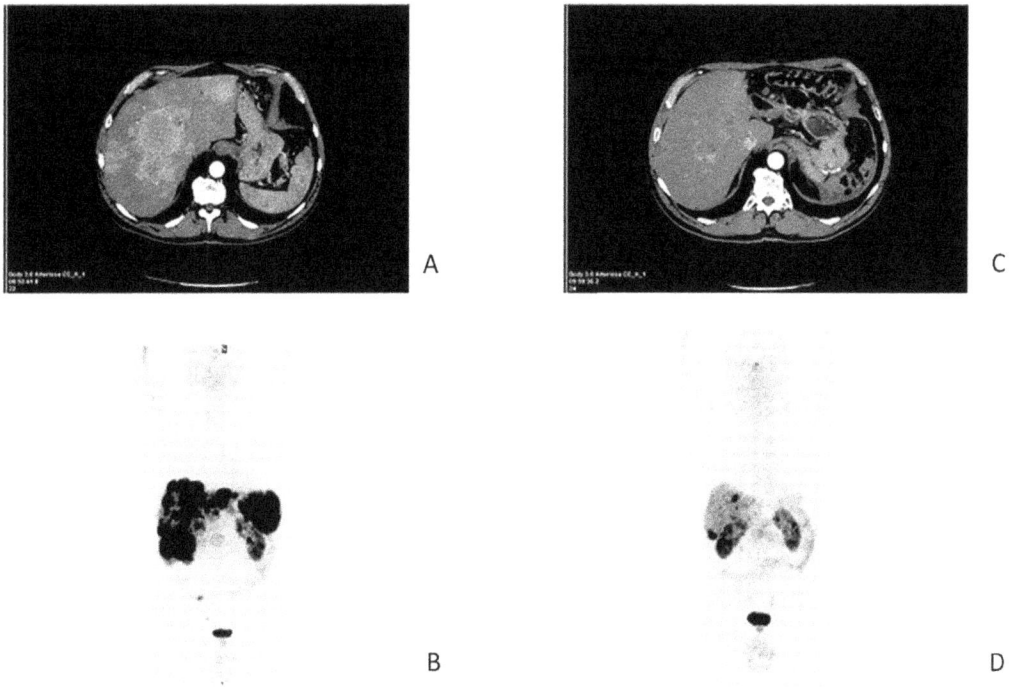

FIGURE 5.4 ^{68}Ga-DOTA-peptides PET/CT (B) and CT (A) before the 1st cycle of PRRT; ^{68}Ga-DOTA-peptides PET/CT (D) and CT (C) after the 5th cycle of PRRT in a 58 y.o. male patient with G2 p-NET. Images from Nuclear Medicine Unit – IRCCS Istituto Romagnolo per lo Studio dei Tumori (IRST) "Dino Amadori", Meldola, Italy.

administration cycles to reduce the likelihood of hematological toxicity, up to the maximum dose to obtain a therapeutic effect without trespassing the dose-limit of 25–27 Gy to the kidneys, which represent the dose-limiting organs. The radiopharmaceutical is infused diluted with saline, via an indwelling catheter, over about 15–30 minutes (because both the total dose and the duration of the infusion influence the dose sparing to the kidneys) and co-administered with an amino-acid solution. Proximal tubular reabsorption of the radiopharmaceutical and the consequent retention can cause high renal irradiation. To reduce the radiation dose to the kidneys, various renal protection protocols are available, including the administration of positively charged amino-acid solutions. The blood clearance, activity elimination, and tumor uptake are not altered by the administration of renal protectors and the absorbed dose to the kidneys is consistently lowered (about 20–30% reduction) [7].

The more frequent acute side effects comprise mild nausea and, rarely, vomiting (mostly related to the co-infused renal protective agents). These symptoms are easily manageable with appropriate anti-nausea pharmaceuticals. About 10% of patients report abdominal pain for a few days in the post-treatment phase. The most frequent subacute effects are fatigue, mild alopecia (10% of patients), and hematological toxicity. All these symptoms are usually mild and transient. Severe toxicities occur in about 10% of patients (more frequently when ^{90}Y-DOTATOC is administered) but are usually reversible and require support in rare cases. Chronic and permanent effects such as loss of renal functionality and reduction of bone marrow reserve are rare. Secondary myeloproliferative diseases (e.g. leukaemia or myelodysplastic syndrome) are extremely rare. The likelihood of these adverse events is significantly reduced by applying appropriate precautions, like the above-mentioned renal protection protocols and personalized dosage and cycling. Dosage tailoring and cycles timing differentiation are under experimental evaluation.

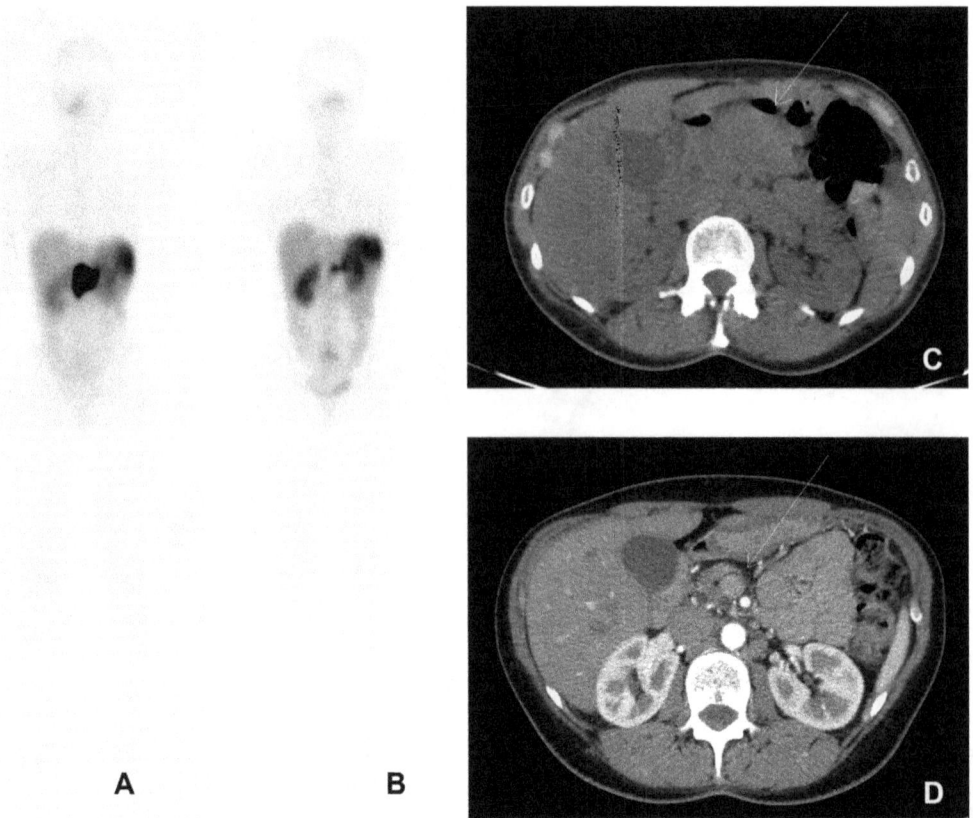

FIGURE 5.5   Whole-body scan (WBS) post-PRRT after the 1st (A) and after the 5th cycle of PRRT (B); CT before the 1st (C) and after the 5th cycle of PRRT (D) in a 42 y.o. female patient with G2 p-NET. Images from Nuclear Medicine Unit – IRCCS Istituto Romagnolo per lo Studio dei Tumori (IRST) "Dino Amadori", Meldola, Italy.

The radiopharmaceutical Lutathera® is administered in 4 cycles every 8 weeks, with a fixed activity per cycle of 7.4 GBq. However, many authors investigated toxicity, safety, and efficacy of different dosage schemes and cycle timing schedule. In a recent paper [8], Paganelli and co-workers analyzed the late toxicity and activity after 10 years follow-up for a cohort of 43 progressive GI-NETs patients who underwent ^{177}Lu-DOTATATE PRRT at two different activities (18.5 GBq and 27.5 GBq, in 5 cycles). The reduced activity of 3.7 GBq per cycle was scheduled for those patients presenting risk factors for hematological or renal toxicity. With an overall 84% disease control rate (DCR), patients were monitored for a median period of 118 months (range 12.6–139.6). The median progression-free survival (mPFS) in patients receiving 18.5 GBq was 59.8 months as the ones treated with 27.5 GBq. On the other hand, the median overall survival (mOS) was 71.0 months in the group that received 18.5 GBq and 97.6 months in the group treated with 27.5 GBq ($P = 0.22$). Remarkably, no late renal or hematological toxicity was observed in either group. The long-term follow-up of the study confirmed that ^{177}Lu-DOTATATE is well tolerated and is effective over time also in patients with renal and bone marrow limited function otherwise excluded from PRRT at standard dosage. In a dosimetric study published in 2008 by the IEO Milan group, [9] the authors analyzed the long-term renal toxicity in patients (23 with ^{90}Y-DOTATOC and 5 with ^{177}Lu-DOTATATE) treated with escalating administered activities. Dosimetric analyses were performed using ^{111}In-DOTATOC as a surrogate of ^{90}Y-DOTATOC and ^{177}Lu-DOTATATE gamma emissions. A linear quadratic method revised for radionuclide therapy was used to evaluate the biological effective dose (BED) to the kidneys. Patients were followed up for a median of 30 months after therapy (range 3–97 months) with periodic measurements of serum creatinine and creatinine clearance. Nine of the patients treated with ^{90}Y-DOTATOC showed creatinine toxicity (7 grade 1, 1 grade 2, 1 grade 3) after 1–5 years of PRRT. Patients who demonstrated a higher risk of developing long-term renal toxicity were those with pre-existing risk factors like elderly age, diabetes mellitus, long-standing or scarcely controlled hypertension, renal abnormalities, and previous chemotherapy with nephrotoxic agents (e.g. platinum). Nephrotoxicity was also statistically correlated with the kidney BED. No significant correlation was observed between toxicity and absorbed dose or cumulative activities. BED threshold for renal toxicity was 28 Gy in patients with risk factors and 40 Gy for those without risk factors. None of the patients treated with ^{177}Lu-DOTATATE showed renal toxicity. Tissues with low α/β ratio values (like kidneys) are more influenced by small changes in the dose per fraction and dose rate and although a statistical correlation between fractionation schedule and occurrence of renal toxicity was not found, the authors observed a tendency to a higher occurrence of creatinine clearance loss in hypofractionated schemes. These results suggested that patients with pre-existing risk factors could benefit from the choice of using ^{177}Lu-DOTATATE and of reduced cumulative and per-cycle activity with a more fractionated schedule and that in these patients the BED threshold of 28 Gy should not be trespassed.

Currently, few trials are ongoing to assess the safety and efficacy of different administration timing. At IRCCS-IRST in Meldola, Italy, the Luthree trial (EUDRACT N. 2015-004727-3; Clinical Trials.Gov N. NCT03454763), a phase II randomized study, has been designed to compare the safety and efficacy of an intensive schedule (every 5 weeks) of PRRT with ^{177}Lu-DOTATATE versus the standard 8 weeks treatment in advanced GEP and pulmonary NETs. Moreover, patients are divided into two cohorts assigned to receive high or reduced activities (5.5 versus 3.7 GBq per cycle) in 5 cycles. Lower activities are reserved for patients with renal or bone marrow toxicity risk factors. Preliminary data demonstrated an optimal safety, without major hematological or kidney toxicity. Patients who received the intensive treatment demonstrated a tendency toward a better overall response rate (ORR), suggesting that ^{177}Lu-DOTATATE PRRT with more intensive schedules has the possibility to obtain better results without further toxicity. The possibility to personalize the dosages, lowering the likelihood of toxicities, can lead to better OS.

5.7 FUTURE PERSPECTIVE IN PRRT

5.7.1 RE-TREATMENT

The hypothesis of a second PRRT treatment is extremely interesting taking into consideration that the majority of patients may relapse after 3–5 years of the first PRRT. The criteria to re-treatment require ^{68}Ga DOTA-peptides PET/CT positivity and a history of good PRRT response at first cycle. Nicolini et al. [10] investigated the use of low-dosage re-treatment with ^{177}Lu-DOTATATE in 26 patients affected by GEP-NETs (with a PFS of at least 12 months) who relapsed after PRRT with ^{90}Y-DOTATOC. All patients received 14.8–18.5 GBq of ^{177}Lu-DOTATATE in 4 or 5 cycles (median total activity 16.5 GBq in 5 cycles). The DCR was 84.6% and the mPFS was 22 months. Toxicity was mild after ^{177}Lu-DOTATATE re-treatment in the majority of the patients. Only two patients had G2 and one had G3 bone marrow toxicity; only one patient had G2 and one had G3 renal toxicity. Therefore, low-dosage ^{177}Lu-DOTATATE resulted to be safe, and DCR and PFS rates were comparable with those observed when ^{90}Y-DOTATOC was used as primary PRRT treatment.

5.7.2 COMBINED ^{90}Y- AND ^{177}LU-DOTA-PEPTIDE PROTOCOLS (TANDEM THERAPY)

As part of specific trials, combination protocols with alternate administration of ^{90}Y-DOTATOC and ^{177}Lu-DOTATATE are under investigation. These "Tandem Therapy" protocols have the purpose of making the most advantages of the different physical properties and receptor affinity of each radiopharmaceutical. In a phase II study, Seregni et al. [11] evaluated the feasibility of combined PRRT in 26 patients with metastatic NETs refractory to conventional therapy. Patients were treated with four therapeutic cycles alternating ^{177}Lu-DOTATATE 5.55 GBq and ^{90}Y-DOTATOC 2.6 GBq, obtaining OR in 42.3% of patients and a longer than 24 months mPFS. Moreover, 90% of patients with carcinoid syndrome showed a symptomatic response and/or a reduction in tumor-associated pain.

5.7.3 COMBINED PRRT AND EBRT

External beam radiotherapy (EBRT), delivered both in fractionated modality or as a single high-dose administration (stereotactic body radiotherapy, SBRT), has a well-established role in the therapeutic management of GI carcinomas and other solid tumors, used either alone or in combination with surgery or chemotherapy. On the contrary, there is no updated strong evidence about the true effect of radiotherapy in NETs, and prospective trials in homogeneous populations are required. Early studies carried out in the 1980s showed a not favorable cost-benefit profile for EBRT in the treatment of intra-abdominal NETs because of the high rate of toxicity; even more, low-grade NETs have classically been considered radio-resistant as a consequence of their slow rate of proliferation. However, the safety profile of radiotherapy has nowadays improved markedly, and the risk of severe acute and late adverse effects can be minimized using appropriate patient immobilization, modern image guidance, and dose-constraint techniques (e.g. SBRT techniques). More updated but numerically limited studies seem to show that EBRT may play a role in reducing symptoms from the primary tumor or metastasis; it may also potentiate systemic therapies by controlling one or a few sites of oligoprogression; moreover, stereotactic radiotherapy or radio-surgery could represent a treatment option for brain metastases from bronchial NETs or for small p-NETs in patients not candidates for surgical resection [12].

Considering the new data about the safety and effectiveness of EBRT, a potential area of interest could be the evaluation of the combined use of PRRT and EBRT in NETs. Due to the above-mentioned lack of an established role of EBRT in GEP-NETs therapy, this kind of "mixed" approach still remains largely unexplored. Meningiomas could be cited as one of the few types of neoplasms in which the use of combined PRRT and EBRT has been investigated in terms of safety and effectiveness (see below).

5.7.4 PRRT IN NON-GEP-NET NEOPLASMS

5.7.4.1 Lung Carcinoids

According to the current WHO classification, bronchopulmonary NETs are divided into typical carcinoids (TC) and atypical carcinoids (AC). Patients with AC typically demonstrate the worst prognosis. About 80% of lung NETs show high expression of SSTR with a prevalence of subtype 2.

Whenever possible, surgery is the treatment of choice even if a standardization for the management of the advanced cases does not exist at present.

In a phase II study published in 2015 by Ianniello et al. [13], 34 consecutive patients with metastatic progressive lung NETs (15 with TC and 19 with AC) were enrolled to receive 4 or 5 cycles of ^{177}Lu- DOTATATE every 6–8 weeks. The planned activity per cycle was 3.7 or 5.5 GBq according to bone marrow functionality and the presence of risk factors for kidney toxicity, with cumulative activities of 18.5 and 27.8 GBq, respectively. The median cumulative administered activity was 21.5 GBq (range 12.9–27.8 GBq). No major (Grade 3 or 4) acute or delayed toxicity occurred in either group. The median follow-up (FUP) was 29 months (range 7–69). Among the 34 patients, 1 showed complete response (CR), 4 partial response (PR) and 16 stable disease (SD), with a DCR of 62%. The mPFS and the mOS were 18.5 and 48.6 months respectively. Patients with TC showed a better DCR, mPFS, and mOS than patients affected by AC. The study also demonstrated a relevant prognostic role of FDG PET/CT in terms of mOS and mPFS. Moreover, in a recently published retrospective study by Zidan and co-workers [14], the researchers demonstrated the efficacy and safety of PRRT in this particular histology. The study included 48 pulmonary NET patients (43 AC and 5 TC) receiving a median cumulative activity of 27.4 GBq of ^{177}Lu-DOTATATE (range 7.1–43.4GBq) administered in up to 4 cycles 6–10 weeks apart. At 3 months follow-up, the DCR was 88%. The mPFS and mOS were, respectively, 23 months and 59 months. PRRT resulted to be well tolerated with a low number of G3/G4 toxicity during treatment, which for the large part reversed to G1/2 after 3 months.

5.7.4.2 Pheochromocytomas and Paragangliomas

Pheochromocytomas (Pheo) and Paragangliomas (Pgl) are rare tumors generally overexpressing SSTRs and therefore susceptible to being treated with PRRT. In a study by Severi et al. [15], 46 progressive Pheo and Pgl patients were consecutively enrolled to receive ^{90}Y-DOTATOC or ^{177}Lu-DOTATATE. All patients showed a positive status for SRI. Twelve patients received ^{90}Y-DOTATOC (cumulative activity range 7.4 to 11 GBq) and 34 patients were treated with ^{177}Lu-DOTATATE (cumulative activity 18.5 or 27.5 GBq). Both radiopharmaceuticals were well tolerated with no significant renal or bone marrow toxicity. The median FUP was 73 months (5–146 months). The overall DCR was 80%. ^{177}Lu-DOTATATE patients showed a longer mOS than those treated with ^{90}Y-DOTATOC and a better DCR was also observed in those who received higher dosages. SDHx mutations did not correlate with the efficacy of the treatment. Hence, the authors concluded that PRRT was safe and effective in patients with progressive Pheo/Pgl, especially at higher dosages.

5.7.4.3 Meningiomas

There are also non-NETs pathologies overexpressing SSTR receptors and PRRT may represent a good therapeutic strategy in those patients. Meningiomas are generally benign neoplasms and surgery is usually effective and curative but in high-grade histotypes or non-completely resected cases, recurrence is quite common.

SSTR are commonly highly expressed on meningioma cell surfaces allowing the treatment with PRRT. Kreissl and co-workers [16] investigated the role of PRRT in association with EBRT in patients with recurring or progressive symptomatic meningiomas with encouraging results, showing that the combination of PRRT and EBRT is well tolerated and can represent an attractive treatment option even in long-term follow-up [17]. Bartolomei et al. [18] also investigated the role of PRRT in the treatment of recurrent meningiomas, demonstrating that it is well tolerated and can interfere with tumor growth.

5.8 DOSIMETRIC ASPECTS IN PRRT

Nowadays, dosimetric evaluation is not routinely performed in the framework of PRRT. Dosimetric data reported in literature normally refer to small patient cohort and the methodologies implemented are not uniform across the different studies. Lack of dosimetric data is due to different factors, some that may be ascribed to the technical aspects (e.g. necessity to acquire several post treatment images/data, patient compliance, reimbursement), other to a cultural bias (e.g. habit to apply fixed or empirical treatment schemes in terms of both number of cycles and activity level instead of treatment schemes tailored at patient level). In any case, there is a broad awareness about the role of dosimetry in the experimental protocols, when the biodistribution and the kinetic of the new radiopharmaceuticals are under investigation, but the clinical implementation of the dosimetry is still struggling to take off even though the European Council Directive (2013/59 EURATOM) requires a personalized dosimetric approach similar to the one widely implemented in EBRT.

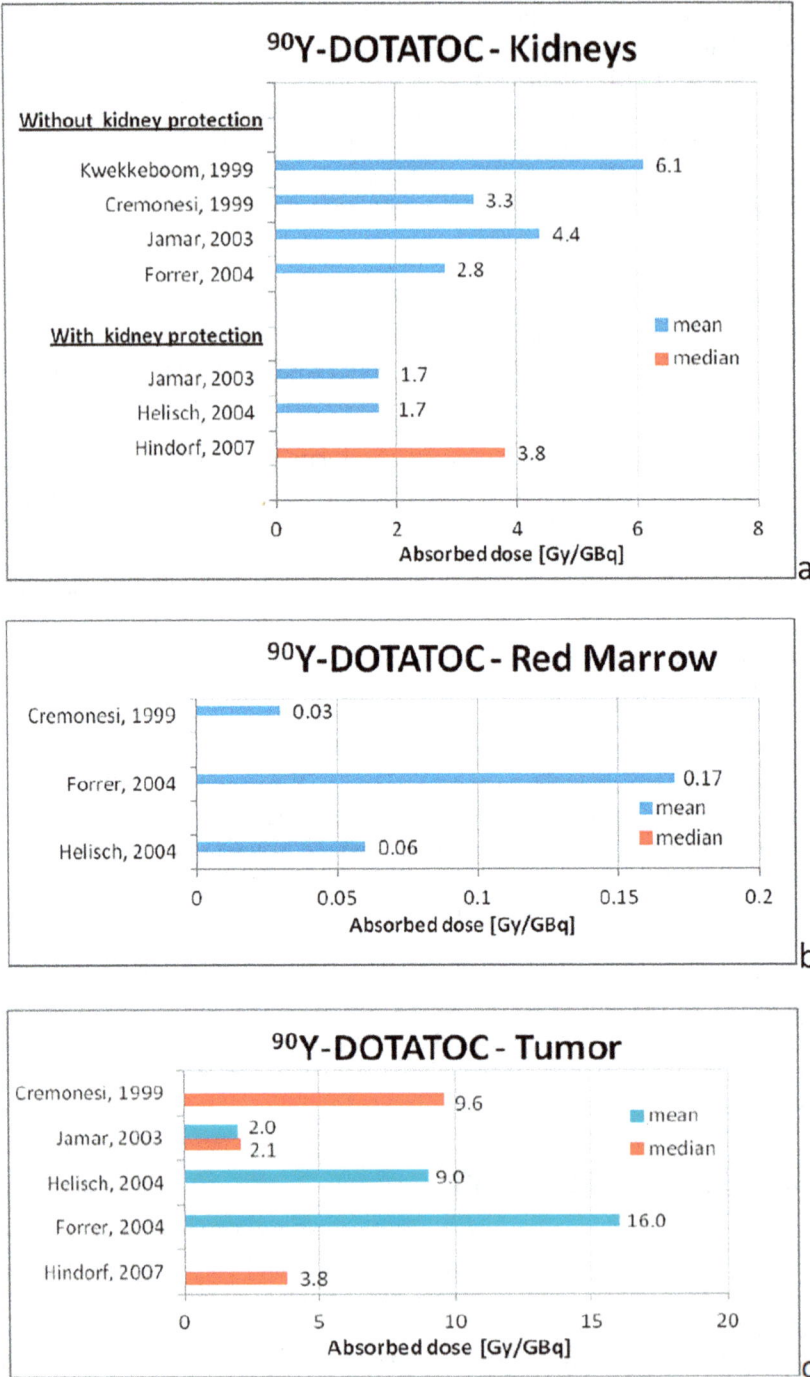

FIGURE 5.6 Absorbed dose of ^{90}Y-DOTATOC per unit activity in the kidneys (a), red marrow (b), and tumor (c). For kidneys, both older and more recent studies with and without kidney protection, respectively, are shown. A 30–60% absorbed dose reduction would be expected with administration of kidney protectors. Blue bars show mean values of absorbed doses per unit activity; red bars show median values. Data kindly granted by M. Cremonesi, taken from Cremonesi et al EJNMMI 2018 (reference n.24) with author's permission.

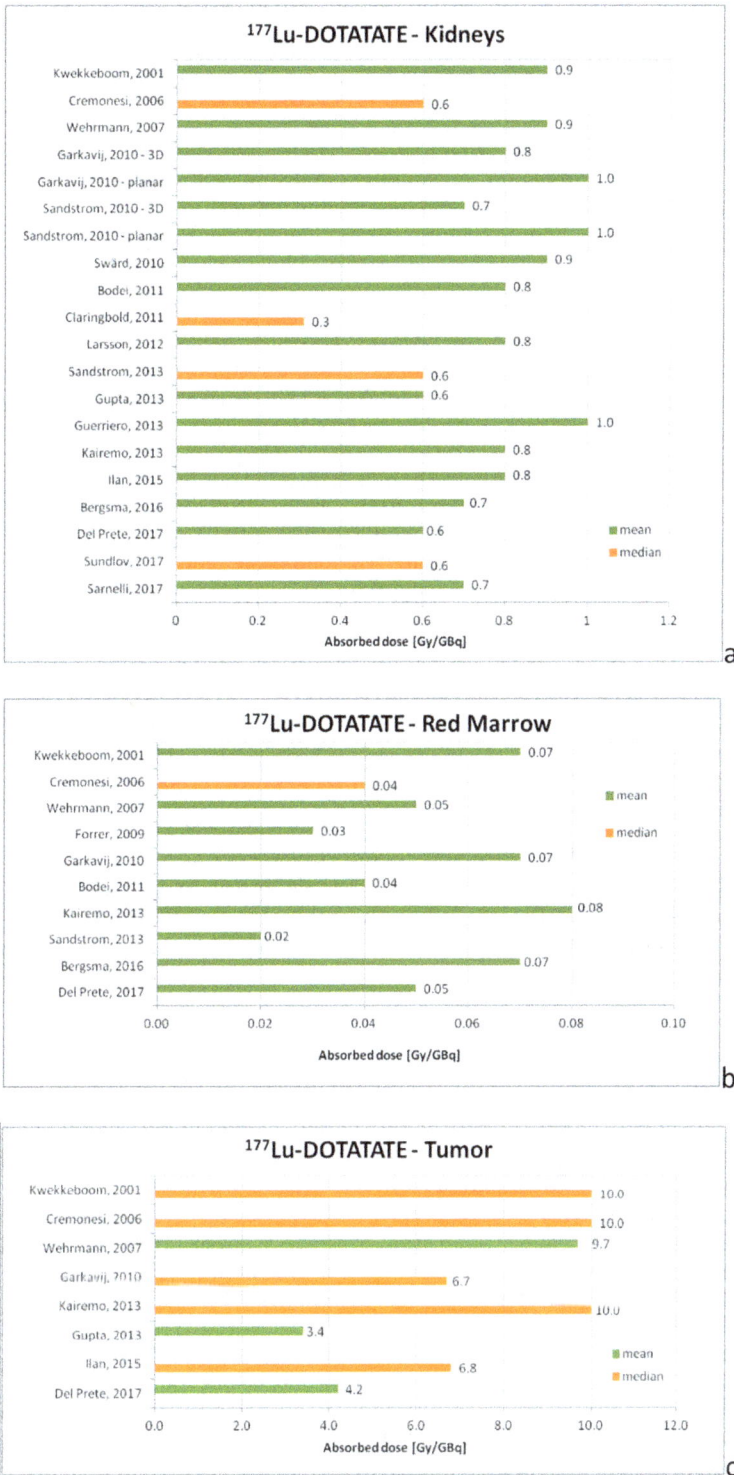

FIGURE 5.7 Absorbed dose of ^{177}Lu-DOTATATE per unit activity in the kidneys (a), red marrow (b), and tumor (c). Green bars show mean values of absorbed doses per unit activity; orange bars show median values. Data kindly granted by M. Cremonesi, taken from Cremonesi et al EJNMMI 2018 (reference n.24) with author's permission.

Different post-injection images are required in order to derive the time activity curve, essential to perform a dosimetric evaluation. Protocols may include only whole-body planar images, multiple planar images, plus a single SPECT/CT 3D image or only SPECT/CT 3D images, namely 2D, hybrid, or 3D dosimetric approaches, respectively. For all methodologies, the acquisition of a late time point (i.e. roughly 3–5 times the effective half-live of radiopharmaceutical [19]) will increase the accuracy of dosimetric evaluation by avoiding overestimation of absorbed dose; this is especially important for the tumor absorbed dose evaluation [20,21].

Since the first pioneering studies [22,23], there was a proliferation of scientific publications reporting data on dosimetric evaluation for PRRT. For sake of simplicity, we report only the last review data [24], summarized in Figures 5.6 and 5.7 and extracted from the main dosimetric studies published in the literature for ^{90}Y-DOTATOC and ^{177}Lu-DOTATATE (24), respectively; the variability among studies is visible. This encourages the requirement to implement a systematic dosimetric evaluation in clinical settings, also in combination with treatment outcome evaluation in terms of efficacy and safety. In this prospective, the harmonization of dosimetric protocols among different centers, following for example national and international guidelines, will help in the promulgation of dosimetric evaluations [25]. Single-point dosimetry that requires a single image acquisition and the application of a pre-determined time activity curve (derived either from literature studies or from a dosimetric evaluation of the same patient performed on a previous therapy cycle) recently gained great interest in the field. While the advantage gained with this methodology and the opportunity to increase dosimetric data available are clear, the accuracy of this evaluation should be confirmed in a large clinical setting. The implementation in the clinical routine of dosimetric evaluation with each aforementioned method will require a stronger collaboration between clinicians and experts in medical physics promoting a culture of team working, as is routinely applied in EBRT [24].

The availability of the dosimetric data as well as the clinical outcome (tumor control and toxicity) are needed [19] at the patient population level, in order to build proper normal tissue complication probability (NTCP) and tumor control probability (TCP) models, as well as [20] at the single patient level, in order to optimize the treatment by modifying the schedule and increase the therapeutic index [21]. In addition to that, the possibility to combine PRRT and EBRT treatment requires dosimetric evaluation of both radiation therapies in order to optimize the efficacy and safety profiles.

REFERENCES

1. Sgouros G, Bodei L, McDevitt MR, Nedrow JR Radiopharmaceutical therapy in cancer: clinical advances and challenges. *Nat Rev Drug Discov.* 2020 Sep; 19(9): 589–608. doi: 10.1038/s41573-020-0073-9. Epub 2020 Jul 29. Erratum in: Nat Rev Drug Discov. 2020 Sep 7;: PMID: 32728208; PMCID: PMC7390460.
2. Hejna M, Schmidinger M, Raderer M The clinical role of somatostatin analogues as antineoplastic agents: much ado about nothing? *Ann Oncol.* 2002. 13: 653–668. 10.1093/annonc/mdf142
3. Naik M, Al-Nahhas A, Khan SR. Treatment of neuroendocrine neoplasms with radiolabeled peptides – where are we now. *Cancers (Basel).* 2022 Feb 1; 14(3): 761. Doi: 10.3390/cancers14030761. PMID: 35159027; PMCID: PMC8833798.
4. Nagtegaal ID, Odze RD, Klimstra D, Paradis V, Rugge M, Schirmacher P, et al. The 2019 WHO classification of tumours of the digestive system. *Histopathology.* 2020; 76: 182–188.
5. Sansovini M, Severi S, Ianniello A, Nicolini S, Fantini L, Mezzenga E, Ferroni F, Scarpi E, Monti M, Bongiovanni A, Cingarlini S, Grana CM, Bodei L, Paganelli G Long-term follow-up and role of FDG PET in advanced pancreatic neuroendocrine patients treated with 177Lu-D OTATATE. *Eur J Nucl Med Mol Imaging.* 2017 Mar; 44(3): 490–499.
6. Kratochwil C, Stefanova M, Mavriopoulou E, Holland-Letz T, Dimitrakopoulou-Strauss A, Afshar-Oromieh A, et al. SUV of [68Ga]DO TATOC-PET/CT predicts response probability of PRR T in neuroendocrine tumors. *Mol Imaging Biol.* 2015; 17: 313–318.

7. Cremonesi M, Ferrari M, Bodei L, Tosi G, Paganelli G Dosimetry in peptide radionuclide receptor therapy: a review. *J Nucl Med*. 2006 Sep; 47(9): 1467–1475. PMID: 16954555.
8. Paganelli G, Sansovini M, Nicolini S, Grassi I, Ibrahim T, Amadori E, et al. 177Lu-PRR T in advanced gastrointestinal neuroendocrine tumors: 10-year follow-up of the IR ST phase II prospective study. *Eur J Nucl Med Mol Imaging*. 2021; 48: 152–160.
9. Bodei L, Cremonesi M, Ferrari M, Pacifici M, Grana CM, Bartolomei M, Baio SM, Sansovini M, Paganelli G Long-term evaluation of renal toxicity after peptide receptor radionuclide therapy with 90Y-DOTATOC and 177Lu-DOTATATE: the role of associated risk factors. *Eur J Nucl Med Mol Imaging*. 2008 Oct; 35(10): 1847–1856. doi: 10.1007/s00259-008-0778-1. Epub 2008 Apr 22. Erratum in: Eur J Nucl Med Mol Imaging. 2008 Oct;35(10):1928. PMID: 18427807.
10. Nicolini S, Severi S, Ianniello A, Sansovini M, Ambrosetti A, Bongiovanni A, et al. Investigation of receptor radionuclide therapy with 177Lu-DOTATATE in patients with GEP-NEN and a high Ki-67 proliferation index. *Eur J Nucl Med Mol Imaging*. 2018; 45: 923–930.
11. Seregni E, Maccauro M, Chiesa C, Mariani L, Pascali C, Mazzaferro V, et al. Treatment with tandem [90Y]DOTA-TATE and [177Lu]DOTATATE of neuroendocrine tumours refractory to conventional therapy. *Eur J Nucl Med Mol Imaging*. 2014; 41: 223–230.
12. Chan DL, Thompson R, Lam M, Pavlakis N, Hallet J, Law C, Singh S, Myrehaug S External beam radiotherapy in the treatment of gastroenteropancreatic neuroendocrine tumours: a systematic review. *Clin Oncol (R Coll Radiol)*. 2018 Jul; 30(7): 400–408.
13. Ianniello A, Sansovini M, Severi S, Nicolini S, Grana CM, Massri K, Bongiovanni A, Antonuzzo L, Di Iorio V, Sarnelli A, Caroli P, Monti M, Scarpi E, Paganelli G Peptide receptor radionuclide therapy with (177)Lu-DOTATATE in advanced bronchial carcinoids: prognostic role of thyroid transcription factor 1 and (18)F-FDG PET. *Eur J Nucl Med Mol Imaging*. 2016 Jun; 43(6): 1040–1046. doi: 10.1007/s00259-015-3262-8. Epub 2015 Nov 27. PMID: 26611427.
14. Zidan L, Iravani A, Oleinikov K, Ben-Haim S, Gross DJ, Meirovitz A, Maimon O, Akhurst T, Michael M, Hicks RJ, Grozinsky-Glasberg S, Kong G Efficacy and safety of 177Lu-DOTATATE in lung neuroendocrine tumors: a bicenter study. *J Nucl Med*. 2022 Feb; 63(2): 218–225. doi: 10.2967/jnumed.120.260760. Epub 2021 May 28. PMID: 34049983; PMCID: PMC8805789.
15. Severi S, Bongiovanni A, Ferrara M, Nicolini S, Di Mauro F, Sansovini M, et al. Peptide receptor radionuclide therapy in patients with metastatic progressive pheochromocytoma and paraganglioma: long-term toxicity, efficacy and prognostic biomarker data of phase II clinical trials. *ESMO Open*. 2021; 6: 100171.
16. Kreissl MC, Hänscheid H, Löhr M, Verburg FA, Schiller M, Lassmann M, et al. Combination of peptide receptor radionuclide therapy with fractionated external beam radiotherapy for treatment of advanced symptomatic meningioma. *Radiat Oncol*. 2012; 7: 99.
17. Hartrampf PE, Hänscheid H, Kertels O, Schirbel A, Kreissl MC, Flentje M, Sweeney RA, Buck AK, Polat B, Lapa C Long-term results of multimodal peptide receptor radionuclide therapy and fractionated external beam radiotherapy for treatment of advanced symptomatic meningioma. *Clin Transl Radiat Oncol*. 2020 Mar 5; 22: 29–32.
18. Bartolomei M, Bodei L, De Cicco C, Grana CM, Cremonesi M, Botteri E, et al. Peptide receptor radionuclide therapy with (90)YDOTATOC in recurrent meningioma. *Eur J Nucl Med Mol Imaging* 2009; 36: 1407–1416.
19. Stabin MG, Wendt RE Flux GD RADAR guide: standard methods for calculating radiation doses for radiopharmaceuticals, Part 1 – collection of data for radiopharmaceutical dosimetry. *J Nucl Med*. 2022; 63(2): 316–322.
20. Huzing DMV, de Wit-van der Veen BJ, Verheij M, Stokkel MPM Dosimetry methods and clinical applications in peptide receptor radionuclide therapy for neuroendocrine tumours: a literature review. *EJNMMI Res*. 2018; 8: 89.
21. Guerriero F Ferrari ME Botta F, Fioroni F, Grassi E, Versari A et al. Kidney dosimetry in 177Lu and 90Y peptide receptor radionuclide therapy: influence of image timing, time-activity integration method, and risk factors. *Biomed Res Int*. 2013; 2013: 935351.
22. Cremonesi M, Ferrari M, Zoboli S, Chinol M, Stabin MG, Orsi F et al. Biokinetics and dosimetry in patients administered with (111)In-DOTA-Tyr(3)-octreotide: implications for internal radiotherapy with (90)Y-DOTATOC. *Eur J Nucl Med*. 1999; 26(8): 877–886.
23. Kwekkeboom DJ, Kooij PP, Bakker WH, Mäcke HR, Krenning EP Comparison of 111In-DOTA-Tyr3-octreotide and 111In-DTPAoctreotide in the same patients: biodistribution, kinetics, organ and tumor uptake. *J Nucl Med*. 1999; 40(5): 762–767.

24. Cremonesi M, Ferrari ME, Bodei L, Chiesa C, Sarnelli A, Garibaldi C et al. Correlation of dose with toxicity and tumour response to 90Y- and 177Lu-PRRT provides the basis for optimization through individualized treatment planning. *Eur J Nucl Med Mol Imaging.* 2018; 45: 2426–2441.

25. Lawhn-Heath C, Hope TA, Martinez J, Fung EK, Shin J, Seo Y et al. Dosimetry in radionuclide therapy: the clinical role of measuring radiation dose. *Lancet.* 2022; 23: e75–e87.

6 Radionuclide-Conjugated Cancer Specific Vectors
Small Molecules and Antibodies

Charles Xian-Yang Goh, Sumbul Zaheer, Yiu Ming Khor, and Chang-Tong Yang

6.1 INTRODUCTION

The concept of personalized medicine and targeted therapies was first introduced in the 1950s. These precision medicines and therapies are designed based on the patients' unique medical profiling, thus optimizing therapeutic efficacy with minimum side effects [1]. This concept has been widely employed in radionuclide therapy by conjugating targeting molecules that are specific to organ or tissue for therapeutic purposes. These molecules include small molecules such as prostate specific membrane antigen (PSMA), fibroblast activation protein (FAP), metaiodo-benzylguanidine (MIBG), antibodies, peptides, and nanoparticles.

Owing to the small size, small molecules are often selected for radioligand therapy as they possess an advantage over biologics (like monoclonal antibodies, polypeptides, antibody–drug conjugates, and nucleic acids) to target not only the extracellular components like cell surface receptors or protein domains attached to the cell membranes like glycoproteins but also the intracellular proteins like different kinases [2]. The binding of radioimmunoconjugates to tumors depends on several factors, including dose, affinity, antigens per cell, and molecular size. It should be noted that the appropriate size of antibodies should be engineered to achieve optimal targeting efficiency [3].

The selection of radioisotopes for target-specific treatments should be based on their physical and biochemical properties. For therapy, radionuclides that emit alpha particles or beta particles with high energy are suitable for internal radiotherapy so that the non-penetrating radiation can inhibit cancerous cells from proliferation or kill cancerous cells locally [4]. In contrast, penetrating radiation such as γ-radiation and X-rays are commonly used for diagnostic purposes.

6.2 RADIOLABELED SMALL MOLECULES

Small molecule drugs are low molecular weight organic compounds that can enter cells easily. They have been the mainstay of the pharmaceutical industry in modern medicine for several decades. Small molecules used for radionuclide therapy have an advantage over macromolecules such as antibodies for specific receptor binding leading to activity inhibition. They are easy to synthesize by chemical reactions and radiolabeling. Examples of small molecules in radio-theranostics include prostate PSMA targeting agents, FAP targeting small molecules, and MIBG.

6.2.1 PSMA

Prostate cancer is the second most common type of cancer in men worldwide, with more than 1.4 million new cases and 375,000 deaths reported in 2020 [5]. While early stage prostate cancer

DOI: 10.1201/9781003250913-8

can be treated with surgery or radiation therapy, a significant proportion of patients subsequently develop biochemical recurrence (BCR), usually detected by rising prostate-specific antigen (PSA) levels. Conventional imaging techniques such as computed tomography (CT) and bone scan have low sensitivity and specificity for the evaluation of nodal disease and distant metastasis, both in the settings of staging and recurrence, limiting their use in guiding therapy [6]. Advanced prostate cancer requires systemic therapy, including androgen deprivation therapy (ADT), chemotherapy, and immunotherapy. These treatments can have significant side effects and may not be effective in all patients. Recent advances in PSMA directed imaging and therapy have enabled significantly more accurate staging and restaging, as well as targeted radionuclide therapy. The extensive research into these techniques and rapid clinical adoption are testament to their immense value in diagnosis and management of prostate cancer.

PSMA, also known as glutamate carboxypeptidase II, N-acetyl-α-linked acidic dipeptidase I, or folate hydrolase 1, is a type II transmembrane glycoprotein. Several characteristics make it an attractive target for theranostics. First, it is overexpressed by 100–1000 times in prostate cancer cells, including primary tumors and metastases, compared to normal prostate cells, increasing its sensitivity and specificity as a biomarker for prostate cancer [7]. Increased PSMA expression has been shown to correlate with higher tumor grade, pathological stage, serum PSA levels, and in the setting of BCR. Second, upon binding with PSMA, ligands are internalized into cancer cells, allowing for effective delivery of radionuclides for the purpose of imaging and therapy [8,9]. Finally, PSMA has a low expression in normal tissues, reducing the risk of off-target effects. It should be noted that PSMA, despite its name, is not specific to prostate cancer. It is also expressed in the neovasculature of several non-prostatic tumors such as breast, lung, hepatocellular, renal, and brain malignancies [10].

6.2.1.1 Development of Small Molecule Inhibitors of PSMA

The development of small molecule inhibitors of PSMA represented a significant step forward in clinical utility, as they have rapid biodistribution and uptake by prostate cancer lesions and rapid clearance from blood pool. They provide excellent lesion to background contrast within a short time after injection of 1 hour. After the initial description of urea-based inhibitors of PSMA by Kozikowski et al. in 2001 [11], numerous PSMA binding radioligands have been developed for imaging and therapy. These radioligands contain a PSMA binding pharmacophore (most in clinical use contain the glutamate-urea-glutamate or glutamate-urea-lysine motif) to target the active binding site of PSMA and are labeled with various radionuclides (including ^{123}I, ^{99m}Tc, ^{111}In, ^{18}F, ^{68}Ga, ^{177}Lu, and ^{225}Ac). The choice of radionuclide determines the mode of imaging or therapy. Gamma-emitting radionuclides (such as ^{123}I or ^{99m}Tc) enable gamma camera imaging, positron emitters (such as ^{18}F or ^{68}Ga) enable PET imaging, while alpha or beta emitters (such as ^{225}Ac or ^{177}Lu) enable targeted therapy.

6.2.1.2 Development of PSMA-Targeted Antibodies

Even before PSMA small molecule inhibitors were introduced, there were attempts to develop a PSMA-targeted agent using radiolabeled monoclonal antibodies. Capromab pendetide (an ^{111}In labeled murine monoclonal antibody), marketed as Prostascint, was the first PSMA-targeted SPECT imaging agent to be approved by the US Food and Drug Administration (FDA) in 1996. However, as Prostascint targets the intracellular epitope of PSMA, it is only taken up in necrotic, non-viable cells and thus suffered from low sensitivity and specificity of 62% and 72%, respectively [12]. Subsequently, the monoclonal antibody J591 was developed, which targeted the extracellular domain of PSMA. ^{111}In labeled J591 showed promise for the imaging of bone and soft tissue lesions in metastatic prostate cancer [13]. However, these radiolabeled antibodies have prolonged soft tissue clearance time, necessitating a 5–7 day wait between injection of the tracer and imaging, and resulting in poor quality images. This severely limits the clinical utility of these tracers.

6.2.1.3 PSMA SPECT Imaging

The development of SPECT imaging using small molecule inhibitors of PSMA began with ^{123}I-MIP-1072 and ^{123}I-MIP-1095 [14]. While these were proven to detect metastatic prostate cancer lesions, in view of the better imaging characteristics and wide availability of ^{99m}Tc, tracers such as ^{99m}Tc-MIP-1404 (trofolastat) were subsequently developed. ^{99m}Tc MIP-1404 is presently undergoing evaluation in a phase III study to determine its ability to identify clinically significant prostate cancer in patients diagnosed with low- or very low-grade prostate cancer [14]. SPECT tracers have clinical utility in many centers that do not have PET imaging facilities available and can also be used to perform radio-guided surgery using intraoperative probe localization. However, currently, PSMA PET tracers have largely superseded SPECT tracers due to higher spatial resolution, sensitivity, and specificity.

6.2.1.4 PSMA PET Imaging

Two small molecule PSMA PET tracers have been FDA approved for the imaging of prostate cancer: ^{68}Ga-PSMA-11 (HBED-CC) and Pylarify (piflufolastat ^{18}F of ^{18}F-DCFPyL). The European Medicines Association has also approved ^{68}Ga-PSMA-11 for use in imaging prostate cancer. These approvals are on the back of several large trials proving the superiority of PSMA PET/CT over conventional imaging modalities, in particular for the staging of high-risk prostate cancer and in BCR. ^{68}Ga-PSMA-11 is the most widely used PSMA PET tracer globally due to its earlier introduction and use in clinical trials, simpler synthesis, and wide availability because of the lack of a controlling patent.

The value of PSMA PET was first demonstrated in low PSA BCR. Following initial radical prostatectomy or radiation therapy for prostate cancer, recurrent disease is most frequently diagnosed based on rising PSA levels on two consecutive determinations, and this is known as BCR. BCR occurs in about 30–50% of patients in the 10 years following radical prostatectomy (depending on risk factors) [15] and salvage radiotherapy (SRT) to the pelvis is the mainstay of treatment. Treatment at low PSA values (< 0.5 ng/ml) has been reported to offer a higher chance of cure [16], but unfortunately, conventional imaging techniques such as bone scan, MRI and CT scans show very low detection rate in this scenario, with reported sensitivity for locoregional recurrence of less than 11% at a PSA value of < 1 ng/ml [17]. Therefore, current guidelines advocate SRT to the pelvis even in the absence of imaging findings of disease. This understandably may result in treatment failure if prostate cancer lesions are outside of the radiotherapy field, and indeed, post SRT, BCR within 5 years can occur in up to 70% of high-risk patients [18].

PSMA PET/CT has been shown in a large prospective study in 635 men to have high detection rate for BCR, even at low PSA values (38% for < 0.5 ng/mL, 57% for 0.5 to < 1.0 ng/mL, 84% for 1.0 to < 2.0 ng/mL), and this allowed for PET-directed focal therapy for these lesions [19].

It was subsequently demonstrated in a prospective study of 302 men that PSMA PET/CT outperformed conventional imaging with bone scan and CT for staging of high-risk prostate cancer (sensitivity 85% versus 38% and specificity 98% versus 91%), with impact on patient management [20].

Other indications for PSMA PET imaging include targeted biopsy in patients with a high suspicion of prostate cancer and previous negative biopsy, and monitoring of systemic therapy in metastatic prostate cancer, though further studies are needed to validate these use cases. Researchers are also studying the use of PSMA PET in imaging other malignancies, as PSMA is known to be overexpressed in the neovasculature of various solid tumors [10].

6.2.1.5 PSMA-Targeted Radioligand Therapy

With the high tumor specific activity demonstrated with PSMA small molecule inhibitor imaging, there was great interest in developing corresponding therapeutic radioligands for the treatment of prostate cancer. Multiple PSMA-targeted radioligands have been developed for the treatment of metastatic castration resistant prostate cancer (mCRPC), which is advanced prostate cancer refractory to hormonal treatment. While initially, ^{131}I labeled ligands such as ^{131}I-MIP-1095 were developed, they have since largely been replaced by ^{177}Lu labeled ligands that have better availability and convenient labeling via kit formulations. The two most commonly used in clinical practice are PSMA I&T and PSMA-617 labeled with ^{177}Lu. Two recently concluded large trials evaluating the use of ^{177}Lu PSMA-617 in patients with mCRPC provided unequivocal evidence of its clinical utility: the phase 2 TheraP trial and the phase 3 VISION trial. The TheraP trial compared ^{177}Lu-PSMA-617 against carbazitaxel (a second-line chemotherapy agent) and found that it led to higher treatment response (in the form of PSA decrease – 66% versus 37%) and fewer high grade adverse events (33% versus 53%) [21]. The VISION trial compared ^{177}Lu-PSMA-617 and standard of care treatment against standard of care alone and demonstrated prolonged progression free survival (8.7 versus 3.4 months) and overall survival (15.3 versus 11.3 months) with ^{177}Lu-PSMA-617 [22]. The results of the VISION trial led to the FDA approval of ^{177}Lu-PSMA-617 (marketed as Pluvicto – ^{177}Lu vipivotide tetraxetan) in March 2022. These trials have cemented the role of PSMA radioligand therapy (RLT) in the treatment of advanced mCRPC. Studies are presently ongoing to evaluate its value earlier in the course of disease. The use of alpha-emitter labeled PSMA ligands (using ^{225}Ac) is also under active research.

6.2.1.6 Clinical Aspects of PSMA Radioligand Therapy

Current clinical practice reserves the use of PSMA RLT for patients with advanced mCRPC that have been previously treated with second-generation antiandrogen therapies (Abiraterone or Enzalutamide) or taxane-based chemotherapy (e.g. docetaxel). Patients must demonstrate high uptake at tumor sites on pre-treatment PSMA PET scan (significantly higher than liver uptake), which predicts good uptake of the therapeutic radioligand during treatment. Figure 6.1 demonstrates the high level of concordance between uptake at tumor sites on pre-treatment PSMA PET and post-therapy planar imaging using the theranostic pair of ^{68}Ga-PSMA-11 and ^{177}Lu-PSMA-I&T. Treatment is well tolerated with a low incidence of grade 3 or 4 adverse events that are mainly hematologic in nature (lymphocytopenia, thrombocytopenia, anemia, and neutropenia), attributable to radiation effects on the bone marrow [21,22].

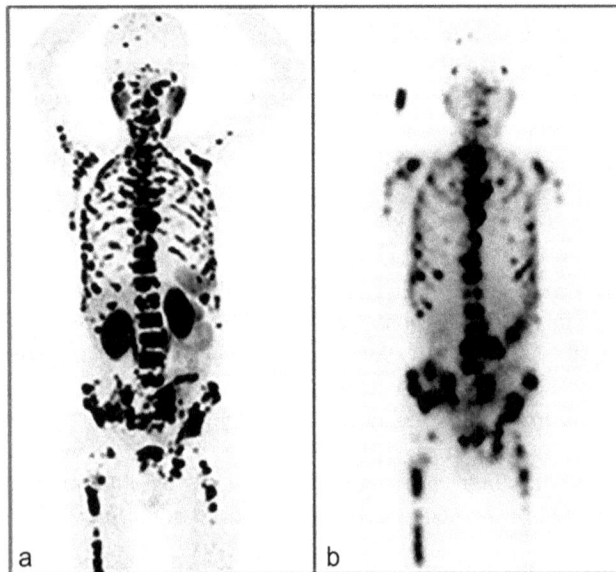

FIGURE 6.1   (a) Maximum intensity projection image of ^{68}Ga-PSMA-11 PET and (b) post-therapy planar image after ^{177}Lu-PSMA-I&T administration in the same patient.

The development and implementation of PSMA directed imaging and therapy is a modern-day success story for the field of nuclear medicine and has demonstrated the strength of the theranostic approach. Identification of an ideal biologic target in PSMA followed by iterative development of targeting ligands and labeling with suitable radionuclides led to the swift deployment and evaluation of multiple candidate radioligands for imaging and therapeutic applications. Today, the use of theranostic pairs such as ^{68}Ga-PSMA-11 and ^{177}Lu-PSMA-617 enables highly accurate detection of prostate cancer recurrence, followed by targeted therapy in suitable candidates.

6.2.2 FAP

FAP is a membrane bound protease that plays a pro-tumorigenic role in cancer-associated fibroblasts [23]. It is highly overexpressed in stromal tissue of various cancers [24]. Since these cells are present in most cancerous tissues and FAP is rarely expressed in healthy tissues, anti-FAP tracers have a potential as pantumor agents. Compared to the standard tumor tracer [^{18}F]FDG, these tracers show better tumor-to-background ratios in many indications, and unlike [^{18}F]FDG, FAP-targeted tracers do not require exhausting patient preparations, such as dietary restrictions, and offer the possibility of RLT in a theragnostic approach [23].

The initial FAP targeting compounds were monoclonal antibodies and peptides; however, the long circulation and slow clearance caused by their high molecular mass hampered their wider adoption. Small molecular compounds targeting FAP have improved pharmacokinetics and tissue penetration [23].

Kratochwil et al. used the quinolone-based tracer ^{68}Ga-FAPI-04 that acts as a FAP inhibitor to demonstrate remarkably high tracer uptake and image contrast in several highly prevalent cancers, as shown in Figure 6.3 of their publication [25]. They concluded that the high and rather selective tumor uptake may open up new applications for non-invasive tumor characterization, staging examinations, or RLT.

Growing numbers of publications on FAPI-based theranostics in 2023 are testament to the growing interest in this field, with the question being raised whether FAPI-PET/CT could replace FDG PET/CT in the next decade, and the conclusion was that FAPI PET/CT will add important complementary diagnostic, phenotypic, and biomarker information to FDG PET/CT and the theranostic use of FAPI can have high value in cancer therapeutics [26].

Reviews of FAP-targeted radionuclide therapy are now available. Privé BM et al. have summarized studies on more than 100 patients with different FAP-targeted radionuclide therapies (TRT) such as [^{177}Lu]Lu-FAPI-04, [^{90}Y]Y-FAPI-46, [^{177}Lu]Lu-FAP-2286 and [^{177}Lu]Lu-DOTA.SA.FAPI [24]. In these studies, FAP TRT has resulted in objective responses in difficult to treat end-stage cancer patients with manageable adverse events. Although no prospective data are yet available, these early data encourage further research.

Sidrak et al. [27] have also published a systematic review of all available articles that included both diagnosis and therapy with FAPI tracers. They have concluded that although FAPI theranostics is still in its infancy and lacks solid grounds to be brought into clinical practice, it does not show any collateral effects that prohibit administration to patients thus far and has good tolerability profiles.

6.2.3 MIBG

The molecular analog of norepinephrine, MIBG labeled with ^{131}I (^{131}I-MIBG), is another classic theranostic agent that is suitable for gamma camera and SPECT imaging, and it has been used in clinical settings since 1981 [28]. ^{131}I-MIBG enters the neuroendocrine cells of the sympathetic nervous system by means of diffusion and remains stored in neurosecretory vesicles. That allows for diagnosis and follow-up assessment (using ^{123}I-MIBG or ^{131}I-MIBG treatment)of tumors [29]. Recent improvements in the field of MIBG theranostics include the use of ^{124}I-MIBG for PET, which yields higher spatial resolution and accuracy.

It has high sensitivity (> 90%) and specificity (> 95%) for the detection of neural crest-derived (neuroectodermic) tumors and their secondary lesions (particularly in neuroblastoma, pheochromocytoma, and paraganglioma), complementing conventional imaging and indicating which

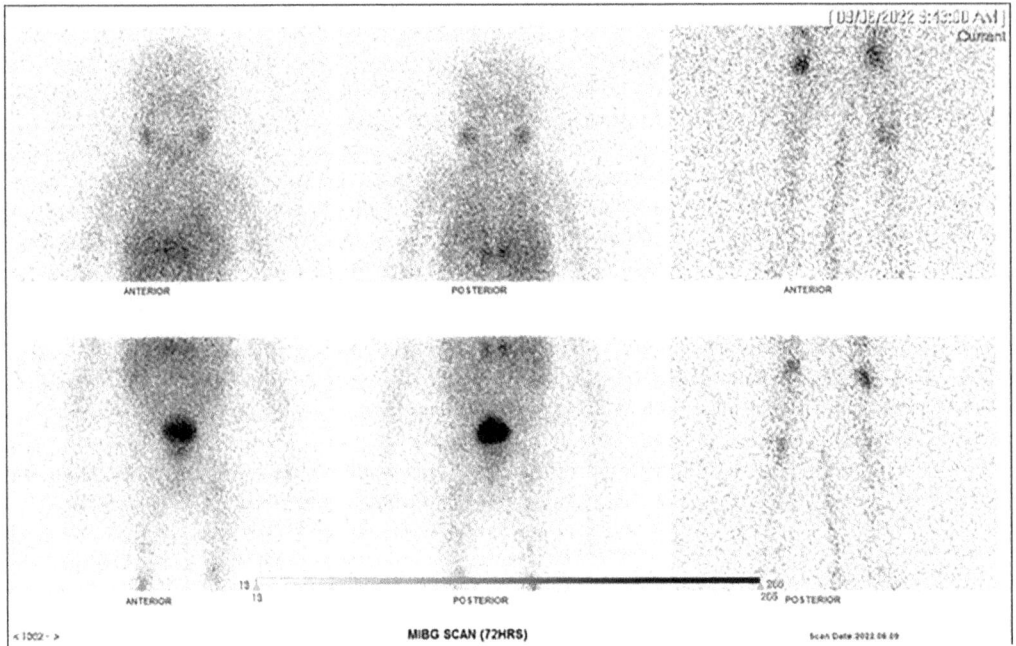

FIGURE 6.2 Diagnostic scan after injection of 37 MBq of ^{131}I-MIBG in a 4-year-old child with neuroblastoma. Anterior and posterior planar views of the upper and lower body and lower limbs show foci of tracer uptake in bilateral femora due to bone metastases.

tumors may benefit from radioisotopic therapy [28]. Like radioiodine, ^{123}I-MIBG facilitates better imaging and is suitable for SPECT and SPECT/CT but is not widely available. ^{123}I-MIBG imaging is the method of choice, particularly in pediatric patients, because of the lower radiation exposure with ^{123}I due to its shorter half-life and the risk of normal thyroid tissue damage from β particles when ^{131}I-MIBG is used for imaging. Therefore, in patients exposed to ^{131}I-MIBG, thyroidal uptake of free ^{131}I should be blocked by saturating the gland with solutions containing non-radioactive iodine, such as potassium iodide, before the procedure.

Shown in Figure 6.2 is the diagnostic scan after injection of 37 MBq ^{131}I-MIBG in a 4-year-old child with neuroblastoma. Figure 6.3 shows the post-therapy scan in the same patient performed 2 months later with a much higher dose of ^{131}I-MIBG (5.62 GBq). Even with the smaller dose of the diagnostic tracer, abnormal foci of tracer uptake are seen in the lower limbs suspicious for bone metastases. The true extent of these lesions is seen in the post-therapy scan in Figure 6.3.

Possible side effects include nausea and vomiting, as well as longer-term effects such as hypothyroidism and myelosuppression, which must be monitored closely during treatment. Although rare, hematologic malignancies may occur after treatment [29]. Indications for therapy are nonresectable, metastatic pheochromocytoma or paraganglioma, neuroblastoma, and recurrent metastatic medullary thyroid cancer, and these are considered here briefly.

6.2.3.1 Neuroblastoma

These are neural crest-derived tumors that exhibit highly variable clinical and pathologic behavior [28]. Most referred patients have high-risk (stage IV) disease at the time of therapy, leading to poor (<50%) disease-free survival at 5 years. There is significant uptake of MIBG in 90% of neuroblastoma cases. Treatment with ^{131}I-MIBG classically has been restricted to only patients with refractory disease, but recent data suggest that it might be a suitable therapeutic agent for induction and consolidation in high-risk patients. Tumor response is around 68% during induction phases versus 32% in cases of recurrent or refractory tumors.

(a)

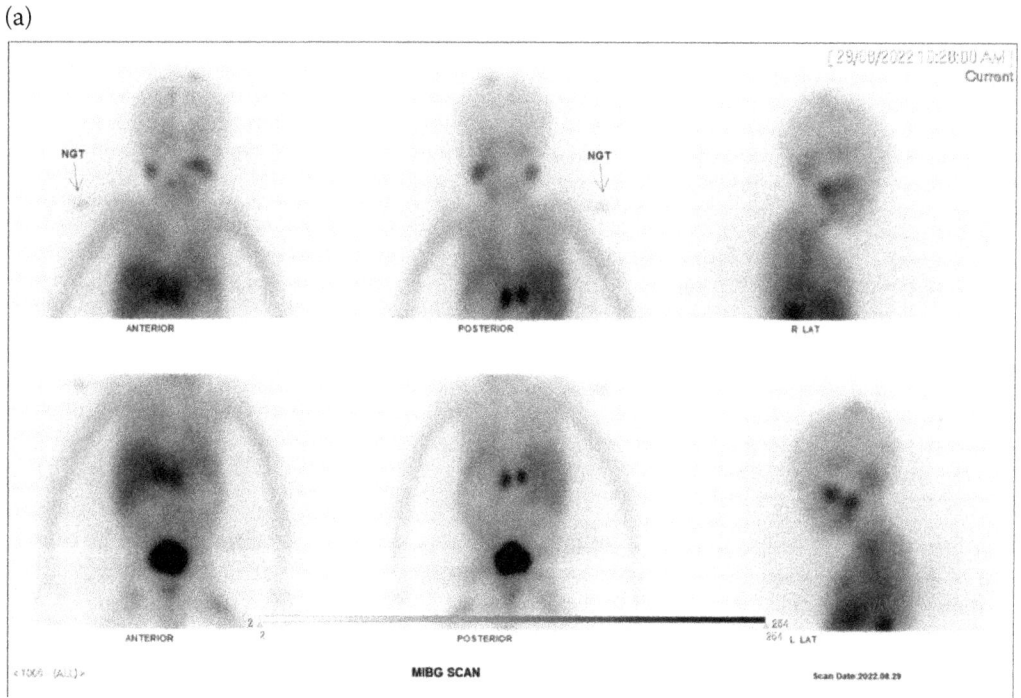

(b)

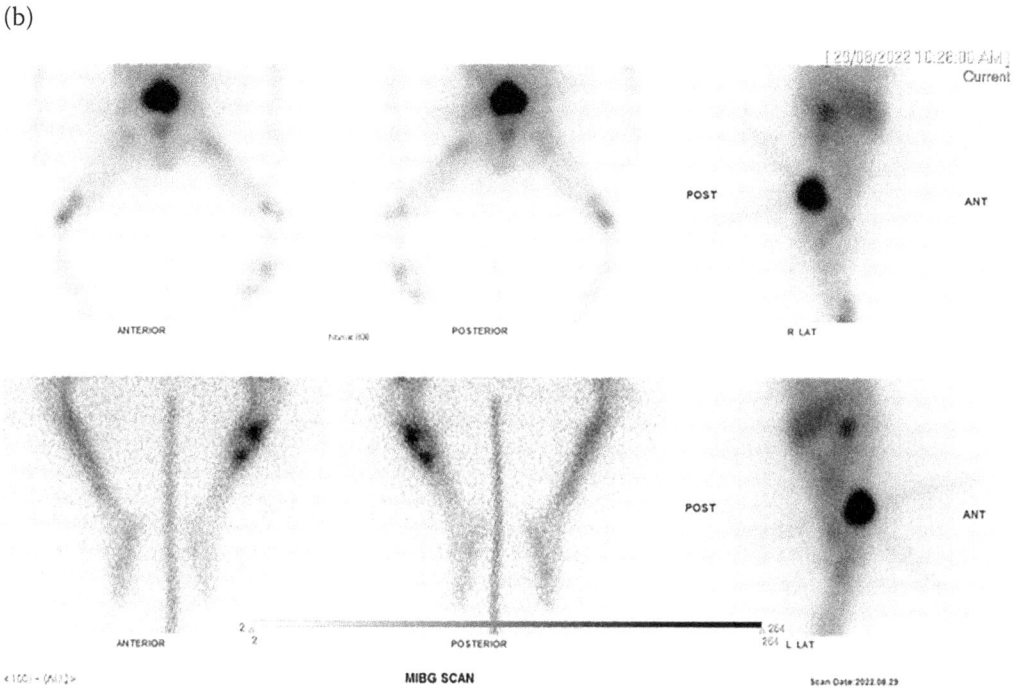

FIGURE 6.3 Post-therapy scan performed after injection of 5.62 GBq of ^{131}I-MIBG. Anterior, posterior, and lateral views of the upper (a) and lower body and lower limbs (b) show more intense tracer uptake and clearer visualization of the bone metastases in the lower limbs. Additional bone metastases can be seen in the skull vault and facial bones. At the right shoulder is the nasogastric tube (NGT) representing tracer outside the body. Physiological tracer activity is seen in the salivary glands, liver, adrenals, urinary tract, and a few bowel loops.

6.2.3.2   Pheochromocytoma and Paraganglioma

There are numerous retrospective studies and a few prospective studies investigating the use of ^{131}I-MIBG for treatment of pheochromocytomas and paragangliomas, which are associated with relatively favorable outcomes [28]. ^{131}I-MIBG is mainly used as an adjunct to surgery, chemotherapy, and tyrosine kinase inhibitors in patients with metastasis. Usually, the therapy alleviates symptoms by lowering the level of circulating catecholamines. Rates of complete or partial treatment response are variable (~7–62%) in different reports, mainly ranging from 25% to 30% of patients, and stable disease is seen in approximately 8% of patients. The activities used also vary considerably among different studies, ranging from 3.7 to more than 74 Gbq.

6.3   RADIOLABELED ANTIBODIES

Radioimmunotherapy (RIT) involves the administration of a radioactive isotope linked to an antibody targeted to a specific cell type. After the radiolabeled antibodies bind to receptors or tumor antigens expressed on the surface of cancerous tissue, the targeted cells that are irradiated absorb high amount of energy in the form of photons or charged particles that promote cell death. Because the ranges of ionizing radiations in tissues are rather large compared with a typical cell size, RIT has an additional crossfire effect to damage cells in close proximity to the site of antibody localization. A tumor's response to radiation is highly dependent on the intrinsic radiosensitivity of the tumor cells; compared to solid organ tumors, lymphoma is more radiosensitive and is the cancer targeted in the only two FDA-approved and commercially available radiolabeled antibodies [3].

RIT of lymphoma with Zevalin and Bexxar was approved by FDA in 2002 and 2003, respectively, for the treatment of relapsed or refractory CD20+ follicular B-cell non-Hodgkin's lymphoma (NHL). Both of them are radiolabeled monoclonal antibodies that target CD20, a protein that is expressed on the surface of B cells, including those found in some types of NHL. Zevalin uses the monoclonal mouse IgG1 antibody ibritumomab in conjunction with the chelator tiuxetan, to which the radioactive isotope yttrium-90 is added. For Bexxar, the monoclonal antibody tositumomab is radiolabeled with iodine-131. By delivering radiation directly to the CD20-expressing cancer cells, these targeted treatments are designed to kill the cancer cells while sparing healthy tissue. Normal B cells express CD20 too and are abundant in the spleen. To minimize binding of radiolabeled antibodies to normal cells, treatments consist of a two-phase process: In the first step, patients receive a dose of non-radiolabeled monoclonal antibody to bind to non-cancerous B-cells in the circulation and the spleen. This is followed by the administration of radiolabeled monoclonal antibody which emits radiation that damages the DNA in the cancer cells and leads to cell death. The radiation also helps to stimulate the immune system to attack the cancer cells.

In phase III trials, Bexxar achieved higher overall objective response rate (ORR) and complete response (CR) compared to non-radiolabeled tositumomab [30] and salvage chemotherapy [31] in patients with transformed or refractory low-grade NHL. In clinical trials, Zevalin treatment in patients with relapsed or refractory NHL resulted in significantly higher ORR and CR compared to unlabeled rituximab therapy alone [32] and longer median progression free survival compared to control [33].

Both treatments were not widely used in clinical practice, partly because of the complexity involving specialized radioactive shielding equipment, the two-phase process, and the coordination between medical oncologists and nuclear physicians, contributing to relatively high cost. Due to a decline in usage, sale of Bexxar had been discontinued since 2014.

Nonetheless, the interest in RIT as a targeted therapy continues to grow with ongoing research and clinical trials involving radiolabeled antibodies targeting solid organ tumors. Recent development includes the use of radiolabeled antibodies in the treatment of glioblastoma that targets the epidermal growth factor receptor, treatment of colorectal cancer with radiolabeled antibodies against carcinoembryonic antigen, and treatment of breast and ovarian cancer using radiolabeled trastuzumab, which is a humanized IgG monoclonal antibody directed against the extracellular domain of the human epidermal growth factor receptor 2 (HER-2)/neu [34].

6.4 CONCLUSION

Because of the advantages of targeted radionuclide therapy, elevated attention has been paid to the development of radiolabeled, targeted molecules in recent years ever since successful clinical application of radionuclide therapy in nuclear medicine. Many radiolabeled targeting molecules including small molecules, antibodies, and peptides are still under clinical evaluation. With adequate understanding of pharmacokinetic characteristics to enhance therapeutic effects of the targeted radionuclide and advanced technologies available in the field, more and more radiolabeled targeting molecules will be approved in the future with this regard to increase patient survival rate.

REFERENCES

1. Akhoon N Precision medicine: a new paradigm in therapeutics. *International Journal of Preventive Medicine* 2021;12:12. 10.4103/ijpvm.IJPVM_375_19.
2. Buvailo A Will biologics surpass small molecules in the pharmaceutical race? *Biopharmatrend.com.* 2022;21:2.
3. Steiner M, Neri D Antibody-radionuclide conjugates for cancer therapy: historical considerations and new trends. *Clinical Cancer Research.* 2011 Oct 15;17(20):6406–6416.
4. Yeong C-H, Cheng M.-h., Ng K-H Therapeutic radionuclides in nuclear medicine: current and future prospects. *Journal of Zhejiang University Science B – Biomedicine and Biotechnology.* 2014;15(10):845–863. 10.1158/1078-0432.CCR-11-0483.
5. Wang L, Lu B, He M, Wang Y, Wang Z, Du L Prostate cancer incidence and mortality: global status and temporal trends in 89 countries from 2000 to 2019. *Frontiers in Public Health.* 2022 Feb 16;10:811044.
6. Perera M, Papa N, Roberts M, Williams M, Udovicich C, Vela I, et al. Gallium-68 prostate-specific membrane antigen positron emission tomography in advanced prostate cancer—updated diagnostic utility, sensitivity, specificity, and distribution of prostate-specific membrane antigen-avid lesions: a systematic review and meta-analysis. *European Urology.* 2020 Apr 1;77(4):403–417.
7. Ristau BT, O'Keefe DS, Bacich DJ The prostate-specific membrane antigen: lessons and current clinical implications from 20 years of research. In Urologic Oncology: Seminars and Original Investigations 2014 Apr 1 (Vol. 32, No. 3, pp. 272–279). Elsevier.
8. Begum NJ, Glatting G, Wester HJ, Eiber M, Beer AJ, Kletting P The effect of ligand amount, affinity and internalization on PSMA-targeted imaging and therapy: A simulation study using a PBPK model. *Scientific Reports.* 2019 Dec 27;9(1):20041.
9. Jeitner TM, Babich JW, Kelly JM Advances in PSMA theranostics. *Translational Oncology.* 2022 Aug 1;22:101450.
10. Fragomeni RA, Amir T, Sheikhbahaei S, Harvey SC, Javadi MS, Solnes LB, et al. Imaging of non-prostate cancers using PSMA-targeted radiotracers: rationale, current state of the field, and a call to arms. *Journal of Nuclear Medicine.* 2018 Jun 1;59(6):871–877.
11. Kozikowski AP, Nan F, Conti P, Zhang J, Ramadan E, Bzdega T, et al. Design of remarkably simple, yet potent urea-based inhibitors of glutamate carboxypeptidase II (NAALADase). *Journal of Medicinal Chemistry.* 2001 Feb 1;44(3):298–301.7.
12. Rosenthal SA, Haseman MK, Polascik TJ Utility of capromab pendetide (ProstaScint) imaging in the management of prostate cancer. *Techniques in Urology.* 2001 Mar 1;7(1):27–37.
13. Bander NH, Trabulsi EJ, Kostakoglu L, Yao D, Vallabhajosula S, Smith-Jones P, et al. Targeting metastatic prostate cancer with radiolabeled monoclonal antibody J591 to the extracellular domain of prostate specific membrane antigen. *Journal of Urology.* 2003 Nov 1;170(5):1717–1721.
14. Afshar-Oromieh A, Babich JW, Kratochwil C, Giesel FL, Eisenhut M, Kopka K, et al. The rise of PSMA ligands for diagnosis and therapy of prostate cancer. *Journal of Nuclear Medicine.* 2016 Oct 1;57(Supplement 3):79S–89S.
15. Stephenson AJ, Scardino PT, Eastham JA, Bianco Jr FJ, Dotan ZA, Fearn PA, et al. Preoperative nomogram predicting the 10-year probability of prostate cancer recurrence after radical prostatectomy. *Journal of the National Cancer Institute.* 2006 May 17;98(10):715–717.
16. Ohri N, Dicker AP, Trabulsi EJ, Showalter TN Can early implementation of salvage radiotherapy for prostate cancer improve the therapeutic ratio? A systematic review and regression meta-analysis with radiobiological modelling. *European Journal of Cancer.* 2012 Apr 1;48(6):837–844.

17. Vargas HA, Martin-Malburet AG, Takeda T, Corradi RB, Eastham J, Wibmer A, et al. Localizing sites of disease in patients with rising serum prostate-specific antigen up to 1 ng/ml following prostatectomy: how much information can conventional imaging provide? In *Urologic Oncology: Seminars and Original Investigations* 2016 Nov 1 (Vol. 34, No. 11, pp. 482–e5). Elsevier.

18. Calais J, Czernin J, Cao M, Kishan AU, Hegde JV, Shaverdian N, et al. ^{68}Ga-PSMA-11 PET/CT mapping of prostate cancer biochemical recurrence after radical prostatectomy in 270 patients with a PSA level of less than 1.0 ng/mL: impact on salvage radiotherapy planning. *Journal of Nuclear Medicine.* 2018 Feb 1;59(2):230–237.

19. Fendler WP, Calais J, Eiber M, Flavell RR, Mishoe A, Feng FY, et al. Assessment of ^{68}Ga-PSMA-11 PET accuracy in localizing recurrent prostate cancer: a prospective single-arm clinical trial. *JAMA Oncology.* 2019 Jun 1;5(6):856–863.

20. Hofman MS, Emmett L, Sandhu S, Iravani A, Joshua AM, Goh JC, et al. [177Lu] Lu-PSMA-617 versus cabazitaxel in patients with metastatic castration-resistant prostate cancer (TheraP): a randomised, open-label, phase 2 trial. *The Lancet.* 2021 Feb 27;397(10276):797–804.

21. Sartor O, De Bono J, Chi KN, Fizazi K, Herrmann K, Rahbar K, et al. Lutetium-177–PSMA-617 for metastatic castration-resistant prostate cancer. *New England Journal of Medicine.* 2021 Sep 16;385(12):1091–1103.

22. Hofman MS, Lawrentschuk N, Francis RJ, Tang C, Vela I, Thomas P, et al. Prostate-specific membrane antigen PET-CT in patients with high-risk prostate cancer before curative-intent surgery or radiotherapy (proPSMA): a prospective, randomised, multicentre study. *The Lancet.* 2020 Apr 11;395(10231):1208–1216.

23. Lindner, T, Giesel, FL, Kratochwil, C, Serfling, SE Radioligands targeting fibroblast activation protein (FAP). *Cancers.* 2021;13:5744. 10.3390/cancers13225744.

24. Privé BM, Boussihmad MA, Timmermans B, van Gemert WA, Peters SMB, Derks YHW, et al. Fibroblast activation protein-targeted radionuclide therapy: background, opportunities, and challenges of first (pre)clinical studies. *European Journal of Nuclear Medicine and Molecular Imaging.* 2023 Feb 23; 50: 1906–1918.

25. Kratochwil C, Flechsig P, Lindner T, Abderrahim L, Altmann A, Mier W, et al. ^{68}Ga-FAPI PET/CT: Tracer uptake in 28 different kinds of cancer. *Journal of Nuclear Medicine.* 2019;60(6):801–805.

26. Calais J, Mona CE Will FAPI PET/CT Replace FDG PET/CT in the next decade? Point—An important diagnostic, phenotypic, and biomarker role. *American Journal of Roentgenology.* 2021;216(2):305–306.

27. Sidrak MMA, De Feo MS, Corica F, Gorica J, Conte M, Filippi L, et al. Fibroblast activation protein inhibitor (FAPI)-based theranostics—Where we are at and where we are heading: A systematic review. *International Journal of Molecular Sciences.* 2023;24(4):3863.

28. Gomes Marin JF, Nunes RF, Coutinho AM, Zaniboni EC, Costa LB, Barbosa FG, et al. Theranostics in nuclear medicine: emerging and re-emerging integrated imaging and therapies in the era of precision oncology. *Radio Graphics.* 2020;40(6):1715–1740.

29. Solnes LB, Werner RA, Jones KM, Sadaghiani MS, Bailey CR, Lapa C, et al. Theranostics: leveraging molecular imaging and therapy to impact patient management and secure the future of nuclear medicine. *Journal of Nuclear Medicine.* 2020;61(3):311–318.

30. Davis TA, Kaminski MS, Leonard J Long-term results of a randomized trial comparing tositumomab and iodine-131 tositumomab with tositumomab alone in patients with relapsed or refractory low-grade or transformed low grade non-Hodgkin's lymphoma. *American Society of Hematology.* 2003;102:405a.

31. Kaminski MS, Zelenetz AD, Press OW, Saleh M, Leonard J, Fehrenbacher L et al. Pivotal study of iodine I-131 tositumomab for chemotherapy-refractory low-grade or transformed low-grade B-cell non-Hodgkin's lymphomas. *Journal of Clinical Oncology.* 2001;19(19):3918–3928.

32. Witzig TE, Gordon LI, Cabanillas F, Czuczman MS, Emmanouilides C, Joyce R et al. Randomized controlled trial of yttrium-90-labeled ibritumomab tiuxetan RIT versus rituximab immunotherapy for patients with relapsed or refractory low-grade, follicular, or transformed B-cell non-Hodgkin's lymphoma. *Journal of Clinical Oncology.* 2002;20(10):2453–2463.

33. Morschauer F, Radford J, Van Hoff A, Vitolo U, Soubeyran P, Tilly H et al. Phase III trial of consolidation therapy with yttrium-90-ibritumomab tiuxetan compared with no additional therapy after first remission in advanced follicular lymphoma. *Journal of Clinical Oncology.* 2008;26(32):5156–5164.

34. Hidekazu K Radioimmunotherapy: A specific treatment protocol for cancer by cytotoxic radioisotopes conjugated to antibodies. *The Scientific World Journal.* 2014, Article ID 492061.

7 Radionuclide-Conjugated Cancer-Specific Vectors
Nanoparticles

Ivan Kempson and Ali Nazarizadeh

7.1 INTRODUCTION

Nanoparticles (NPs), in their various forms, offer unique properties for delivering therapeutics to improve treatment outcomes in terms of disease control and reduction of treatment-induced morbidity. For oncolytic therapeutic delivery, NPs most commonly have dimensions on the order of approximately 5–200 nm in diameter. Sometimes, firm measures of dimensions are recommended for defining specifically what a "nanoparticle" is; however, regardless of particular definitions, the intention is that the size scale promotes accumulation within the tumor and can be internalized by cells (which are on the order of ~10–20 microns in diameter). From an efficacy perspective, there is greater capacity for cells to internalize more NPs if their size is on the order of a few to 10s of nanometers diameter compared to larger particles. Many NPs have sizes comparable to proteins and subcellular structures which make them highly recognizable by cells and able to be internalized via conventional biological processes. While several NP formulations have reached clinical use (e.g. Doxil® and Hensify®) for chemotherapy and radiosensitization, their state of development for radionuclide delivery in treatment of cancer is largely limited to preclinical studies. This chapter overviews key examples of literature separated by broad classifications of NP types with the aim of highlighting the state of progress in the development of nano-formulated radionuclides, highlighting potential advantages over free or targeted radionuclides. It concludes with a discussion around biodistribution and potential limitations. First however, the following section explains the allure of using NP-formulated radionuclides and the benefits they offer.

7.2 WHY NANOPARTICLES?

NPs can be synthesized from a broad range of materials such as metals and their oxides, polymers and biological molecules. Their structure can be varied to act as a substrate for binding radionuclides or other moieties to the surface, or they can have a porous, sponge-like structure or act as nano-sized capsules, loaded with a therapeutic agent. For radiopharmaceutical treatment of cancer, the intention of using a nano-formulation is to improve pharmacokinetics and delivery to the tumor, provide a carrier with known pharmacokinetics which can be used for multiple diagnostic or therapeutic functions, and/or provide additional functions to complement the radionuclides' action. Additional functions most often involve the binding of a targeting ligand to facilitate the NP's preferential uptake by cancer cells overexpressing specific receptors. While this is largely analogous with a receptor targeted radionuclide conjugate, the diverse chemical and physical properties of NPs can be useful in broadening the range of possible targeting moieties compared to what can be conjugated directly to radionuclides. Points of distinction where NPs offer further advantage are mentioned below.

DOI: 10.1201/9781003250913-9

- The ability to load multiple radionuclides. Consequently, the pharmacokinetics and bio-distribution can be directed by the NP properties rather than the individual radionuclide product. In this case, a NP could be developed with favorable properties and then used for different radionuclides whether they be for diagnostics or therapeutics and the same biodistribution is achieved regardless of the radionuclide used. This assists in ensuring therapeutic isotopes have the same biodistribution as diagnostic isotopes.
- NPs can have other beneficial properties such as providing contrast for complementary imaging modalities such as CT, MRI, PET and ultrasound. In this way, NPs can provide insight into where the radionuclide formulation goes, providing information useful for biodistribution and dosimetry. Fluorescent properties can also be useful for visually tracking NPs where possible.
- Formulation of combinatorial treatments is possible, for example, by loading the same NPs simultaneously with radionuclides and chemotherapy agents. The chemo agent is administered simultaneously with radionuclides, and both will have a fate directed by the NP properties, and not by each component. With respect to pharmacokinetics and bio-distribution, the "cocktail" can be considered as a monotherapy rather than a co-therapy mixture which conventionally have distinct differences in their biological fate.
- NPs can reduce the breakage of bonds tethering the radionuclide to targeting agents, thus improving biodistribution.

The major benefit highlighted in this chapter, based on preclinical data, is improved tumor retention of nano-formulations compared to free radionuclide molecules. NPs are easily extravasated into tumor volumes due to the leaky nature of the tumor microstructure. Free radionuclides can easily drain out of tumor volumes via lymphatic flow; however, NPs exhibit far superior retention (also known as enhanced permeability and retention (EPR) effect) and can increase the radiation dose delivered to the tumor.

7.3   RADIONUCLIDE NANOPARTICLE FORMULATIONS

In a generalized sense, NPs comprise a core, structural material which may be solid, porous or capsule-like (Figure 7.1A). There is commonly a surface coating (often polyethylene glycol, PEG) to promote colloidal stability and reduce the binding of proteins to the NPs. This prevents NP aggregation and increases blood circulation. NPs are often bound with a targeting ligand (e.g. peptides, antibodies) which has a high affinity for a receptor over-represented on tumor cells (e.g. cancer cells, and cancer-associated fibroblasts) compared to normal cells. The NP will also have the therapeutic agent(s) physically incorporated (loaded), or chemically bound, within the particle or on its surface. NPs have well-defined synthetic routes, reliable preparation, generally acceptable biosafety profiles and controlled shapes and sizes which make them highly amenable for following good manufacturing processes and quality-by-design principles. A range of different NP types exist. Some are represented in Figure 7.1B–F and those that dominate the research literature for radionuclide treatment of cancer are described in the following sections.

7.3.1   METAL AND METALLOID NANOPARTICLES

This section considers inorganic NPs comprising a metal or metalloid and their oxides. These NPs are often spherical and used as a substrate to bind other moieties on their surface. They are often made from a relatively biologically inert metal such as gold, or a material which is ultimately biodegradable such as silica. They have very well-defined surface chemistry and are able to provide strong covalent bonding for the conjugation of other molecules used for formulation stability, functional targeting or binding radionuclides. Gold NPs (AuNPs) have dominated research. Prolonged circulation in vivo and delayed clearance from tumor tissues can lead to

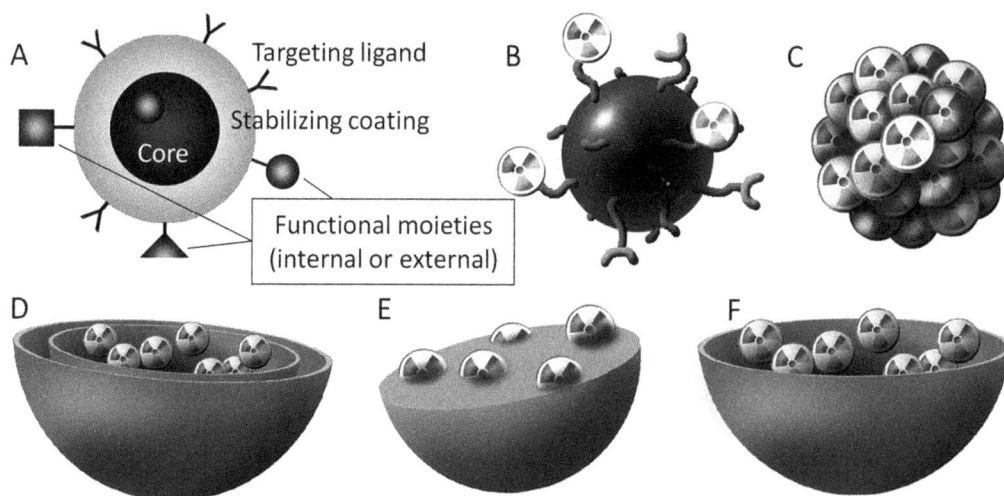

FIGURE 7.1   (A) A generalized scheme of a nanoparticle. (B) A solid metal nanoparticle with surface bound radionuclides and targeting ligands. (C) A nanoparticle constructed from a radionuclide. (D) A liposome. (E) A nanoparticle which could be a porous, polymer or biomolecular structure (F) A micelle. Note that no stabilizing or targeting moieties are indicated in C–F although they are generally used.

improved tumor control and survival in mice. ^{211}At is an example of an alpha emitter for which standard methods of conjugation to monoclonal antibodies produce unstable products. However, chemisorption onto targeted AuNPs can produce a highly stable formulation [1]. In other examples, both ^{177}Lu-DOTA and ^{99m}Tc-HYNIC have been bound to AuNPs with tumor-targeting peptides [2]. The system was highly stable and pure (radiochemical purity ~96%). Following intratumor injection in a mouse model, >40% of the isotopes were retained in the tumor at 24 hours. The ^{177}Lu-absorbed dose per injected activity was 7.9 Gy/MBq, more than double that for the formulation without the targeting peptide. However, absorbed doses to the kidney, liver and spleen were reported as 0.80 ± 0.11, 0.18 ± 0.04 and 0.49 ± 0.09 Gy/MBq, respectively.

NPs can simultaneously be loaded with additional targeted therapeutics. For example, ^{177}Lu labeled 15 nm AuNPs have been conjugated with cetuximab, a targeted anticancer drug [3]. Dose distribution and biodistribution in a mouse model showed reasonably homogenous distribution in the tumor; however, the liver and spleen had the highest content. Intratumoral injection in a mouse model with ^{177}Lu labeled AuNPs conjugated with panitumumab not only showed superior antitumor behavior compared to the nontargeted formulation but also accumulated in liver and spleen [4].

Metal-based NPs can provide complementary properties themselves, in addition to the transport of radionuclides. For instance, their density can give rise to contrast in CT. Magnetic NPs can provide contrast in magnetic resonance imaging (MRI) [5], enable magnetic guidance (see Figure 7.3) and hyperthermia [6]. Targeted, ^{131}I labeled 14 nm superparamagnetic iron oxide nanoparticles (SPIONs) intratumorally injected in a mouse model were retained at the injection site even after 14 days while free ^{131}I distributed throughout the body after 6 hours and was observable in the thyroid only at day 8 [6]. The combination of magnetic hyperthermia with radionuclide therapy resulted in better tumor control than the radiotherapy alone.

Silicon and silica NPs (SiNPs) have been widely explored in nanomedicine because of their amenability for diverse silane chemistry modifications and biocompatibility. Mesoporous structures in particular have provided highly flexible platforms for enabling drug delivery and controlled release. Surface chemical-modifications allow diverse moieties to bind for therapeutics and targeting molecules [7]. Silicon and silica are also biodegradable, which facilitates longer-term clearance.

7.3.2 LIPOSOMES

Liposomes are spherical vesicles made with a lipid bilayer "shell" and typically range in size upwards from ~100 nm in diameter [8]. Liposomes have slightly different characteristics compared to other NPs in that they act like capsules which can encapsulate solutions of drug or radionuclide, or both. Delivery of their active component is also slightly different in that the lipid bilayer of the liposome fuses with the cell membrane and then releases its content directly into the cytoplasm, compared to other NPs that are internalized most often via endocytic pathways and can be retained within vesicles. This difference in delivery can be important for chemical agents with a specific intracellular site of action, but may not influence therapeutic effects of radionuclides which can deliver dose beyond the confines of intracellular vesicles. Liposomal formulations are established clinically for chemotherapy delivery such as DOXIL®.

A PEG-stabilized, tumor-cell-targeting liposome loaded with ^{125}I-labeled anthracyclines (~100 nm) demonstrated a twofold longer survival in a mouse model than those administered with a nontargeted formulation [9]. More than half the mice were tumor-free at the end of the study. However, accumulation of the radioisotope in the liver and spleen together with slight histologic damages to the spleen were noticed. Similar observations have also been recorded for a [188]Re-liposome [10]. Another study with [188]Re-liposomes however reported no obvious toxicity [11].

Of particular note is a [188]Re-loaded PEGylated nanoliposome that has reached clinical trials (Figure 7.2A) [12], registered in 2012 and reported in 2019. This formulation has progressed through a variety of preclinical studies reviewed elsewhere [13]. Consistently, [188]Re-liposomes have significantly prolonged survival in mice. While SPECT/CT images showed free [188]Re was rapidly washed out, the [188]Re-liposome was still detectable after 48 hours in the tumor, spleen and liver [14]. The phase 0 clinical study concluded that the "nanocarrier [188]Re-liposome achieves favorable tumor accumulation and tumor to normal organ uptake ratios for a subset of cancer patients. The clinical pharmacokinetic, biodistribution, and dosimetry results justify a further dose-escalating phase 1 clinical trial".

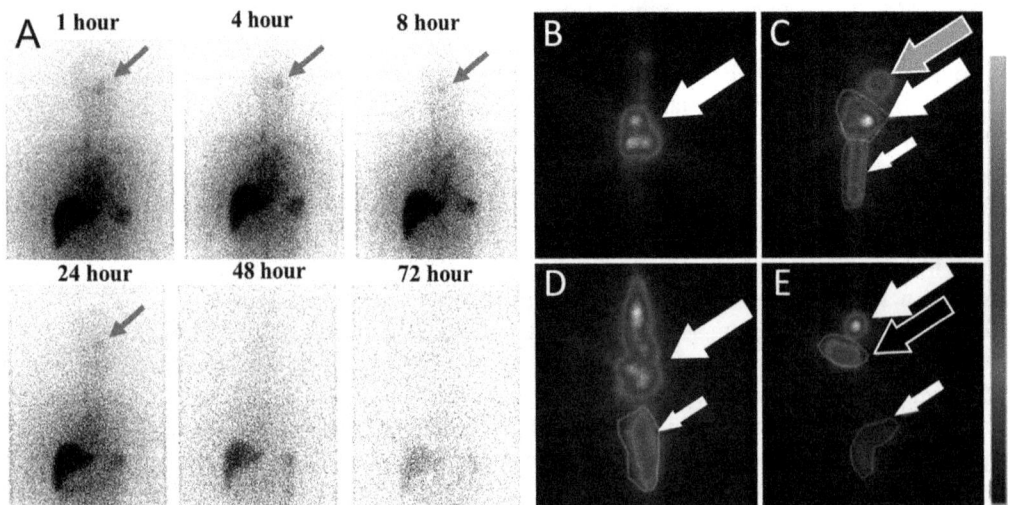

FIGURE 7.2 (A) Accumulation of a [188]Re-liposome in a lesion in the nasopharynx (indicated by the arrows) at six time points after injection. Adapted from Shyh-Jen Wang et al., 2019, Copyright © 2019, The Authors [12]. (B–E) Scintigraphic images recorded within 30 min post injection of gum arabic-coated [198]AuNPs in dogs with spontaneous prostate cancer. Images show AuNPs within the prostate post-injection as indicated by the large white arrows; multiple injection points in the tumor are clearly seen in dog (B). Leakage of NPs into bladder, urethra and extra prostate region following injection is indicated by the gray, small white and black arrows, respectively. International Journal of Nanomedicine 2014 9(1) 5001-5011, Originally published by, adapted and used with permission from Dove Medical Press Ltd. [15]. Copyright © 2014 Axiak-Bechtel et al.

7.3.3 MICELLES

Nanomicelles are an interesting carrier for therapeutics, made of surfactants analogous to common soaps. They comprise long-chain molecules that have a hydrophilic head and hydrophobic tail. A micelle is a construct of these molecules with the hydrophobic tails orientated inwards creating a hydrophobic environment; yet the hydrophilic surface of the micelle means it can be suspended in aqueous solutions. These structures are especially useful for loading lipophilic materials (such as chemotherapeutic agents and photodynamic agents). The micelle can be suspended in aqueous solvents, whereas the free therapeutic would conventionally be challenging to disperse. Many free radionuclide compounds do not have miscibility issues; however, micelles provide opportunity to encapsulate additional materials within the same "capsule". The resulting biodistribution and pharmacokinetics are dictated by the micelle properties, rather than the individual traits of each component. For example in the formulation of ^{90}Y, the biodistribution of the fabricated lactosome was assessed using ^{111}In (replaced with ^{90}Y) following intravenous injection [16]. They are also useful for co-delivery, such as in an example of loading a micelle with doxorubicin (size: ~107–194 nm) and ^{188}Re [17], or ^{125}I with a photosensitizer [18]. While free ^{125}I had almost no therapeutic effects, the nanomicelle efficiently suppressed tumor growth. Moreover, the laser irradiation further enhanced the therapeutic effects through action of the photosensitizer. No significant pathologic changes were detected in blood and major organs.

7.3.4 NANO-RADIONUCLIDES

NPs exhibit pharmacokinetics and biodistributions substantially different to small molecules or free ions. As demonstrated in a number of preclinical studies, retention within the tumor is much more favorable for particles. In this sense, there is potential advantage of radionuclides being prepared in particulate form. This has been demonstrated clinically, at least for microparticles, where ^{32}P particles are injected directly into pancreatic adenocarcinoma under ultrasound-guided endoscopy [19]. The particulate nature can facilitate local retention and improved therapeutic outcomes. It has also been proposed, and tested preclinically, to scale down the size of low dose-rate brachytherapy seeds for what has been termed nano-brachytherapy. A number of preclinical studies have explored this concept using ^{198}Au-NPs in mouse models of prostate cancer [20]. A similar study, but using a ^{103}Pd coating on hollow gold spheres (~150 nm diameter), achieved >80% tumor growth inhibition after 5 weeks [21].

The use of NPs constructed from radionuclides is dominated by research considering brachytherapy. The advantage is that a colloidal solution uses narrower gauge needles for delivery compared to conventional seeds and reduces discomfort and local inflammation [22]. It is important to note that research to date makes little direct comparison between nano- and conventional-seeds, so potential therapeutic benefits are not clear. The synthesis of these nanostructures is more sophisticated compared to the conventional seeds and is a further barrier for translation. Nanobrachytherapy is challenged by the leakage of radionuclides away from the tumor. The diffusion of NPs in the tumor which is of a highly heterogeneous nature makes dosimetry and planning much more challenging than for conventional seeds. This has been highlighted in dogs presenting spontaneous prostate cancer (Figure 7.2B–E) [15]. That study concluded "localization of radioactivity within the prostate was lower than anticipated and likely due to normal vestigial prostatic ducts. Therefore, further study of retention, dosimetry, long-term toxicity, and efficacy of this treatment is warranted prior to Phase I trials" [15].

7.3.5 ORGANIC NANOPARTICLES

NPs can be prepared from various naturally occurring biomolecules such as polymers, proteins and lipids, and have been developed preclinically driven by their biocompatible nature. Most comprise serum albumin coupled with a targeting ligand for delivery of [131]I [23,24]. Compared to free ^{131}I, these NPs also show improved tumor accumulation in mouse models and can also be conjugated with other therapeutics such as paclitaxel [25]. Other examples of these NPs include reconstituted high-density lipoproteins that recognize a specific receptor overexpressed in several types of cancer cells, as a vehicle for delivery of [225]Ac [26]. Melanin is another interesting biomolecule. It is an amorphous, natural and biodegradable pigment found in a variety of tissues, including human skin and hair [27]. ^{64}Cu-labeled melanin NPs for PET/CT of mice showed tumor uptake peaked 8 hours post injection (~14% of the administered activity); however, the liver and spleen had relatively high uptake as well [28].

7.3.6 Synthetic Polymeric Nanoparticles

Polymer-based NPs are colloidal systems made up of natural or synthetic polymers. Polymer NPs are highly stable in biological fluids and their surface is easily functionalized to modulate polymer degradation and the release of loaded compound(s) as a function of specific stimuli [29]. These NPs are highly diverse and can be constructed in numerous ways giving rise to many other sub-classifications of polymer NPs such as dendrimers, which are nano-sized, radially symmetric molecules with well-defined, homogeneous and monodisperse structures [30]. Polymers provide what is probably the most flexibility in chemistry options that provide the broadest range of physicochemical properties. These can provide biodegradability, stimuli-responsiveness (e.g. to pH or hypoxia) and the ability to bind any radionuclide. An example is an ultrasmall hyperbranched semiconducting polymer NP (~5 nm) modified with PEG acting as a vehicle for diagnostic (^{99m}Tc and ^{125}I) or therapeutic (^{131}I) radionuclides [31].

7.4 BIODISTRIBUTION

Preclinical research shows consistently that NPs, especially targeted NPs, can promote significant improvements in animal survival. This has been demonstrated for a broad range of NP types, radionuclides and cancer models. NPs are much more effective at being retained in the tumor which promotes efficacious delivery by intravenous or intratumor injection. This is highlighted in Figure 7.3A–D where free [188]ReO$_4$ injected into tumor rapidly leached out and distributed throughout mice [32]. A magnetic nano-formulation showed strong retention within the tumor tissue. The nano-formulation was only injected into one tumor, while a tumor on the opposing side exhibited accumulation of the nano-formulation due to the use of an external magnetic field. The free isotope was unable to demonstrate substantial oncolytic action while the nano-formulation did. Other studies concur with similar findings showing greater than ~15% of the administered activity being retained in the tumor even after 24 hours compared to less than 0.5% for the free [188]Re compound [33]. Intratumoral injection is not always a practical route of administration though. Intravenous injection of NPs still leads to retention in tumors for several days [34].

Nano-formulations can increase systemic circulation, leading to additional risks to organs. Even though NPs are small, their relatively large size compared to most biomolecules, and scavenging by macrophages, leads to accumulation in kidney, liver and spleen (Figure 7.3E and F). While doses reported of 0.92 ± 0.35, 0.32 ± 0.09 Gy/GBq in liver and kidney, respectively, for a non-targeted liposome in human patients (Figure 7.2A) [12] are acceptable, other preclinical studies report much higher doses. Different NPs will distribute differently, however, depending on size, targeting ligands and other factors, but is a major consideration for development and translation of NP radionuclide formulations. Renal excretion can be the primary route of clearance when NPs are sufficiently small, as shown for ~6 nm silica NPs, with approximately 40% of the activity excreted at 24 hour post injection and roughly 80% excreted at 96 hour post injection in animal models [34]. Also, NPs offer the ability to respond to the local tumor microenvironment [32,35]. For example, a

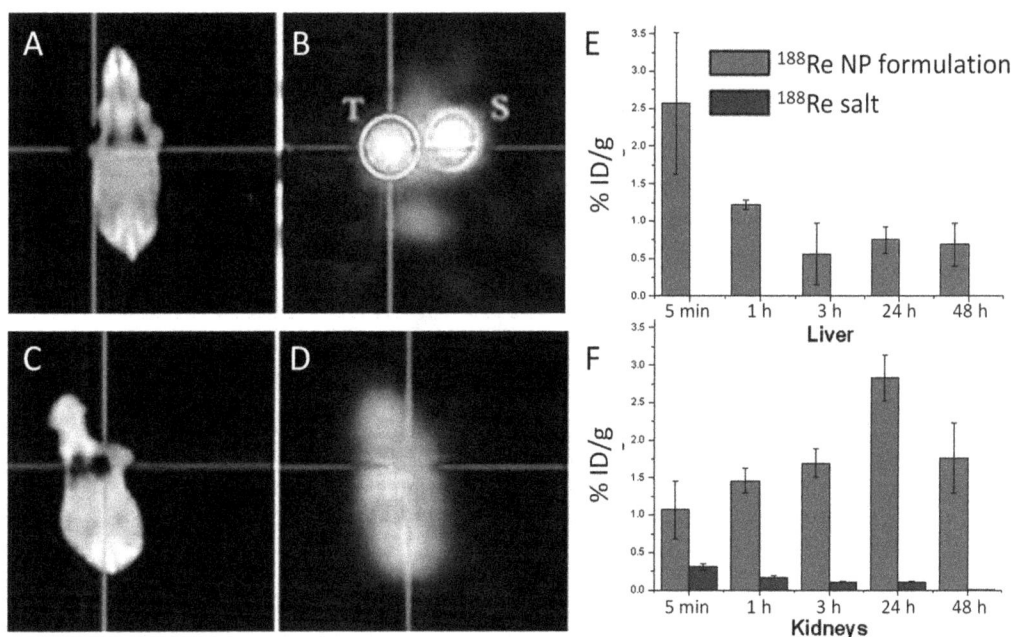

FIGURE 7.3 (A–D). (A,C) CT images of mice and (B,D) SPECT images 1 hour after injection of [188]Re formulations. Mice bearing tumors on both forelimbs received injection of [188]Re into the left tumor. A magnet was positioned next to the right tumor. (B) A large portion of a [188]Re iron oxide NP formulation remains within the left tumor. NPs that leak out from the left tumor are magnetically guided to accumulate in the right tumor. (D) In contrast, the [188]Re salt rapidly leaks out of the tumor and is uniformly distributed through the mouse. Adapted with permission from [32]. Copyright 2017 American Chemical Society. (E,F) Biodistribution of [188]Re after systemic administration in Wistar rats with a NP-based [188]Re conjugate or as a salt. The NP formulation leads to much greater accumulation in liver and kidneys. Copyright © 2019, The Authors [33].

graphene oxide modified core–shell Fe_3O_4/SiO_2 NP could carry [188]Re and release it preferentially in the acidic tumor microenvironment. This may help with delivering the radionuclide but then also enable faster clearance.

Another approach to prevent leakage after intratumoral injection is to co-inject a biocompatible polymer, such as alginate, to sequester NPs at the site of injection [22]. In this example, NPs reduced tumor volume after 4 weeks by 56% and by 75%, compared to controls, for [103]Pd-based and [103]Pd[198]Au-based NPs, respectively. Biodistribution assessments within 30–50 days revealed that still around 16% and 3% of the administered activity was associated with liver and spleen, respectively [22]. Most toxicity assessments are currently at a basic level and more detailed long-term assessments should be considered in future studies.

Receptor-targeting conjugates can experience bond breakage during the parent decay. The daughter product, which can still be radioactive, then no longer has targeting functionality and may also change biodistribution. There is scope that NPs can reduce this issue. On the other hand though, there is limited knowledge on how the decay of radionuclides can degrade or compromise the NP structure and functionality.

7.5 CONCLUSION

Many different types of nano-formulations have consistently shown therapeutic advantages in preclinical models compared to free radionuclides. However, little is known about how targeted

NPs compare with targeted radionuclide compounds. Few studies compare NPs with targeted radionuclides, rather than just their salts. Compared to free radionuclides, NPs have greater accumulation in other organs such as the kidney, liver and spleen in addition to the tumor. There is a lack of understanding currently as to what long-term impact this may have on these organs. However, formulations can be designed to reduce doses to organs at risk. The full potential of nano-formulations offers many advantages that are currently evolving and being developed. There are very notable advantages for creating formulations amenable for a range of isotopes for diagnostic or therapeutic purposes while exhibiting identical biodistribution directed by NP characteristics.

REFERENCES

1. Dziawer, L., et al., Gold nanoparticle bioconjugates labelled with 211At for targeted alpha therapy. *RSC Advances*, 2017. 7(65): pp. 41024–41032.
2. Jimenez-Mancilla, N., et al., Multifunctional targeted radiotherapy system for induced tumours expressing gastrin-releasing peptide receptors. *Current Nanoscience*, 2012. 8(2): pp. 193–201.
3. Shabbir, R., et al., EGFR targeting of [177Lu] gold nanoparticles to colorectal and breast tumour cells: affinity, duration of binding and growth inhibition of cetuximab-resistant cells. *Journal of King Saud University – Science*, 2021. 33(7): p. 101573.
4. Yook, S., et al., Intratumorally injected 177Lu-labeled gold nanoparticles: gold nanoseed brachytherapy with application for neoadjuvant treatment of locally advanced breast cancer. *Journal of Nuclear Medicine*, 2016. 57(6): pp. 936–942.
5. Cedrowska, E., et al., Trastuzumab conjugated superparamagnetic iron oxide nanoparticles labeled with (225)Ac as a perspective tool for combined alpha-radioimmunotherapy and magnetic hyperthermia of HER2-positive breast cancer. *Molecules*, 2020. 25(5): p. 1025.
6. Stankovic, A., et al., Aminosilanized flower-structured superparamagnetic iron oxide nanoparticles coupled to (131)I-labeled CC49 antibody for combined radionuclide and hyperthermia therapy of cancer. *International Journal of Pharmaceutics*, 2020. 587: p. 119628.
7. Watermann, A. and J. Brieger, Mesoporous silica nanoparticles as drug delivery vehicles in cancer. *Nanomaterials*, 2017. 7(7): p. 189.
8. Kostarelos, K. and D. Emfietzoglou, Liposomes as carriers of radionuclides: from imaging to therapy. *Journal of Liposome Research*, 1999. 9(4): pp. 429–460.
9. Gedda, L., et al., Experimental radionuclide therapy of HER2-expressing xenografts using two-step targeting nuclisome particles. *Journal of Nuclear Medicine*, 2012. 53(3): pp. 480–487.
10. Shen, Y.A., et al., Intraperitoneal (188)Re-liposome delivery switches ovarian cancer metabolism from glycolysis to oxidative phosphorylation and effectively controls ovarian tumour growth in mice. *Radiotherapy and Oncology*, 2016. 119(2): pp. 282–290.
11. French, J.T., et al., Interventional therapy of head and neck cancer with lipid nanoparticle-carried rhenium 186 radionuclide. *Journal of Vascular and Interventional Radiology*, 2010. 21(8): pp. 1271–1279.
12. Wang, S.J., et al., A phase 0 study of the pharmacokinetics, biodistribution, and dosimetry of 188Re-liposome in patients with metastatic tumors. *EJNMMI Research*, 2019. 9: pp. 1–13.
13. Chang, C.H., et al., Translating research for the radiotheranostics of nanotargeted 188re-liposome. *International Journal of Molecular Sciences*, 2021. 22(8): p. 3868.
14. Lin, L.T., et al., Evaluation of the therapeutic and diagnostic effects of PEGylated liposome-embedded 188Re on human non-small cell lung cancer using an orthotopic small-animal model. *Journal of Nuclear Medicine*, 2014. 55(11): pp. 1864–1870.
15. Axiak-Bechtel, S.M., et al., Gum arabic-coated radioactive gold nanoparticles cause no short-term local or systemic toxicity in the clinically relevant canine model of prostate cancer. *International Journal of Nanomedicine*, 2014. 9: pp. 5001–5011. Originally published by, adapted and used with permission from Dove Medical Press Ltd.
16. Kurihara, K., et al., Inflammation-induced synergetic enhancement of nanoparticle treatments with DOXIL® and 90Y-lactosome for orthotopic mammary tumor. *Journal of Nanoparticle Research*, 2016. 18(5): pp. 1–11.
17. Shih, Y.-H., et al., Therapeutic and scintigraphic applications of polymeric micelles: combination of chemotherapy and radiotherapy in hepatocellular carcinoma. *International Journal of Nanomedicine*, 2015; 10: p. 7443.

18. Qin, Y., et al., Photo-driven delivery of (125)I-labeled nanomicelles for nucleus-targeted internal conversion electron-based cancer therapy. *ACS Applied Materials & Interfaces*, 2021. 13(42): pp. 49671–49681.
19. Naidu, J., et al., Combined chemotherapy and endoscopic ultrasound-guided intratumoral 32P implantation for locally advanced pancreatic adenocarcinoma: a pilot study. *Endoscopy*, 2022. 54(1): pp. 75–80.
20. Chanda, N., et al., Radioactive gold nanoparticles in cancer therapy: therapeutic efficacy studies of GA-198AuNP nanoconstruct in prostate tumor–bearing mice. *Nanomedicine: Nanotechnology, Biology and Medicine*, 2010. 6(2): pp. 201–209.
21. Moeendarbari, S., et al., Theranostic nanoseeds for efficacious internal radiation therapy of unresectable solid tumors. *Scientific Reports*, 2016. 6(1): p. 20614.
22. Laprise-Pelletier, M., et al., Low-dose prostate cancer brachytherapy with radioactive palladium-gold nanoparticles. *Advanced Healthcare Materials*, 2017. 6(4): p. 1601120.
23. Li, W., et al., Radionuclide therapy using (1)(3)(1)I-labeled anti-epidermal growth factor receptor-targeted nanoparticles suppresses cancer cell growth caused by EGFR overexpression. *Journal of Cancer Research and Clinical Oncology*, 2016. 142(3): pp. 619–632.
24. Lin, M., et al., Hepatoma-targeted radionuclide immune albumin nanospheres: (131)I-antiAFPMcAb-GCV-BSA-NPs. *Analytical Cellular Pathology (Amsterdam)*, 2016. 2016: p. 9142198.
25. Tian, L., et al., Radionuclide I-131 labeled albumin-paclitaxel nanoparticles for synergistic combined chemo-radioisotope therapy of cancer. *Theranostics*, 2017. 7(3): pp. 614–623.
26. Hernandez-Jimenez, T., et al., (225)Ac-rHDL nanoparticles: a potential agent for targeted alpha-particle therapy of tumors overexpressing SR-BI proteins. *Molecules*, 2022. 27(7): p. 2156.
27. Xia, L., et al., A highly specific multiple enhancement theranostic nanoprobe for PET/MRI/PAI image-guided radioisotope combined photothermal therapy in prostate cancer. *Small*, 2021. 17(21): p. e2100378.
28. Zhou, H., et al. (64)Cu-labeled melanin nanoparticles for PET/CT and radionuclide therapy of tumor. *Nanomedicine*, 2020. 29: p. 102248.
29. Gagliardi, A., et al., Biodegradable polymeric nanoparticles for drug delivery to solid tumors. *Frontiers in Pharmacology*, 2021. 12: p. 601626.
30. Abbasi, E., et al., Dendrimers: synthesis, applications, and properties. *Nanoscale Research Letters*, 2014. 9(1): p. 247.
31. Yi, X., et al., Ultrasmall hyperbranched semiconducting polymer nanoparticles with different radio-isotopes labeling for cancer theranostics. *ACS Nano*, 2018. 12(9): pp. 9142–9151.
32. Yang, Y., et al., Rational design of GO-modified Fe3O4/SiO2 nanoparticles with combined Rhenium-188 and gambogic acid for magnetic target therapy. *ACS Applied Materials & Interfaces*, 2017. 9(34): pp. 28195–28208.
33. Petriev, V.M., et al., Nuclear nanomedicine using Si nanoparticles as safe and effective carriers of (188)Re radionuclide for cancer therapy. Science Reports, 2019. 9(1): p. 2017.
34. Zhang, X., et al., Targeted melanoma radiotherapy using ultrasmall (177)Lu-labeled alpha-melanocyte stimulating hormone-functionalized core-shell silica nanoparticles. *Biomaterials*, 2020. 241: p. 119858.
35. Zhu, C., et al., Alpha-particle radiotherapy: for large solid tumors diffusion trumps targeting. *Biomaterials*, 2017. 130: pp. 67–75.

8 Introduction to Clinical Trials and Drug Development for Radionuclide Therapies

Nicole Lin, Jarey H. Wang, Angela Y. Jia, and Ana P. Kiess

8.1 INTRODUCTION

Medical physicists are key members of the clinical team for delivery of radionuclide therapies (RNTs). RNT agents have an expanding role in oncology with multiple recent regulatory agency approvals, including ^{223}Ra, ^{177}Lu-DOTATATE, ^{131}I-MIBG, and ^{177}Lu-PSMA-617, as well as many other agents in development. Figure 8.1 demonstrates the increasing number of RNT publications per year across various cancer disease sites [1]. Thus, it is increasingly important for medical physicists to learn about RNT development and clinical trials. In this chapter, we will first describe the general process of drug development, including in the United States and Europe. We will summarize the key registry trials that led to regulatory agency approval of recent RNT agents. Finally, we will emphasize some of the unique opportunities and challenges of RNT development.

8.2 PRECLINICAL STUDIES

Before testing in humans, a newly discovered drug candidate must undergo tests to assess its antitumor efficacy, biochemical properties, and potential toxicities both in cells and in animals. This includes collecting information about the RNT agent's pharmacokinetics, biodistribution, dosimetry, and toxicology. In this way, the data can establish a predictable and consistent relationship between the administered dose and response in tumor and normal tissues, as well as assess molecular targeting, clearance, and other characteristics. Frequently, lack of efficacy and/or high toxicity in preclinical studies can lead to early discontinuation of drug development. In fact, for academic drug development projects, there is only a 32% success rate for preclinical studies [2]. To provide guidance on preclinical RNT development, organizations such as the Food and Drug Administration (FDA), European Medicines Agency (EMA), and Health Canada have individual recommendations, and have also adopted consensus recommendations by the International Conference on Harmonization guideline M3 (R2). In particular, the FDA has provided special guidance on microdose compounds ($\leq$ 100 µg administered) to accelerate approval and reduce preclinical expenditures and resource utilization [3].

Data collected on the molecule's pharmacokinetic (PK) properties characterize what the body does to the drug. This is influenced by factors such as absorption, distribution, metabolism, and excretion. Absorption depends on how the material or drug is administered, typically intravenously but sometimes via other routes such as intra-arterial or oral. Distribution refers to how the drug travels to its effector site, which is most commonly via the bloodstream. Metabolism refers to how the body transforms or breaks down compounds. This can result in toxic byproducts being formed, so specific metabolic pathways and mechanisms of toxicity must be understood. For RNT agents, this includes the potential production of "free" daughter radionuclides that may have distinct toxicities. Excretion refers to how the body rids itself of substances, primarily via the kidneys for

DOI: 10.1201/9781003250913-10

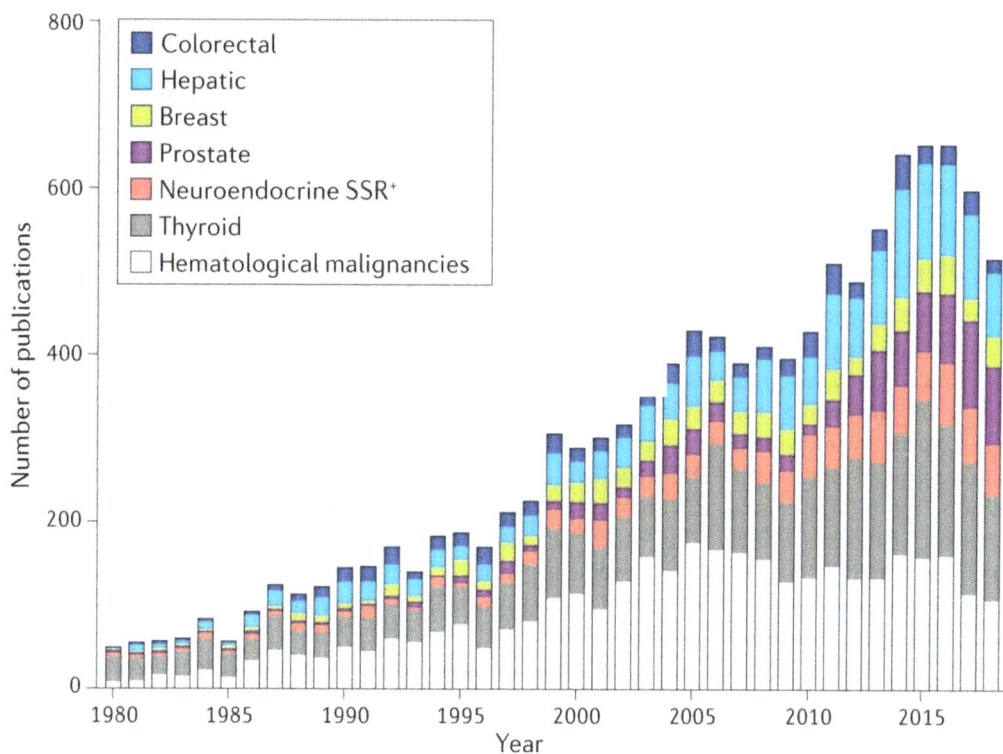

FIGURE 8.1   Publications per year related to RNT by cancer disease site [1].

radionuclides. The combination of these four PK factors greatly impacts how an RNT agent behaves in the body. For instance, the physical half-life of a radioactive material (RAM) is the time it takes for the activity of the agent "on the shelf" to decrease by half. The biological half-life alternatively describes the time for the body to eliminate half of the agent. The effective half-life of an agent takes both into consideration. For ^{177}Lu-PSMA-617, an RNT for prostate cancer, the physical half-life is 6.7 days but the effective half-life is approximately 2 days due to rapid renal clearance [4].

To assess an agent's pharmacokinetics and biodistribution, various experiments are done. For instance, biodistribution experiments can use blood or *ex vivo* tissue samples to assess activity or use in vivo functional imaging to assess tissue activity. For radionuclides, most are amenable to direct imaging of biodistribution via PET or SPECT imaging. Even alpha-emitting RNT agents with very low gamma energy and frequency (such as ^{223}Ra and ^{227}Th) can now be imaged by quantitative SPECT with advanced reconstruction algorithms [5]. Time activity curves, or graphs of activity or dose rate versus time, can then be generated for regions of interest. Dosimetric models such as those based on the International Commission on Radiological Protection (ICRP) 103 guidelines are used to calculate absorbed dose to the regions of interest [6]. For microdose studies (including RNTs), a single mammalian species (both sexes included) suffices. The type of data collected also depends on the type of RNT agent and whether it is intended for therapeutic and/or diagnostic purposes [7].

After establishing PK properties in animal models, experiments must also investigate the agent's dosage and its direct relationship with potential toxicities, including organ-specific toxicities. These experiments on pharmacodynamics find the range of doses estimated to be safe and tolerable for human subjects, compiling information about the agent's concentration and physiologic effects in various tissues. Such studies benefit especially from incorporation of imaging. In the case of RNT agents, pharmacodynamics and pharmacokinetics experiments often overlap, since the concentration of the agent is directly related to the radioactivity, absorbed dose, and physiologic effects of the agent. Unacceptable toxicity in animal models may prevent the agent from continuing to be developed. After toxicity profiles are determined, tolerable doses can be extrapolated to humans based on models taking into consideration parameters like organ to body weight ratios or body surface area ratios.

8.3   IND APPLICATION/APPROVAL

After conducting sufficient preclinical studies, novel RNT agents can be submitted for approval through regulatory agencies. The specific policies vary across countries, particularly regarding non-clinical safety requirements and standards for clinical trial authorization and marketing. For purposes of consistency, this section will discuss the specifics of approval through the FDA in the United States, with discussion on approval via European and Canadian agencies at the end.

In the United States, new FDA guidelines from 2018 onward are allowing for more streamlined pathway for first in human RNTs by changing the requirements for compliance with Good Laboratory Practices (GLP). This policy update now enables in-house preclinical toxicology studies in controlled laboratory environments prior to submitting an Investigational New Drug (IND) or exploratory IND (eIND) application to the FDA. Application submission is done by a sponsor or sponsor-investigator after preclinical studies and is required before human clinical trials. This proposal contains the investigator qualifications, investigational clinical plan, pre-clinical data (including toxicology and dosimetry), as well as any available clinical data. Details of the clinical trial must be proposed, including selection criteria, sample size, trial duration, controls, drug dose, method of delivery, assessments/tests to be collected, and method of analysis.

Another important factor that must be determined before starting the trial is how to assess for success and when to end the trial. The primary endpoint of a clinical trial is the main result that is measured, which varies from safety endpoints for a phase I trial to efficacy endpoints for a phase II or III trial. The primary efficacy endpoint(s) for RNTs may depend on patient population, and common endpoints include overall survival (OS), progress-free survival (PFS), and overall response rate (ORR). Surrogate endpoints, which are measurements related to the primary endpoint that may be easier to measure, can also be utilized to enhance study efficiency for some clinical trials. For instance, blood pressure can be used to predict cardiovascular related mortality as the two factors are strongly correlated [8]. However, these must be applied with care and validated.

Other aspects of a clinical trial that must be established prior to IND approval include manu-facturing details. When producing the RNT agent to use in human studies, it must be produced with good laboratory/manufacturing practice (GLP/GMP). Under these regulations, laboratory management must approve standard operating procedures (SOPs) for each process that could affect the quality of the product, and there must be documentation of the process for every batch of product. The drug must also be the same drug that was tested in the animal preclinical studies, and sterility regulations may require special equipment. These measures can be cost-intensive and time-intensive.

As the RNT agent moves into clinical trials in humans, additional regulations and checks are implemented to protect the human subjects of the research. Human research requires Institutional Review Board (IRB) approval to protect the rights of the subjects. IRB criteria involve minimizing risk to subjects, equitable selection of subjects, informed consent, and provisions to monitor subject safety and confidentiality. Data and Safety Monitoring Boards are usually created by the sponsor and principal investigator and are tasked with enforcing the criteria of IRB approvals and monitoring data and safety results from the study.

The pathway to initiating use of RNTs in the clinical setting in Europe follows either national regulations or EU-Clinical Trial regulations. There is ongoing effort by the EMA to harmonize existing regulations (both preclinical and clinical) into a single framework for submitting clinical trials for RNTs as Investigational Medical Products. The submission processes both via individual national systems and through the centralized EU system are similar. The required documentation has elements similar to the IND application, including components such as details of the study protocol (clinical document) and information on manufacturing specifications and preclinical safety studies (central document). In Canada, the clinical trial application process for new RNTs also follows similar requirements to those in the United States and the European Union [3].

8.4 PHASE I CLINICAL TRIALS

After approving the IND and IRB applications, the phase I clinical trial(s) may begin. The purpose of phase I is to evaluate safety and toxicity at different doses (or administered activities), as well as human pharmacokinetics and pharmacodynamics and early evidence of efficacy. The maximum tolerated dose (MTD) is often determined through dose escalation, where the dose is administered at increasing levels to determine the highest dose that does not cause serious adverse events. All the data from the phase I trial are used to determine the recommended dose for phase II trials (RP2D) to optimize potential efficacy versus toxicity. As such, phase I trials have many pre-determined components to accomplish these goals such as the starting dose, how to increment and escalate the dose, and criteria for dose-limiting toxicities (DLTs) and MTD [9]. Of note, for most RNT trials, the "dose" in these terms is the fixed administered activity.

Since DLTs are vital for determining MTD and RP2D, their definition is usually standardized through the Common Terminology Criteria for Adverse Events (CTCAE, currently version 5.0) [10]. Typical DLTs may include CTCAE grade 4+ hematological toxicities such as life-threatening neutropenia, anemia, leukopenia, and/or thrombocytopenia or grade 3+ non-hematologic toxicities. Many hematologic DLT criteria also include duration or sequelae such as grade 3 thrombocyto-penia with bleeding or grade 3 neutropenia with fever [11].

The method of incrementing and escalating the dose can vary with the design of the phase I trial. In the standard 3 + 3 phase I design, an initial three patient cohort is recruited and is allocated to the lowest dose level. If there are no DLTs, then another cohort is recruited with a higher dose level. If two or three patients develop DLTs, then the trial is stopped and the MTD is determined to be the previous dose. If only one patient has a toxic response, then another cohort is recruited at the same dose level to see if they also develop DLTs before considering further dose escalation. In this way, the MTD is traditionally defined according to the proportion of patients experiencing DLTs [12]. However, there are limitations in this form of study design, noted even by the FDA [13], which may prevent the accurate determination of MTD for early phase trials, so alternative methods can be used such as the Continual Reassessment Method, Bayesian Logistic Regression Method, or Modified Toxicity Probability Interval Design. For RNTs, there is additional concern regarding potential late radiation toxicities that would not be detectable during the acute DLT period. Given the ability to directly measure radiation absorbed dose through dosimetry techniques, many RNT phase I studies are currently designed to stop escalation of administered activity at a maximum absorbed dose to normal organs such as kidney or bone marrow. For example, the current FDA guidelines refer to the whole kidney absorbed dose limit of less than 23 Gy based on historic external beam X-ray tolerance data [14–16]. For this reason, phase I RNT trials are often stopped before clinical DLTs are reached, and the trial design may also incorporate alternative methods as noted above. The need for accepted normal organ toxicity avoidance dose limits for RNTs is widely recognized, and an international workshop on Radiopharmaceutical Therapy Normal Tissue Effects in the Clinic (RPT-TEC) was convened on this topic in September 2022 [17].

8.5 PHASE II CLINICAL TRIALS

If the RPT agent passes the predetermined checkpoints for phase I, it may move to phase II trials. These trials typically have accrual targets of several hundred patients, and the purpose of these trials is to determine drug effectiveness. In oncology, the primary endpoint depends on the patient population and may commonly be PFS, OS, or ORR. Radiographic PFS is often standardized using the Response Evaluation Criteria in Solid Tumors (RECIST), which is a set of rules that assess the response of tumors and categorize them into complete response, partial response, stable disease, or progressive disease. Biomarkers such as prostate-specific antigen for prostate cancer are also frequently incorporated into PFS endpoints (e.g. Prostate Cancer Working Group definitions). Initial or preliminary evidence of efficacy can be determined by comparing the RNT agent with previously published trials, comparing different dosing arms, or randomizing subjects to different treatment arms. Due to the small sample size for phase II trials, statistical power calculations are critical for study design.

Secondary endpoints may assess other characteristics of the RNT agent such as its mechanism, biochemical properties, adverse effects, minimum clinically effective dose, and optimal dose and dose frequencies. Key elements for informative phase II trials involve evidence that the molecule is present at the hypothesized site of action, that it binds to the therapeutic target, and that it triggers a pharmacodynamic downstream biological effect (radiation dose response). Again, imaging and dosimetry facilitate these investigations for RNT agents.

8.6   PHASE III CLINICAL TRIALS

Once the predetermined checkpoints are met for phase II trials, the RNT agent may move on to phase III trials with a larger sample size of the patient population of interest. These phase III trials, or "pivotal trials," can include up to thousands of patients with the condition to be studied and last around 2–4 years. The purpose of a phase III RNT trial is to compare the safety and efficacy of the new RNT agent (or combination therapy) to the current standard of care. The most common types of phase III trials are randomized controlled trials of comparative efficacy, which are designed to reduce potential errors associated with bias, confounding, or chance. If the RNT agent shows significant benefit over standard of care in phase III trials, then a New Drug Application may be submitted to the FDA. If FDA approval is granted, the drug may be marketed and may often become the new standard of care for its approved indication. For RNT agents, post-marketing studies (e.g. phase IV trials) are often required for surveillance for rare late effects such as late renal toxicity, myelodysplastic syndrome, or leukemia that may occur many years after therapy. Long-term safety studies of ^{177}Lu-DOTATATE are underway [18,19]. Additional phase II and III trials may investigate new disease indications, earlier line or earlier stage indications, combination therapies, biomarkers, and/or other research questions.

8.7   KEY PHASE III TRIALS

8.7.1   ALSYMPCA

ALSYMPCA or ALpharadin in SYMPtomatic Prostate Cancer is a phase III clinical trial that assessed the efficacy and safety of radium-223 dichloride in patients with metastatic castrate-resistant prostate cancer (mCRPC) and symptomatic skeletal metastases [20]. ^{223}RaCl$_2$ is an alpha emitter and calcium mimetic targeting hydroxyapatite in regions of high bone turnover due to metastasis. The study was a randomized, double-blind controlled trial that randomized 921 patients in a 2:1 ratio. Treatment consisted of six intravenous administrations of 50 kBq per kg body weight every 4 weeks of either the experimental RNT agent or placebo in addition to the best standard of care (BSOC). The primary endpoint was predetermined to be OS. At the final updated analysis, the experimental arm had a higher median OS of 14.9 months compared to the BSOC/placebo arm of 11.3 months. FDA approval of ^{223}RaCl$_2$ was granted in 2013 [20].

8.7.2   NETTER-1

NETTER-1 is a phase III clinical trial that evaluated ^{177}Lu-DOTATATE in patients with inoperable, progressive, somatostatin receptor (SSR)-positive midgut neuroendocrine tumors. ^{177}Lu-DOTATATE is a beta emitter that targets somatostatin-receptor positive tumors and is paired with ^{68}Ga-DOTAT-ATE for PET imaging. The NETTER-1 study was a randomized trial that randomized 229 patients in a 1:1 ratio. The experimental arm consisted of ^{177}Lu-DOTATATE at an activity of 7.4 GBq intra-venously every 8 weeks (plus best supportive care including 30 mg octreotide long-acting repeatable [LAR] intramuscularly), and the control arm was octreotide LAR alone at a dose of 60 mg every 4 weeks. The RNT agent was administered with concomitant amino acids to protect the kidneys, which were predicted to be potential dose-limiting organs. The primary endpoint was PFS defined using RECIST and assessed with CT/MRI scans. At the predetermined time for the primary endpoint, the estimated rate of PFS at month 20 was 65.2% in the ^{177}Lu-DOTATATE group compared to 10.8% in the control group [21]. FDA approval of ^{177}Lu-DOTATATE was granted in 2018.

8.7.3   VISION

VISION is a phase III study that evaluated [177]LuPSMA-617 in patients with mCRPC who received previous treatment with at least one androgen-receptor-pathway inhibitor and one or two taxane regimens. The study consisted of 831 patients randomized in a 2:1 ratio. Patients in the experimental group received treatment with 7.4 GBq ^{177}Lu-PSMA-617 intravenously every 6 weeks plus protocol-permitted standard care, and the control group received standard care alone. The alternate primary endpoints were OS and radiographic progression-free survival (rPFS). Median OS was 11.3 months for patients receiving standard care and 15.3 months with the addition of ^{177}Lu-PSMA-617. There was also prolongation of median rPFS from 3.4 months to 8.7 months [22] (Figure 8.2).

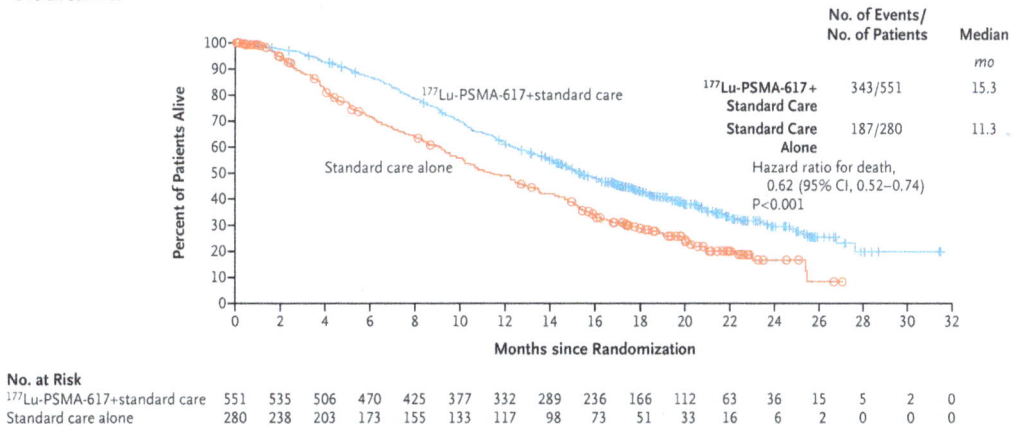

FIGURE 8.2   Overall survival among 831 patients in VISION phase III trial randomized to ^{177}Lu-PSMA-617 plus standard care versus standard care alone [22].

8.8   ADDITIONAL TRIALS

8.8.1   New Indications

For the RNT agents tested in the key phase III trials above, additional applications are currently being developed and tested. ^{177}Lu-DOTATATE is currently in trials for other SSR-positive diseases including a phase II trial for SSR-positive advanced bronchial neuroendocrine tumors and another for inoperable pheochromocytoma/paraganglioma [23,24]. ^{223}RaCl$_2$ has also been tested for other cancers with bone metastases such as hormone receptor-positive, bone-dominant metastatic breast cancer [25].

8.8.2 COMBINATION THERAPIES

The above FDA-approved RNTs have also been tested in combination with other therapies. ^{177}Lu-DOTATATE and the immunotherapy nivolumab have recently completed phase I/II trials for patients with small cell lung cancer or advanced NET of the lungs with overexpressed SSRs [26]. The combination of ^{223}RaCl$_2$ and the immunotherapy pembrolizumab is under investigation in an ongoing phase I/II trial for stage IV non-small cell lung cancer [27]. PARP inhibitors such as olaparib have been combined with ^{223}RaCl$_2$ in phase I/II trials for mCRPC and ^{177}Lu-DOTATATE in various SSR+ cancers [28–30].

8.8.3 EARLIER STAGE/LINE

Trials are also underway to test new RNTs and approved agents at earlier stages of cancer. For patients with oligometastatic hormone-sensitive prostate cancer, stereotactic body radiation therapy (SBRT) is being tested with or without ^{223}RaCl$_2$ in the multi-institutional RAVENS trial [31,32], and the LUNAR trial is testing SBRT with or without ^{177}Lu-PSMA-PNT2002 [33]. Another trial is testing ^{223}RaCl$_2$ alone for biochemically recurrent prostate cancer [34]. Multiple ongoing trials are investigating ^{177}Lu-PSMA-radioligand therapies in earlier line and earlier stage prostate cancer. ^{177}Lu-DOTATATE has also been in phase II trials as a neoadjuvant treatment before surgery for resectable pancreatic neuroendocrine tumors [35].

8.9 RNT IMAGING AND DOSIMETRY

Currently, the prescription for most RNTs is based on fixed activity (e.g. 7.4 GBq for ^{177}Lu-DOTATATE or ^{177}Lu-PSMA-617) or weight-based activity like for ^{223}RaCl$_2$. However, there is widely recognized potential for personalized treatment planning. Pharmacokinetics and pharmacodynamics vary between individuals, influenced by levels of target expression, body weight, tumor burden, and kidney function. These variables can be assessed via imaging and dosimetry with SPECT or planar imaging of the therapeutic agent or by SPECT, planar, or PET imaging using a paired agent such as ^{68}Ga-DOTATATE or sodium iodide-123. In the case of thyroid cancer, Na^{123}I therapy to allow for dose estimates to be calculated and prescription activity to be adjusted before treatment is administered [36]. Currently, PET imaging agents are used for patient selection for ^{177}Lu-DOTATATE and ^{177}Lu-PSMA-617 therapy, but there is much more potential for imaging in terms of response assessment, dosimetry, and personalized treatment planning. The results of the DOSISPHERE-01 trial (randomized, multicenter, open-label phase 2) suggest that personalized dosimetry may be crucial for efficacy [37]. In the study, patients ($n = 60$) were randomized to standard dosimetry (120±20 Gy) or personalized dosimetry (≥205 Gy to index lesion). A significantly greater proportion of patients in the personalized dosimetry arm showed an objective response with comparable toxicity rates.

Overall, this topic is of key importance to medical physicists and is discussed in more detail in other chapters of this book.

8.10 UNIQUE ASPECTS OF RNT CLINICAL TRIALS

8.10.1 RADIOACTIVE MATERIALS AND PRODUCTION

RAMs require a license and specialized facilities for production, distribution, storage, use, and disposal. Prior to conducting clinical research or standard of care treatment, a RAM license must be obtained or amended to include the specific radioisotope(s) and amount, and authorized users must be approved. Each cycle of RNT for each patient must be ordered days to weeks in advance in coordination with the medical physicist and radiation safety officer, and the treatment schedule cannot usually be altered at the last minute due to the decay and shelf life. Furthermore, access to certain radionuclides for research is currently affected by production limitations such as ^{211}At which has a short half-life of 7.2 hours and requires a medium-energy cyclotron [36].

8.10.2 FACILITIES AND RADIATION PRECAUTIONS

Facilities where treatment is given must often include a specialized treatment room shielded for radiation and a separate bathroom. Furthermore, measures must be taken for radiation safety precautions during and after administration. Additional documentation is required such as standard operating procedures, written directive, activity calibration and quality assurance documents, medical physics checklist, treatment summary, and patient discharge instructions. Different RNTs also have different radiation precautions and accompanying logistical requirements. ^{223}RaCl$_2$ is an almost pure alpha emitter and therefore has simpler safety precautions. Administration can usually be completed in 30 minutes in an outpatient treatment room with a preloaded syringe. In comparison, ^{177}Lu-DOTATATE and ^{177}Lu-PSMA-617 have more significant gamma emissions and more complex logistical arrangements. Treatment is typically done by infusion in a shielded or separate room with its own bathroom.

8.10.3 RESEARCH INFRASTRUCTURE

Research infrastructure for oncology is more complex when using RAMs. For instance, radioactive biosamples such as blood may not be permitted for research phlebotomy scheduling or core lab testing, and sample waste management or regulated shipping may be required. Research nurses must be trained in radiation safety and precautions. RNT trials also require review and approval from the radiation review committee as part of the IRB process.

8.11 CONCLUSION

Many promising RNTs are in development for a variety of oncologic targets and disease sites, and there are exciting clinical trial opportunities for patients and clinical care teams. We have described the basic process of clinical development from preclinical testing to phase I-III trials, including regulatory considerations and unique aspects of RNTs at each step. We also noted several important future directions for RNT clinical research, including the potential for expanded imaging and dosimetry applications and the need for updated normal organ toxicity avoidance dose limits.

8.12 DISCLOSURES

APK: Insitutional clinical trials funding from Bayer, Novartis, Lanthcus, and Merck. Unpaid advisory boards and steering committee for Novartis.

REFERENCES

1. Sgouros G, Bodei L, McDevitt MR, Nedrow JR (2020) Radiopharmaceutical therapy in cancer: clinical advances and challenges. *Nature Reviews Drug Discovery* 19:589–608. 10.1038/s41573-020-0073-9
2. Takebe T, Imai R, Ono S (2018) The current status of drug discovery and development as originated in United States academia: the influence of industrial and academic collaboration on drug discovery and development. *Clinical and Translational Science* 11:597–606. 10.1111/cts.12577

3. Schwarz SW, Decristoforo C, Goodbody AE, et al (2019) Harmonization of U.S., European Union, and Canadian first-in-human Regulatory requirements for radiopharmaceuticals: is this possible? *Journal of Nuclear Medicine* 60:158–166. 10.2967/jnumed.118.209460

4. Kurth J, Krause BJ, Schwarzenböck SM, et al (2018) External radiation exposure, excretion, and effective half-life in 177Lu-PSMA-targeted therapies. *EJNMMI Research* 8:32. 10.1186/s13550-018-0386-4

5. Ghaly M, Sgouros G, Frey E (2019) Quantitative dual isotope SPECT imaging of the alpha-emitters Th-227 and Ra-223. *Journal of Nuclear Medicine* 60:41–41

6. Vennart J (1991) The 1990 recommendations of the International Commission on Radiological Protection. *Journal of Radiological Protection* 11:199–203. 10.1088/0952-4746/11/3/006

7. Sunderland JJ, Ponto LB, Capala J (2021) Radiopharmaceutical delivery for theranostics: pharmacokinetics and pharmacodynamics. *Seminars in Radiation Oncology* 31:12–19. 10.1016/j.semradonc.2020.07.009

8. Lassere MN, Johnson KR, Schiff M, Rees D (2012) Is blood pressure reduction a valid surrogate endpoint for stroke prevention? an analysis incorporating a systematic review of randomised controlled trials, a by-trial weighted errors-in-variables regression, the surrogate threshold effect (STE) and the biomarker-surrogacy (BioSurrogate) evaluation schema (BSES). *BMC Medical Research Methodology* 12:27. 10.1186/1471-2288-12-27

9. Le Tourneau C, Lee JJ, Siu LL (2009) Dose escalation methods in Phase I cancer clinical trials. *JNCI: Journal of the National Cancer Institute* 101:708–720. 10.1093/jnci/djp079

10. U.S. Department of Health and Human Services (2017) Common Terminology Criteria for Adverse Events (CTCAE).

11. Paoletti X, Le Tourneau C, Verweij J, et al (2014) Defining dose-limiting toxicity for phase 1 trials of molecularly targeted agents: results of a DLT-TARGETT international survey. *European Journal of Cancer* 50:2050–2056. 10.1016/j.ejca.2014.04.030

12. Chevret S (2014) Maximum tolerable dose (MTD). In: *Wiley StatsRef: Statistics Reference Online*. John Wiley & Sons, Ltd.

13. U.S. Department of Health and Human Services Food and Drug Administration Guidance for Industry, Clinical Considerations for Therapeutic Cancer Vaccines.

14. Emami B, Lyman J, Brown A, et al (1991) Tolerance of normal tissue to therapeutic irradiation. *International Journal of Radiation Oncology*Biology*Physics* 21:109–122. 10.1016/0360-3016(91)90171-Y

15. U.S. Department of Health and Human Services Food and Drug Administration Center for Drug Evaluation and Research (CDER) (2011) Nonclinical Evaluation of Late Radiation Toxicity of Therapeutic Radiopharmaceuticals. *Pharmacology and Toxicology*.

16. U.S. Department of Health and Human Services Food and Drug Administration Center for Drug Evaluation and Research (CDER), Oncology Therapeutic Radiopharmaceuticals: Nonclinical Studies and Labeling Recommendations Guidance for Industry.

17. Corfu Summer School and Workshops on Elementary Particle Physics and Gravity. In: Google My Maps. https://www.google.com/maps/d/viewer?mid=137MVM1GxutbVloFmTi0WMtlk9la_LY02. Accessed 22 Feb 2023

18. Brabander T, van der Zwan WA, Teunissen JJM, et al (2017) Long-term efficacy, survival, and safety of [177Lu-DOTA0,Tyr3]octreotate in patients with gastroenteropancreatic and bronchial neuroendocrine tumors. *Clinical Cancer Research* 23:4617–4624. 10.1158/1078-0432.CCR-16-2743

19. Sitani K, Parghane RV, Talole S, Basu S (2021) Long-term outcome of indigenous 177Lu-DOTA-TATE PRRT in patients with metastatic advanced neuroendocrine tumours: a single institutional observation in a large tertiary care setting. *The British Journal of Radiology* 94:20201041. 10.1259/bjr.20201041

20. Bayer (2016) A Double-blind, Randomised, Multiple Dose, Phase III, Multicentre Study of Alpharadin in the Treatment of Patients with Symptomatic Hormone Refractory Prostate Cancer with Skeletal Metastases. *clinicaltrials.gov*

21. Advanced Accelerator Applications (2022) A Multicentre, Stratified, Open, Randomized, Comparator-controlled, Parallel-group Phase III Study Comparing Treatment with 177Lu-DOTA0-Tyr3-Octreotate to Octreotide LAR in Patients with Inoperable, Progressive, Somatostatin Receptor Positive Midgut Carcinoid Tumours. *clinicaltrials.gov*

22. Sartor O, de Bono J, Chi KN, et al (2021) Lutetium-177–PSMA-617 for metastatic castration-resistant prostate cancer. *New England Journal of Medicine* 385:1091–1103. 10.1056/NEJMoa2107322

23. National Cancer Institute (NCI) (2023) Randomized Phase II Trial of Lutetium Lu 177 Dotatate Versus Everolimus in Somatostatin Receptor Positive Bronchial Neuroendocrine Tumors. *clinicaltrials.gov*
24. National Cancer Institute (NCI) (2023) Lu-177-DOTATATE (Lutathera) in Therapy of Inoperable Pheochromocytoma/Paraganglioma. *clinicaltrials.gov*
25. M.D. Anderson Cancer Center (2021) Phase II Trial of Ra-223 Dichloride in Combination with Hormonal Therapy and Denosumab in the Treatment of Patients with Hormone-Positive Bone-Dominant Metastatic Breast Cancer. *clinicaltrials.gov*
26. (2016) Nivolumab and Lutetium Lu 177-DOTA-TATE in Treating Patients with Relapsed or Refractory Extensive-Stage Small Cell Lung Cancer or Grade I-II Lung Neuroendocrine Tumors That Are Advanced or Cannot Be Removed by Surgery – NCI. https://www.cancer.gov/about-cancer/treatment/clinical-trials/search/v?id=NCI-2017-02485. Accessed 22 Feb 2023
27. Reck M, Mileham KF, Clump DA, et al (2020) 1420TiP A phase I/II trial of radium-223 (Ra-223) in combination with pembrolizumab in patients (pts) with stage IV non-small cell lung cancer (NSCLC). *Annals of Oncology* 31:S897–S898. 10.1016/j.annonc.2020.08.1734
28. National Cancer Institute (NCI) (2022) A Phase 1/2 Study of Combination Olaparib and Radium-223 in Men with Metastatic Castration-Resistant Prostate Cancer with Bone Metastases (COMRADE). *clinicaltrials.gov*
29. National Cancer Institute (NCI) (2023) Phase I/II Study of Lu-177-DOTATATE (Lutathera) in Combination with Olaparib in Inoperable Gastroenteropancreatico Neuroendocrine Tumors (GEP-NET). *clinicaltrials.gov*
30. Peter MacCallum Cancer Centre, Australia (2022) 177Lu-PSMA-617 Therapy and Olaparib in Patients with Metastatic Castration Resistant Prostate Cancer. *clinicaltrials.gov*
31. Sidney Kimmel Comprehensive Cancer Center at Johns Hopkins (2022) A Phase II Randomized Trial of RAdium-223 and SABR Versus SABR for oligoMEtastatic Prostate caNcerS (RAVENS). *clinicaltrials.gov*
32. Hasan H, Deek MP, Phillips R, et al (2020) A phase II randomized trial of RAdium-223 dichloride and SABR versus SABR for oligoMEtastatic prostate caNcerS (RAVENS). *BMC Cancer* 20:492. 10.1186/s12885-020-07000-2
33. Jonsson Comprehensive Cancer Center (2022) 177-Lutetium-PSMA Neoadjuvant to Ablative Radiotherapy for Oligorecurrent Prostate Cancer (Lunar). *clinicaltrials.gov*
34. National Cancer Institute (NCI) (2023) Phase II Trial of Radium-223 in Biochemically Recurrent Prostate Cancer. *clinicaltrials.gov*
35. Falconi M (2022) A Prospective Phase II Single-Arm Trial on Neoadjuvant Peptide Receptor Radionuclide Therapy with 177Lu-DOTATATE Followed by Surgery for Resectable Pancreatic Neuroendocrine Tumors. *clinicaltrials.gov*
36. Kunos CA, Mankoff DA, Schultz MK, et al (2021) Radiopharmaceutical chemistry and drug development—what's changed? *Seminars in Radiation Oncology* 31:3–11. 10.1016/j.semradonc.2020.07.006
37. Garin E, Tselikas L, Guiu B, et al (2021) Personalised versus standard dosimetry approach of selective internal radiation therapy in patients with locally advanced hepatocellular carcinoma (DOSISPHERE-01): a randomised, multicentre, open-label phase 2 trial. *The Lancet Gastroenterology & Hepatology* 6:17–29. 10.1016/S2468-1253(20)30290-9

9 Epidemiologic Studies of Cancer Risk among Patients Administered Radionuclides

John D. Boice Jr. and Lawrence T. Dauer

9.1 INTRODUCTION

Since the 1930s, patients have been administered radioactive nuclides to diagnose or treat malignant and nonmalignant diseases [1–4]. This chapter covers epidemiologic studies of patients administered radionuclides. Radioactive iodine-131 is used to diagnose thyroid disorders and treat both hyperthyroidism and thyroid cancer. Large epidemiologic studies have found no evidence that leukemia is a late effect following iodine-131 therapy for hyperthyroidism, and the evidence that thyroid cancer, breast cancer and total cancers are increased is controversial [5–18]. Leukemia, however, is reported to be increased among patients administered high doses of iodine-131 to treat thyroid cancer [19–21]. Radioactive phosphorus-32 was used to treat polycythemia vera (PV) and excesses of leukemia reported [22–25]. Thorium dioxide, a component of the colloid Thorotrast, was used for cerebral angiography and convincing evidence was found for excesses of leukemia, liver cancer, and mesothelioma, but not bone cancer [26–30]. Radium-224 was used to treat ankylosing spondylitis, and studies in Germany found clear evidence of excesses of bone cancer but inconsistent evidence for leukemia [31–36]. Radium-226 needles and applicators were used to treat skin hemangiomas in Sweden and France and excesses of thyroid cancer and breast cancer, but not leukemia, were reported from this external (not internal) source of radiation [37–40]. New radiopharmaceuticals are part of a developing and exciting area in nuclear medicine where radiotherapy at the cellular level can occur, sparing other tissues and reducing healthy tissue complications [41–43]. Radium-223 dichloride is used to treat metastatic prostate cancer. Lutetium-177 DOTATATE is used to treat neuroendocrine tumors. Samarium-153 lexidronam is used to relieve bone pain due to cancer. Gallium-67 citrate is used to diagnose lymphomas. Technetium-99m continues to be used to image the skeleton and heart muscle and other organs and is the most widely used diagnostic radioisotope in nuclear medicine. Because, with the exception of radiogenic leukemia, the time between exposure and cancer development is generally many decades on average, it is important to be mindful of the potential late effects of the new radiopharmaceuticals in light of their widespread use [44]. Long-term consequence research can influence the choice of effective and less toxic therapies as was seen for phosphorus-32 and chlorambucil in PV [45].

9.2 EPIDEMIOLOGIC STUDIES

Epidemiologic studies conducted over the past 60 years have shown that radionuclides used to diagnose and treat malignant and nonmalignant diseases can result in adverse health effects, and cancer in particular. Epidemiologic studies will be discussed that provide evidence for or against increased cancer risk following radionuclide administrations (Table 9.1). Radionuclides discussed include phosphorus-32, iodine-131, Thorotrast (thorium dioxide), and radium-224. Radium-226, as a source of external radiation, will be covered in the context of low dose and low dose rate effects.

DOI: 10.1201/9781003250913-11

TABLE 9.1

Epidemiologic Studies of Patient Populations Administered Radionuclides

Radionuclide	Patient Population	Main Finding	Main Reference
Phosphorus-32	Polycythemia vera	Leukemia excess	[22–25]
Iodine-131 diagnosis	Swedish scintillation examinations for thyroid conditions	Adults, no excess of thyroid cancer; confounding by indication a concern; no excess of leukemia	[7,46–48]
Iodine-131 therapy	Hyperthyroidism	No evidence for an excess of leukemia. Inconsistent evidence for an excess of thyroid cancer. Small overall cancer risk possible. Confounding by indication a concern. Current controversy on late effects.	[5,7–9,11,13,14,49–53]
	Thyroid cancer	Leukemia excess	[19–21]
Thorium (Thorotrast)	Cerebral angiography	Leukemia excess, liver cancer excess, mesothelioma excess, no excess of bone cancer	[26–30,34,54]
Radium-224	Ankylosing spondylitis	Bone cancer excess; inconsistent evidence whether leukemia in excess	[31–36,55]
Radium-226 (external)	Skin hemangioma	Excess of thyroid cancer; excess of breast cancer	[37–40]

9.2.1 PHOSPHORUS-32

PV is a blood disease characterized by the overproduction of red cells. In the past, PV was treated with phosphorus-32, X-rays, and cytotoxic drugs. In a study of 1,222 patients with PV, 11% of 228 patients treated with phosphorus-32 developed leukemia in contrast to 1% of 133 patients who received no radiation therapy [22,23]. Conceivably, the bone marrow of patients with PV may be unusually sensitive to radiation or perhaps biological factors determining treatment, e.g., spleen size, rather than the treatment itself could be associated with leukemia. A randomized clinical trial, however, found that 9 of 156 (6%) patients treated with phosphorus-32 developed leukemia compared with 1 of 134 (1%) treated by phlebotomy [56]. Subsequent studies confirmed the association between phosphorus-32 and leukemia and reported an enhancement of risk with chemotherapy maintenance [24,25,57]. Because of the studies confirming the leukemia risk of phosphorus-32, coupled with the availability of effective and less toxic forms of treatment, phosphorus-32 is rarely used today [45].

9.2.2 DIAGNOSTIC USE OF IODINE-131

A comprehensive epidemiologic study of over 35,000 Swedish patients given diagnostic doses of ^{131}I for existing or suspected thyroid conditions found no evidence for an increased risk of radiation-related thyroid cancer [46]. Medical records were abstracted to obtain information on thyroid size, administered amounts of radioactive iodine, and perhaps most important, the reason why the scintillation scan was requested by the referring physician. Given the high dose to the thyroid (mean 0.94 Gy), a substantial excess of thyroid cancer was anticipated. Explanations for the absence of a radiation risk included the possibility that [131]I (half-life = 8 days) might be less effective than external X-rays in causing thyroid cancer because of the protracted nature of the exposure, or that the markedly heterogeneous dose distribution from internal beta emitters played a role [10]. Subsequently, however, it was learned that the adult thyroid gland is much less radiosensitive than the childhood gland [10,58], and the few number of children and adolescents in the Swedish study was not sufficient to detect a risk had there been one. Up until the studies following the Chernobyl reactor accident in 1986, there was little convincing evidence that radioactive iodine caused thyroid cancer. The Chernobyl environmental exposure studies of children who ingested contaminated milk now provide clear evidence that following childhood, but not adult, exposure to radioactive iodine, the risk of thyroid cancer development is increased following a mean dose on the order of 1 Gy [47,59]. It is now generally accepted that chromosomal abnormalities induced by high doses of radioactive iodine can cause thyroid cancer [60,61].

The Swedish imaging study of diagnostic ^{131}I to identify any thyroid abnormalities indicated the importance of knowing the reasons behind the requested medical examinations. It was clear that patients examined *because of a suspicion of a thyroid tumor* were at subsequent risk of developing thyroid cancer independent of any ^{131}I exposure, whereas patients examined for other reasons such as hyperthyroidism were at no radiation risk [47,62,63]. In other words, if the *suspicion of thyroid cancer* had not been known as the reason for the examination and considered in the analysis, spurious associations between thyroid cancer and ^{131}I would have occurred. Confounding by indication can occur when clinical or biological factors, e.g., nodules or hyperthyroidism [48], determine the "exposure", i.e., in this case the ^{131}I scintillation scan. The underlying conditions that prompted a referral to evaluate a "suspicion of tumor" caused both the exposure (^{131}I) and the outcome (thyroid cancer). Confounding by indication remains a plausible explanation for the increase in brain cancer, leukemia, and other cancers reported in computed tomography (CT) studies of children where the clinical reasons behind the referring physician request for examination were not generally known. The immediate increase in brain cancer and leukemia seen following CT exams was much too soon to be related to radiation and strongly suggested the likelihood of confounding by indication [62–64]. In observational studies, unfortunately there are no adjustment methods that can fully resolve confounding by indication [65], so care always must be taken in interpreting associations when such confounding is plausible, e.g., in imaging studies.

9.2.3 Therapeutic Uses of Iodine-131

Patients with hyperthyroidism and thyroid cancer have been treated for over 60 years with high doses of radioactive [131]I. Early studies of over 35,000 patients with thyrotoxicosis in the Cooperative Thyrotoxicosis Therapy Follow-up Study (TTFUS) revealed no evidence that leukemia was increased following ^{131}I therapy [5,8,49]. The dose to bone marrow was estimated to average between 80 and 160 mGy delivered at a low dose rate. Subsequent follow-up of TTFUS patients treated with ^{131}I also failed to observe an increased risk of leukemia [11], consistent with other studies conducted in different countries [7,9,50,51] and with recent meta-analyses [66,67]. Higher doses of radioactive iodine to treat thyroid cancer, however, have been associated with excess occurrences of leukemia in patient populations [19–21] and in meta-analyses [68].

The 1989 comprehensive follow-up of the TTFUS failed to link radioactive iodine to total cancer deaths or to any specific cancer with the exception of thyroid cancer [8]. The authors were cautious in concluding whether the link between thyroid cancer and ^{131}I was causal, because the high excess risk seen within 5 years of therapy was too short a radiation latency period; there was no evidence of a dose response based on administered activities after excluding early deaths within 5 years of treatment; the inconsistency with other radiation studies finding no evidence of a radiogenic thyroid cancer effect among exposed adults; the likelihood that such doses of the order of 100 Gy to the thyroid would predominantly kill cells and not transform them; the underlying disease itself, hyperthyroidism, might have been responsible for some of the thyroid cancer excess; and, more likely, that some thyroid cancers may have been present before ^{131}I therapy (see also [10]). The recent 2019 follow-up of TTFUS patients [11,13] evaluated a subset of 18,805 of the 20,949 patients treated with ^{131}I, also found thyroid cancer to be increased at doses of the order of 100 Gy but there was no evidence of a dose response. Stomach cancer and breast cancer mortality was associated with ^{131}I therapy organ doses in the 2019 TTFUS report [11,13], but such increases were not seen in the earlier mortality report [8] nor in most other mortality and incidence studies [6,7,9,50–52]. The Swedish study is of interest because both cancer incidence and mortality were evaluated and the number of patients was large (n = 10,554) [6,7,52]. Thyroid cancer incidence was not linked to ^{131}I therapy, nor was breast cancer or leukemia. Thyroid cancer mortality was significantly increased overall, but not once the first year of follow-up was excluded. Stomach cancer, but not breast cancer, incidence and mortality were associated with ^{131}I therapy in Sweden. The Finnish study is also of interest because they were able to address patient risk factors and concluded "Based on this large-scale, long-term follow-up study, the increased cancer risk in hyperthyroid patients is attributable to hyperthyroidism and shared risk factors, not the treatment modality" [50]. A recent Israeli study also failed to find increases in any cancer, except non-Hodgkin lymphoma, and is unique in being able to account for possible confounders, i.e., both demographic and clinical parameters, including age, sex, smoking history, body mass index, health care residential district, socioeconomic status, history of diabetes mellitus, history of hypertension, and pharmacy administration of at least three prescriptions of aspirin and of statins at the year before cohort entry date [51].

9.2.3.1   The 2019 Thyrotoxicosis Therapy Follow-Up Study

The recent publications from the TTFUS [11,13] generated an enormous number of comments in scientific journals and the press [14] that focused on the rationale and purpose behind the study, and its conduct, interpretation, and patient treatment implication. This tsunami of comments occurred in the original journal [12,69,70], and in other clinical and nuclear medicine journals [14–18,71–76]. An informative statement was prepared by the Executive Committees of the Society for Endocrinology and the British Thyroid Association, covering most of the issues that have raised considerable concern [17]. The many comments questioned the validity of the study analyses, dosimetry and interpretation, including somewhat surprisingly, a separate publication by two of the coauthors [14] of the initial publication [11] – who also were not coauthors on the two subsequent TTFUS publications in 2019 [12,13]. One of the authors for this chapter (JDB) followed the many exchanges with interest; he was the senior author of the Ron et al. 1998 TTFUS article [8] and had directed the reactivation of the TTFUS [5,77] but was not involved with the new follow-up. The new follow-up, dosimetry, analyses, and publications are a *tour de force* and included an additional 24 years of follow-up mortality data [11], a novel approach to organ-dose dosimetry [78], and attempts to address the many potential limitations that might lead to spurious results and interpretations [12,13].

The criticisms, however, were legion including:

- limitations of mortality studies (compared with incidence) and the likelihood that cancers (especially of the thyroid but others) were present at the time of treatment and may not all have been identified fully from the medical record abstracts of the 26 clinics participating in the study;
- the selection of patients for therapy (e.g., whether nodules were present or not; Graves' disease versus toxic goiter; age and antithyroid medications) for whom different cancer predispositions exist (perhaps the most extensive and informative discussion of these clinical issues can be found in Dobyns et al. [77]);
- similarly, *confounding by indication* might be an issue in light of known selection of patients for different treatments based on clinical and demographic characteristics as well as the known associations between hyperthyroidism and shared risk factors with increased cancer risk [17,50,51,76];
- important unknown confounding factors such as smoking, obesity, diabetes, and reproductive history which could influence outcomes;

- the early increases of some cancer deaths after therapies (short latencies for radiogenic cancers are unlikely) and the excess mortality early on may also suggest non-treatment factors responsible for the excess later on;
- the uncertainties in estimated organ doses from radioiodine administrations and the models applied. The authors summarized these issues: "There are multiple sources of uncertainty associated with the dose estimates. The uncertainties related to model structure, parametric least squares fitting, extrapolation of estimated doses and anthropometric-based calculation of the S values are expected to be the most important" [78]. Further, the dosimetry apparently was based on 197 patients and was used to estimate organ doses for 18,805 of the 20,949 patients treated with radioiodine, considering "sex, age, thyroid uptake, anti-thyroid drug treatment, type of disease, severity of the disease, pulse rate, cardiac rhythm, basal metabolic rate, protein bound iodide (PBI) and ophthalmopathy". That so few patients were used to estimate organ doses for so many, *without validation*, was an issue raised by critics [14,16,17,72,73];
- the use of stomach dose as a surrogate for whole-body dose for *all cancer* analyses is questioned [14,15], in part because the specific organ doses were so heterogeneous, e.g., from 18 mGy (mean) for rectum to 1600 mGy (mean) for esophagus and that applying a stomach dose (170 mGy, mean) to represent all organs having known different doses and different etiologies is of questionable validity (a broader question is whether combining cancers with low to no radiosensitivity with cancers of high radiosensitivity has biological or statistical meaning); interestingly, the site with the largest number of deaths, the lung ($n = 437$) had one of the highest organ doses (310 mGy, mean);
- previous treatments with ^{131}I or other therapies were unknown in some patients and thus not accounted for [77];
- an unusual distribution of excess cancer risks associated with radioiodine, e.g., stomach, breast, and all cancers, but not for equally radiosensitive organs with comparable dose estimates such as bone marrow (leukemia) and esophagus;
- an overinterpretation of the statistical results;
- the absence of a comparison population of hyperthyroid patients not treated with radio-iodine such as those treated with thionamides or surgery [14,16,17,76];
- and that because of the rather large number of statistical comparisons made, chance (as mentioned by the authors) remains a possible explanation ("some results may be because of chance; therefore, the results should be interpreted with caution" [11]).

For the interested reader, these and other issues are covered in several publications [14–18,69–76]. The authors to their credit attempted to address many of the concerns but the rather large number made it impossible to address them all and some, frankly, could not be addressed because the information was not available, e.g., on confounding factors such as smoking [11–13]. We provide just a few thoughts on the possible causal nature of the radioactive iodine associations reported in the recent 2019 TTFUS.

(1) The TTFUS is a mortality study and not a cancer incidence study. It is unlikely that all cancers existing before the ^{131}I and other therapies for hyperthyroidism were identified and excluded, particularly given the early years of treatment, 1946–1964, and the 26 medical clinics involved. A Swedish study of 10,554 patients [6,52] and a Finnish study of 4,334 patients evaluated both mortality and incidence [50]. The mortality findings in both studies indicated a risk of thyroid cancer, whereas the cancer incidence findings did not. The authors of the earlier TTFUS studies suggested that pre-existing thyroid cancers were the likely reason why thyroid cancer deaths were increased within 5 years of treatment among these adult patients given therapeutic doses of [131]I [8,77]. Conceivably, other cancer deaths in excess shortly after treatment might be partially the

result of existing cancers that were unknown at the time of treatment and could not be excluded in analyses. Further, cancer deaths later on, and not just early on, might also be related to unidentified cancers present at the time of treatment. Mortality studies are of great value, but limitations include the weakness in studying rare cancers, the possibility that some cancers were present at the time of exposure and that subsequent deaths occurred unrelated to treatment, the likelihood that important co-factors are unknown, at least in years past, and might confound results, and the difference in the quality of diagnoses compared with cancer incidence studies.

(2) The hallmark for radiation effects is leukemia. Radiogenic leukemia occurs early and at a high rate following exposure. It is somewhat remarkable that no study of patients treated with ^{131}I for hyperthyroidism indicates an excess of leukemia, including studies conducted in the United States [5,8,11,13,49], Sweden [7,52], the United Kingdom [9], Finland [50], and Israel [51]. Meta-analyses of patients treated for hyperthyroidism also reveal no leukemia excess [66,67]. A meta-analyses of patients treated for thyroid cancer at higher administrations of radioiodine indicated a leukemia excess but, interestingly, not of breast cancer, stomach cancer, or all cancers [68]. It might be noted that meta-analyses that include the 2019 TTFUS [11,13], such as those by Shim et al. [66] and Yan et al. [67], are not independent with the 2019 TTFUS study since it is included in the meta-analysis. Be that as it may, it is interesting that Shim et al. [66] reported a significant risk of breast cancer and total cancer related to radioiodine, whereas Yan et al. [67] did not; these differences add caution to interpreting meta-analyses and different criteria used for including studies. The new and novel estimated dose to the bone marrow in the TTFUS were sufficiently high (mean 160 mGy, SD 160 mGy) so that the absence of a leukemogenic effect is noteworthy, and perhaps argues against a causal interpretation for the reported excess of breast cancer, a site of lower radiosensitivity especially among older women, but with similar estimated dose (mean 150 mGy, SD 160 mGy).

There is an apparent inconsistency between the new and novel dosimetry [78] and the Ron et al. dosimetry [8,79]. Ron et al. [8] reported a mean dose to the red bone marrow of 42 mGy, or a factor of 4 times lower than reconstructed in the new follow-up (160 mGy). Further, Ron et al. [8] estimates were apparently confirmed by a reconstruction based on 468 original patients [79], which apparently included 271 more patients than the 197 evaluated for the new biokinetic dosimetry [78]. Interestingly, two authors were the same in both of these dosimetry reconstructions. It might be informative to learn why the differences were so great.

(3) The absorbed dose to breast tissue was estimated to be moderately high (mean 150 mGy, SD 160 mGy), and a breast cancer dose response reported. As above, there is an apparent inconsistency between the novel dosimetry [78] and the Ron et al. 1989 dosimetry for breast dose [8]. Ron et al. [8] reported a mean dose to breast of 32 mGy, or a factor of 5 lower than based on the new biokinetic model. Regardless, an association between radiation and breast cancer has been frequently reported [80,81]. However, what seems to be missed, or at least not mentioned, is that the association between radiation and breast cancer is strongest among young women exposed under the ages of 40–45 years and there is little evidence for exposures among older women. About 25% of all 18,805 TTFUS patients (n = 4,788), both men and women, were under age 40 years when treated with radioiodine; 78.0% were women; 38.2% were treated only with ^{131}I; 61.8% were treated with ^{131}I and with antithyroid drugs, surgery, or both; and 93.7% were treated for Graves' disease [11,77]. It would be informative to learn the age-specific risks for females. Young patients with hyperthyroidism are less likely to receive ^{131}I treatments than older patients because of the concern over possible radiation risks, and thyroidectomy was more common among the young [77]. Large-scale comprehensive studies of women with breast

cancer treated with radiation find no evidence for an increased risk of radiation-induced contralateral breast cancer among women over the age of 45 years at mean doses between 500 mGy and 2,000 mGy, although there was clear evidence for a risk among women under the age of 45 [82,83]. Based on the TTFUS authors linear model [11], the relative risk (RR) at 1 Gy might be estimated as 13 and very much higher than seen in other studies, especially when age at exposure is considered [34,81]. The increased excess of breast cancer 1 to <5 years after treatment [8] is unlikely to be related to radiation but to unknown hormonal, pregnancy-related, or other factors [50,51,84–86]. Thus, the excess of breast cancer attributed to radioiodine appears inconsistent with the scientific literature and may be a chance or a confounded observation.

Over the years, radioactive iodine at dose levels used to treat hyperthyroidism was assumed to be related, at most, to a small increased cancer risk. The new follow-up study is controversial in concluding that the risk, while small, is demonstrated, but many disagree [17]. Nonetheless, these exchanges point to the importance of constant vigilance and evaluation of therapies used in nuclear medicine and to the open exchange of ideas! These exchanges raised many important issues related to observational studies of patient populations administered radionuclides, and not just of thyroid conditions. If there is a cancer risk associated with ^{131}I therapy for hyperthyroidism, it appears low as reported in practically all studies conducted around the world, including recent evaluations of cancer incidence with information on patient characteristics, prior medical conditions, lifestyle factors, and potential confounding factors [16,50,51]. Recently, Kim [18] provided a thoughtful overview of the issues surrounding the TTFUS publications, and made several suggestions on ways forward, including the initiation of new epidemiologic studies [18]. One possibility might be to conduct a large-scale cooperative incidence study in countries with high-quality cancer registries and hospital discharge registries [87] such as in Sweden [88], Finland [50], Norway [89], Denmark [84,90], and other countries [53] where details on radioiodine administrations, co-factor information, and long follow-up are possible. Another possibility is to consider including studies in the United States using the Medicare beneficiary claims folder information which could provide information on cancer occurrence and time-dependent co-factor information following chronic conditions such as hyperthyroidism [91–93].

9.2.4 THOROTRAST

Thorotrast is a colloidal solution of thorium dioxide and was used between 1928 and 1955 as a contrast media for cerebral angiography [3,94,95]. Thorium is a heavy metal and was an excellent contrast agent, but it also is radioactive and emits alpha particles. Thorotrast remained in the body for life and continued to expose tissues to alpha-particle radiation at a low dose rate. A typical injection would be 25 ml, and would result in cumulative doses of about 250 mGy to the liver and 160 mGy to the bone marrow. Epidemiologic studies in Denmark, Germany, Portugal, Sweden, and the United States revealed substantial increases in liver cancer and acute myeloid leukemia [26–30,34,54]. Mesothelioma was also increased. The evidence for a radiation bone cancer risk was weak.

Thorium, like radium and plutonium, has an affinity to deposit in bone and is termed a *bone-seeker*. However, Thorotrast due to its colloidal nature, did not deposit in bone but rather was engulfed by macrophages and taken into the bone marrow directly irradiating stem cells. Accordingly, Thorotrast was found to carry a high risk of leukemia and low to no risk of bone cancer. In contrast, radium and plutonium at sufficient doses are linked to high risks of bone cancer but low to no risk of leukemia [34,96]. This comparison shows the importance of the chemical nature of the radionuclides administered which determines the subsequent dose to specific body organs and tissue, and the potential for late health effects.

Very high rates of brain cancer followed Thorotrast injections. However, the interpretation for a radiation association was noncausal because of confounding by indication. In studies where "the suspicion of brain tumor" was known as the reason why the Thorotrast examination was requested, brain cancer death was elevated. However, in studies where the indication was not for brain tumor, e.g., seizures after automobile accidents, and in studies that used a nonradioactive contrast agent instead of Thorotrast, e.g., Diodrast, there was no evidence for increased risks of brain cancer. Confounding by indication is related to the time sequence between exposure and outcome. That the exposure must come before the outcome is an absolute requirement for a causal inference [97]. In the subgroups of Thorotrast patients under suspicion of brain tumor, nascent or overt, the tumors preceded the administration of Thorotrast for cerebral angiography, i.e., the exposure occurred after the indications for brain cancer. This example of confounding by indication, i.e., by factors that led to the exposure [98] in imaging studies, similar to the ^{131}I scintillation studies, adds additional caution to interpreting associations between pediatric CT imaging examinations and brain tumor increase when an increase in brain tumor was detected immediately after the CT examination and there was no to limited information on why the examination was requested [48, 62–64].

9.2.5 RADIUM THERAPY

9.2.5.1 Radium-224 Therapy for Benign Disease

Radium-224 was used to manage bone tuberculosis and ankylosing spondylitis in Germany. Among 899 patients repeatedly injected with ^{224}Ra (half-life = 3.62 days), 56 malignant bone tumors developed versus <1 expected [3,31–33]. The risk of radiogenic bone cancer peaked at 6–8 years and decreased to normal levels after about 33 years. The estimated alpha-particle dose to the bone surface was very high, 30.6 Gy, and children had a higher risk than adults. The average dose to the bone volume (mean skeletal dose) was estimated to be 4.2 Gy and the risk per unit dose to bone volume was about 10 times greater than seen in occupational studies of ^{226}Ra and ^{228}Ra [3,32], reflecting the different dose distributions in bone surface compared with bone volume. The half-life for ^{224}Ra is short (3.62 days) and most of the energy is released on the bone surface where the relevant cells for osteosarcoma induction, the endosteal cells, are located. ^{226}Ra is a bone volume-seeker with a long half-life (1,600 years) and distributes its energy more uniformly throughout the bone including dose distributed to the matrix which is of little consequence to risk. In another series of German patients given ^{224}Ra to treat spondylitis, but at smaller doses (avg 560 mGy), no osteosarcomas occurred but an increase of leukemia was suggested [35,55]. It was unclear, however, what role phenylbutazone, taken to relieve pain and linked to leukemia, might have played. Further, leukemia also developed in 1,462 patients with spondylitis not treated with ^{224}Ra. Lower doses of injections of ^{224}Ra, not surprisingly, were associated with a lower risk of cancer and any excesses were not readily detectable [36]. The nonuniform distribution of dose from ^{224}Ra, the influence of the bone diseases being treated, perhaps enhancing the susceptibility of irradiated cells, and the possible effect of other medications raise caution in interpreting the precise nature of the risk of radiogenic bone cancer.

9.2.5.2 Radium-226 Therapy for Skin Hemangiomas

In Sweden, France, and several other countries in the 1920s–1950s, tens of thousands of infants with skin hemangioma (mainly strawberry hemangiomas) were treated with ^{226}Ra [10,37–40,99,100]. While the ^{226}Ra needles, tubes, and applicators provided external photon treatments for skin hemangiomas and thus not comparable to the administration of radionuclides used in "nuclear medicine", the contrast with studies discussed above is notable. In bygone eras, radiation was considered a cure-all for any ailment and skin hemangioma was not an exception, although it is a benign condition that often resolves without treatment. The average dose to the thyroid was 1 Gy and significant increases of thyroid cancer were observed [37,39]. In contrast to studies of radiotherapy for tinea capitis or thymic enlargement during infancy, the thyroid cancer risk from protracted exposure from [226]Ra applicators were about 2–6 times lower [10,34,58] and hinted that low doses at a low rate of delivery may be less carcinogenic than high dose-rate exposures. For infants with hemangiomas on the chest region, an increased risk of breast cancer was reported that was related to estimated breast doses on the order of several Gy [40,100]. The breast cancer increases were consistent with other studies of irradiation during childhood but also suggested that the protracted nature of the [226]Ra treatments for hemangioma was about 7 times less carcinogenic than the acute radiotherapy exposures for thymic enlargement, another benign disease which resolved without treatment [34,81]. The average dose to the active bone marrow was 130 mGy (max. 4,600 mGy), and no significant association with leukemia was observed [38].

9.3 CURRENT THERAPY WITH RADIOPHARMACEUTICALS

In the 1940s, reports of the use of radioactive iodine to treat thyroid diseases and radioactive phosphorus to treat leukemias were enthusiastically received by the medical profession and have spawned an ongoing series of expanding uses and development of radioactive "magic bullets" worldwide [2,101]. Similar therapies are emerging as a safe and effective targeted approach for treatment of many diseases, especially cancers [42]. Historically, nuclear medicine administrations have been performed as therapies for cancers, targeted radioimmunotherapy of cancer (particularly leukemias and lymphomas), myeloproliferative diseases, palliation of bone pain secondary to skeletal metastases, intracavitary therapy of malignant effusions and ascites, intracranial infusions for residual disease, and other systemic and regional disease therapies. As such, therapeutic radio-pharmaceuticals are employed for treating a variety of disease conditions including ankylosing spondylitis [36], hyperthyroidism and other benign thyroid conditions [102], differentiated thyroid cancer [103,104], PV and essential thrombocythemia [105], B-cell lymphoma [106], skeletal metastases [107,108], neuroblastoma [109], neuroendocrine tumors with peptide receptor [110], prostate cancer, prostate-specific membrane antigen, and folate receptor ligands [111,112], radio-immunotherapy using radiolabeled antibodies that target and bind to tumor-specific antigens [41,113–115], arthritis (radionuclide synovectomy) [116,117], and intra-arterial treatment of hepa-tocellular carcinoma and liver metastases [118]. A compilation of the current and developing radioactive materials used for therapeutic treatment is listed in Table 9.2.

There is continued development of novel radiopharmaceuticals, tagging agents, and immuno-therapy approaches. In addition, there are emerging [119] and re-emerging [120] integrated nuclear imaging and therapies (e.g., theranostics) wherein there is a pairing of diagnostic biomarkers with therapeutic agents sharing particular targets within diseased systems, organs, tissues, and/or cells. These will likely prove important along with the growth in both molecular imaging and personalized medicine, and with the targeted specificity of the therapeutic component of theranostic treatments (i.e., with potentially reduced healthy tissue impacts and associated risks) along with the exquisite information from the diagnostic component (e.g., positron emission tomography [PET] and single-photon emission computed tomography [SPECT]). While diagnostic uses of radioactive materials for general and targeted imaging typically utilize much lower administered activities, the development of ^{18}F-labeled imaging agents and the expanding uses of novel PET radionuclides and labeled materials point toward increased vigilance [121–124]. The discovery of specific tumor-associated targets, better radiochemistry techniques, along with increasing availability of alpha-particle emitters (and other radionuclides) with additional preclinical and clinical studies of nuclear medicine therapies alongside adjuvant treatment modalities will continue over time [42]. These developments come with the increasing ability to image and quantitatively characterize potential biological outcomes.

Overall, the management of patients who have received diagnostic and therapeutic amounts of radionuclides is becoming increasingly complex [125,126]. With both current and developing diagnostics and treatments, it is also important to consider follow-up and long-term epidemiologic studies of patients treated with current and emerging nuclear medicine therapies.

TABLE 9.2

Selected List of Radioactive Materials Used for Therapeutic Treatment

Radionuclide	Typical Activity Range	Chemical Form	Medical Use
^{32}P	111–185 MBq Various 296–444 MBq 370–555 MBq	Sodium phosphate Sodium phosphate Chromic phosphate Colloid Sodium phosphate Chromic phosphate	Polycythemia vera Essential thrombocytosis Synovectomy Intraperitoneal metastases Bone pain, skeletal mets Malignant effusions
^{131}I	185–740 MBq 2.59–3.7 GBq 1.11–14.8 GBq Activity required to deliver 65–75 Gy 555–666 MBq kg^{-1}	Sodium iodide Sodium iodide Sodium iodide Iodine-labeled antibody Tositumomab Metaiodobenzylguanidine	Hyperthyroidism and other benign Thyroid ablation Thyroid cancer Lymphoma therapy Neuroblastoma Neuroblastoma
^{89}Sr	148 MBq	Strontium chloride	Bone pain, skeletal mets
^{153}Sm	37 MBq kg^{-1} of body weight	Samarium lexidronam, a chelate	Bone pain, skeletal mets
^{90}Y	11.1–14.8 MBq kg^{-1} up to 1.19 GBq	Yttrium-labeled antibody ibritumomab tiuxetan Glass or resin microspheres	Lymphoma therapy
^{177}Lu	2.78–7.4 GBq over several cycles 7.4 GBq over several cycles	DOTATATE/DOTATOC Vipivotide textraxetan	Neuroendocrine tumors Prostate cancer, PSMA
^{225}Ac	Developing	Radioimmunotherapy	Various
^{211}At	Developing	Radioimmunotherapy	Various
^{212}Bi (from ^{224}Ra)	Developing	Radioimmunotherapy	Various
^{213}Bi (from ^{225}Ac)	Developing	Radioimmunotherapy	Various
^{223}Ra	55 kBq kg^{-1} over several cycles	Radium dichloride	Bone pain, skeletal mets, castration-resistant prostate cancer
^{224}Ra	5.6–11.1 MBq	Radium dichloride	Ankylosing spondylitis
^{227}Th	Developing	Radioimmunotherapy	Various

9.4   CONCLUSIONS

Studies of patients administered radionuclides for diagnostic or therapeutic purposes have contributed to both patient care and scientific understanding. Phosphorus-32 was an effective treatment for polycythemia vera, but the late consequence of leukemia contributed to a change in therapeutic modalities. Thorotrast was an exceptional contrast media for cerebral angiography. However, the late effects of liver cancer and leukemia resulted in it being abandoned. Diagnostic doses of 1 Gy to the adult thyroid gland following ^{131}I administrations were not linked to deleterious late effects, confirming that the adult thyroid gland is relatively radio-resistant. High therapeutic doses of ^{131}I to treat hyperthyroidism did not cause detectable increases in leukemia, despite a relatively large dose to the bone marrow. It is noteworthy that leukemia is one of the hallmarks following radiation exposure seen in many exposed populations, occurs at all ages of exposure, and has one of the highest risk coefficients of all radiogenic cancers. This finding of a consistent absence of leukemia in all studies of hyperthyroidism following radioiodine therapy provides evidence that low doses administered at a low dose rate may be less leukemogenic than higher doses delivered at a high dose rate. Much higher doses of radioiodine to treat thyroid cancer are linked to increases in leukemia, which suggest, also, a nonlinearity in the dose response. Whether high doses of radioactive iodine to treat hyperthyroidism are causally related to other cancers or all cancers combined is a matter of current controversy, sparked by the most recent follow-up of the Cooperative Thyrotoxicosis Therapy Follow-up Study of patients treated 1946–1964. Other recent high-quality studies of hyperthyroidism attempted to address treatment selection, confounding by indication, demographic and clinical co-factors associated with both hyperthyroidism and outcome found little evidence to support either an increase of individual cancers or of all combined cancer following [131]I. Radium-224 to treat ankylosing spondylitis has been linked to bone cancer but not leukemia, indicating the importance of dose distribution, i.e., dose to bone was high but dose to bone marrow was small. Studies of children receiving external radiotherapy for benign conditions suggest a lower risk of thyroid cancer and of breast cancer when exposures were protracted. Confounding by indication was present in imaging studies using diagnostic ^{131}I and of Thorotrast, raising caution in interpreting the associations reported in some studies of CT imaging examinations in childhood and early onset leukemia, brain, and other cancers. The expanding use of radionuclides in targeted therapies as well as diagnostic procedures continues to support the importance of nuclear medicine in patient care. As in the past, constant vigilance, including epidemiologic evaluations, should continue to measure any possible late effects from new radiation applications, keeping in mind the benefits and improvements afforded in patient care.

REFERENCES

1. Becker, D. V., and C. T. Sawin. 1996. "Radioiodine and thyroid disease: the beginning." *Seminars in Nuclear Medicine* 26 (3): 155–164. doi: 10.1016/s0001-2998(96)80020-1.
2. Wagner, H. N., Jr. 2006. *A Personal History of Nuclear Medicine*. New York: Springer.
3. Boice, J. D., Jr. 2006. "Ionizing radiation." In *Cancer Epidemiology and Prevention, 3rd Edition*, edited by D. Schottenfeld, and J. F. Fraumeni, Jr., 259–293. New York: Oxford University Press.
4. Fahey, F. H., and F. D. Grant. 2021. "Celebrating eighty years of radionuclide therapy and the work of Saul Hertz." *Journal of Applied Clinical Medical Physics* 22 (1): 4–10. doi: 10.1002/acm2.13175.
5. Saenger, E. L., G. E. Thoma, and E. A. Tompkins. 1968. "Incidence of leukemia following treatment of hyperthyroidism. Preliminary report of the Cooperative Thyrotoxicosis Therapy Follow-Up Study." *Journal of the American Medical Association* 205 (12): 855–862.
6. Holm, L. E., P. Hall, K. Wiklund, G. Lundell, G. Berg, G. Bjelkengren, et al. 1991. "Cancer risk after iodine-131 therapy for hyperthyroidism." *Journal of the National Cancer Institute* 83 (15): 1072–1077. doi: 10.1093/jnci/83.15.1072.
7. Hall, P., J. D. Boice, Jr., G. Berg, G. Bjelkengren, U. B. Ericsson, A. Hallquist, et al. 1992. "Leukaemia incidence after iodine-131 exposure." *The Lancet* 340 (8810): 1–4. doi: 10.1016/0140-6736(92)92421-b.

8. Ron, E., M. M. Doody, D. V. Becker, A. B. Brill, R. E. Curtis, M. B. Goldman, et al. 1998. "Cancer mortality following treatment for adult hyperthyroidism. Cooperative Thyrotoxicosis Therapy Follow-up Study Group." *Journal of the American Medical Association* 280 (4): 347–355. doi: 10.1001/jama.280.4.347.

9. Franklyn, J. A., P. Maisonneuve, M. Sheppard, J. Betteridge, and P. Boyle. 1999. "Cancer incidence and mortality after radioiodine treatment for hyperthyroidism: a population-based cohort study." *The Lancet* 353 (9170): 2111–2115. doi: 10.1016/S0140-6736(98)12295-X.

10. National Council on Radiation Protection and Measurements. 2008. *Risk to the Thyroid from Ionizing Radiation*. NCRP Report No. 159. Bethesda: NCRP.

11. Kitahara, C. M., A. Berrington de Gonzalez, A. Bouville, A. B. Brill, M. M. Doody, D. R. Melo, et al. 2019. "Association of radioactive iodine treatment with cancer mortality in patients with hyperthyroidism." *JAMA Internal Medicine* 179 (8): 1034–1042. doi: 10.1001/jamainternmed.2019.0981.

12. Kitahara, C. M., A. Berrington de González, and D. L. Preston. 2019. "Safety of the use of radioactive iodine in patients with hyperthyroidism-reply." *JAMA Internal Medicine* 179 (12): 1739. doi: 10.1001/jamainternmed.2019.5123.

13. Kitahara, C. M., D. L. Preston, J. A. Sosa, and A. Berrington de Gonzalez. 2020. "Association of radioactive iodine, antithyroid drug, and surgical treatments with solid cancer mortality in patients with hyperthyroidism." *Journal of the American Medical Association Network Open* 3 (7): e209660. doi: 10.1001/jamanetworkopen.2020.9660.

14. Tulchinsky, M., and A. B. Brill. 2019. "Spotlight on the association of radioactive iodine treatment with cancer mortality in patients with hyperthyroidism is keeping the highest risk from antithyroid drugs in the blind spot." *Clinical Nuclear Medicine* 44 (10): 789–791. doi: 10.1097/RLU.0000000000002792.

15. Hindié, E., K. B. Ain, S. Zerdoud, and A. M. Avram. 2020. "Association of radioactive iodine treatment of hyperthyroidism with cancer mortality: an unjustified warning?" *The Journal of Clinical Endocrinology & Metabolism* 105 (4): dgz305. doi: 10.1210/clinem/dgz305. PMID: 31875905.

16. Evron, J. M., N. H. Esfandiari, and M. Papaleontiou. 2020. "Cancer incidence and mortality following treatment of hyperthyroidism with radioactive iodine." *Current Opinion in Endocrinology, Diabetes and Obesity* 27 (5): 323–328. doi: 10.1097/MED.0000000000000561.

17. Taylor, P. N., O. E. Okosieme, K. Chatterjee, and K. Boelaert; Executive Committees of the Society for Endocrinology and the British Thyroid Association. 2020. "Joint statement from the Society for Endocrinology and the British Thyroid Association regarding 'Association of Radioactive Iodine Treatment with cancer mortality in patients with hyperthyroidism'." *Clinical Endocrinology (Oxford)*. 92 (3): 266–267. doi: 10.1111/cen.14136.

18. Kim, B. W. 2022. "Does radioactive iodine therapy for hyperthyroidism cause cancer?" *The Journal of Clinical Endocrinology & Metabolism* 107 (2): e448–e457. doi: 10.1210/clinem/dgab700.

19. Brincker, H., H. S. Hansen, and A. P. Andersen. 1973. "Induction of leukemia by 131-I treatment of thyroid carcinoma." *British Journal of Cancer* 28 (3): 232–237. doi: 10.1038/bjc.1973.142.

20. Teng, D. J., Y. W. Hu, S. C. Chen, C. M. Yeh, H. L. Chiang, T. J. Chen, et al. 2016. "Use of radioactive iodine for thyroid cancer and risk of second primary malignancy: a nationwide population-based study." *Journal of the National Cancer Institute* 108 (2): djv314. doi: 10.1093/jnci/djv314.

21. Molenaar, R. J., S. Sidana, T. Radivoyevitch, A. S. Advani, A. T. Gerds, H. E. Carraway, et al. 2018. "Risk of hematologic malignancies after radioiodine treatment of well-differentiated thyroid cancer." *Journal of Clinical Oncology* 36 (18): 1831–1839. doi: 10.1200/JCO.2017.75.0232.

22. Modan, B., and A. M. Lilienfeld. 1964. "Leukaemogenic effect of ionising-irradiation treatment in polycythaemia." *Lancet* 284 (7357): 439–441. 10.1016/S0140-6736(64)90330-7

23. Modan B., and A. M. Lilienfeld. 1965. "Polycythemia vera and leukemia -- the role of radiation treatment. A study of 1222 patients." *Medicine (Baltimore)* 44: 305–344. doi: 10.1097/00005792-196507000-00003.

24. Najean, Y., J. D. Rain, C. Dresch, A. Goguel, F. Lejeune, M. Echard, et al. 1996. "Risk of leukaemia, carcinoma, and myelofibrosis in 32P- or chemotherapy-treated patients with polycythaemia vera: a prospective analysis of 682 cases. The 'French Cooperative Group for the Study of Polycythaemias'." *Leukemia & Lymphoma* 22 (Suppl 1): 111–119. doi: 10.3109/10428199609074368.

25. Najean, Y., and J. D. Rain. 1997. "Treatment of polycythemia vera: use of 32P alone or in combination with maintenance therapy using hydroxyurea in 461 patients greater than 65 years of age. The French Polycythemia Study Group." *Blood* 89 (7): 2319–2327.

26. Andersson, M., and H. H. Storm. 1992. "Cancer incidence among Danish Thorotrast-exposed patients." *Journal of the National Cancer Institute* 84 (17): 1318–1325. doi: 10.1093/jnci/84.17.1318.

27. Andersson, M., B. Carstensen, and H. H. Storm. 1995. "Mortality and cancer incidence after cerebral arteriography with or without Thorotrast." *Radiation Research* 142 (3): 305–320.

28. Andersson, M., H. Wallin, M. Jönsson, L. L. Nielsen, J. Visfeldt, M. Vyberg, et al. 1995. "Lung carcinoma and malignant mesothelioma in patients exposed to Thorotrast: incidence, histology and p53 status." *International Journal of Cancer* 63 (3): 330–336. doi: 10.1002/ijc.2910630304.

29. Travis, L. B., C. E. Land, M. Andersson, U. Nyberg, M. B. Goldman, L. Knudson Gaul, et al. 2001. "Mortality after cerebral angiography with or without radioactive Thorotrast: an international cohort of 3,143 two-year survivors." *Radiation Research* 156 (2): 136–150. doi: 10.1667/0033-7587(2001) 156[0136:macawo]2.0.co;2.

30. Travis, L. B., M. Hauptmann, L. K. Gaul, H. H. Storm, M. B. Goldman, U. Nyberg, et al. 2003. "Site-specific cancer incidence and mortality after cerebral angiography with radioactive Thorotrast." *Radiation Research* 160 (6): 691–706. doi: 10.1667/rr3095.

31. Chmelevsky, D., A. M. Kellerer, C. E. Land, C. W. Mays, and H. Spiess. 1988. "Time and dose dependency of bone-sarcomas in patients injected with radium-224." *Radiation and Environmental Biophysics* 27 (2): 103–114. doi: 10.1007/BF01214600. PMID: 3164868.

32. Nekolla, E. A., L. Walsh, and H. Spiess. 2010. "Incidence of malignant diseases in humans injected with radium-224." *Radiation Research* 174 (3): 377–386. doi: 10.1667/RR1955.1.

33. Spiess, H. 2010. "Life-span study on late effects of 224Ra in children and adults." *Health Physics* 99 (3): 286–291. doi: 10.1097/HP.0b013e3181cb857f.

34. United Nations Scientific Committee on the Effects of Atomic Radiation. 2008. *Effects of Ionizing Radiation, UNSCEAR 2006 Report (Scientific Annex A, Epidemiological Studies of Radiation and Cancer)* Vol I.: Publication E.08.IX.6. New York: United Nations.

35. Wick, R. R., M. J. Atkinson, and E. A. Nekolla. 2009. "Incidence of leukaemia and other malignant diseases following injections of the short-lived alpha-emitter 224Ra into man." *Radiation and Environmental Biophysics* 48 (3): 287–294. doi: 10.1007/s00411-009-0227-y.

36. Priest, N. D., L. T. Dauer, and D. G. Hoel. 2020. "Administration of lower doses of radium-224 to ankylosing spondylitis patients results in no evidence of significant overall detriment." *PLoS One* 15 (4): e0232597. doi: 10.1371/journal.pone.0232597.

37. Lundell, M., T. Hakulinen, and L. E. Holm. 1994. "Thyroid cancer after radiotherapy for skin hemangioma in infancy." *Radiation Research* 140 (3): 334–339.

38. Lundell, M., and L. E. Holm. 1996. "Mortality from leukemia after irradiation in infancy for skin hemangioma." *Radiation Research* 145 (5): 595–601.

39. Haddy, N., T. Andriamboavonjy, C. Paoletti, M. G. Dondon, A. Mousannif, A. Shamsaldin, et al. 2009. "Thyroid adenomas and carcinomas following radiotherapy for a hemangioma during infancy." *Radiotherapy and Oncology* 93 (2): 377–382. doi: 10.1016/j.radonc.2009.05.011.

40. Haddy, N., M. G. Dondon, C. Paoletti, C. Rubino, A. Mousannif, A. Shamsaldin, et al. 2010. "Breast cancer following radiotherapy for a hemangioma during childhood." *Cancer Causes & Control* 21 (11): 1807–1816. doi: 10.1007/s10552-010-9607-5.

41. Sgouros, G., J. C. Roeske, M. R. McDevitt, S. Palm, V. J. Allen, D. R. Fisher et al., 2010. "MIRD Pamphlet No. 22 (abridged): radiobiology and dosimetry of alpha-particle emitters for targeted radio-nuclide therapy." *Journal of Nuclear Medicine* 51 (2): 311–328. doi:10.2967/jnumed.108.058651.

42. Sgouros, G., L. Bodei, M. R. McDevitt, and J. R. Nedrow. 2020. "Radiopharmaceutical therapy in cancer: clinical advances and challenges." *Nature Reviews Drug Discovery* 19 (9): 589–608. doi: 10.1038/s41573-020-0073-9.

43. Yonekura, Y., S. Mattsson, G. Flux, W. E. Bolch, L. T. Dauer, D. R. Fisher, et al. 2019. "Radiological protection in therapy with radiopharmaceuticals. ICRP Publication 140." *Annals of the ICRP* 48 (1): 5–95. doi: 10.1177/0146645319838665.

44. Adelstein, S. James. 2014. "Radiation risk in nuclear medicine." *Seminars in Nuclear Medicine* 44 (3): 187–192. doi: 10.1053/j.semnuclmed.2014.03.003.

45. Tefferi, A., A. M. Vannucchi, and T. Barbui. 2018. "Polycythemia vera treatment algorithm 2018." *Blood Cancer Journal* 8 (1): 3. doi: 10.1038/s41408-017-0042-7.

46. Dickman, P. W., L. E. Holm, G. Lundell, J. D. Boice, Jr., and P. Hall. 2003. "Thyroid cancer risk after thyroid examination with 131I: a population-based cohort study in Sweden." *International Journal of Cancer* 106 (4): 580–587. doi: 10.1002/ijc.11258.

47. Boice, J. D., Jr. 2017. "From Chernobyl to Fukushima and beyond – a focus on thyroid cancer." Chap. 3 in *Thyroid Cancer and Nuclear Accidents – Long-Term After Effects of Chernobyl and Fukushima*, edited by S. Yamashita, and G. Thomas, 21–32. Tokyo: Elsevier.
48. Boice, J. D., Jr. 2015. "Radiation epidemiology and recent paediatric computed tomography studies." *Annals of the ICRP* 44 (Suppl 1): 236–248. doi: 10.1177/0146645315575877.
49. Tompkins, E. 1970. "Late effects of radioiodine therapy." In *Medical Radionuclides: Radiation Dose and Effects*, edited by R. J. Cloutier, C. L. Edwards, and W. S. Snyder, 431–440. Washington, DC: Atomic Energy Commission.
50. Ryödi, E., S. Metso, P. Jaatinen, H. Huhtala, R. Saaristo, M. Välimäki, et al. 2015. "Cancer incidence and mortality in patients treated either with RAI or thyroidectomy for hyperthyroidism." *The Journal of Clinical Endocrinology & Metabolism* 100 (10): 3710–3717. doi: 10.1210/jc.2015-1874.
51. Gronich, N., I. Lavi, G. Rennert, and W. Saliba. 2020. "Cancer risk after radioactive iodine treatment for hyperthyroidism: a cohort study." *Thyroid* 30 (2): 243–250. doi: 10.1089/thy.2019.0205.
52. Hall, P., G. Berg, G. Bjelkengren, J. D. Boice, Jr., U. B. Ericsson, A. Hallquist, et al. 1992. "Cancer mortality after iodine-131 therapy for hyperthyroidism." *International Journal of Cancer* 50 (6): 886–890. doi: 10.1002/ijc.2910500611.
53. Franklyn, J. A., P. Maisonneuve, M. C. Sheppard, J. Betteridge, and P. Boyle. 1998. "Mortality after the treatment of hyperthyroidism with radioactive iodine." *New England Journal of Medicine* 338 (11): 712–718. doi: 10.1056/NEJM199803123381103.
54. dos Santos Silva, I., F. Malveiro, M. E. Jones, and A. J. Swerdlow. 2003. "Mortality after radiological investigation with radioactive Thorotrast: A follow-up study of up to fifty years in Portugal." *Radiation Research* 159 (4): 521–534. doi: 10.1667/0033-7587(2003)159[0521:mariwr]2.0.co;2.
55. Wick, R. R., E. A. Nekolla, W. Gössner, and A. M. Kellerer. 1999. "Late effects in ankylosing spondylitis patients treated with 224Ra." *Radiation Research* 152 (6 Suppl): S8–S11.
56. Berk, P. D., J. D. Goldberg, M. N. Silverstein, A. Weinfeld, P. B. Donovan, J. T. Ellis, et al. 1981. "Increased incidence of acute leukemia in polycythemia vera associated with chlorambucil therapy." *New England Journal of Medicine* 304 (8): 441–447. doi: 10.1056/NEJM198102193040801.
57. Parmentier, C. 2003. "Use and risks of phosphorus-32 in the treatment of polycythaemia vera." *European Journal of Nuclear Medicine and Molecular Imaging* 30 (10): 1413–1417. doi: 10.1007/s00259-003-1270-6.
58. Ron, E., J. H. Lubin, R. E. Shore, K. Mabuchi, B. Modan, L. M. Pottern, et al. 2012. "Thyroid cancer after exposure to external radiation: a pooled analysis of seven studies. 1995." *Radiation Research* 178 (2): AV43–60. doi: 10.1667/rrav05.1.
59. Brenner, A. V., M. D. Tronko, M. Hatch, T. I. Bogdanova, V. A. Oliynik, J. H. Lubin, et al. 2011. "I-131 dose response for incident thyroid cancers in Ukraine related to the Chornobyl accident." *Environmental Health Perspectives* 119 (7): 933–939. doi: 10.1289/ehp.1002674.
60. Tuttle, R. M., and D. V. Becker. 2000. "The Chernobyl accident and its consequences: update at the millennium." *Seminars in Nuclear Medicine* 30 (2): 133–140. doi: 10.1053/nm.2000.5412.
61. Morton, L. M., D. M. Karyadi, C. Stewart, T. I. Bogdanova, E. G. Dawson, M. K. Steinberg, et al. 2021. "Radiation-related genomic profile of papillary thyroid carcinoma after the Chernobyl accident." *Science* 372 (6543): eabg2538. doi: 10.1126/science.abg2538.
62. National Council on Radiation Protection and Measurements. 2012. *Uncertainties in the Estimation of Radiation Risks and Probability of Disease Causation*. NCRP Report No. 171. Bethesda: NCRP.
63. United Nations Scientific Committee on the Effects of Atomic Radiation. 2013. *Sources, Effects and Risks of Ionizing Radiation. UNSCEAR 2013 Report (Scientific Annex B, Effects of Radiation Exposure of Children)*. Vol. II. Publication E.14.IX.2. New York: United Nations.
64. Yavuz, S., and Y. Puckett. 2022. *Iodine-131 uptake study*. Treasure Island, FL: StatPearls Publishing.
65. Bosco, J. L., R. A. Silliman, S. S. Thwin, A. M. Geiger, D. S. Buist, M. N. Prout, et al. 2010. "A most stubborn bias: no adjustment method fully resolves confounding by indication in observational studies." *Journal of Clinical Epidemiology* 63 (1): 64–74. doi: 10.1016/j.jclinepi.2009.03.001.
66. Shim, S. R., C. M. Kitahara, E. S. Cha, S. J. Kim, Y. J. Bang, and W. J. Lee. 2021. "Cancer risk after radioactive iodine treatment for hyperthyroidism: A systematic review and meta-analysis." *Journal of the American Medical Association Network Open* 4 (9): e2125072. doi: 10.1001/jamanetworkopen.2021.25072.
67. Yan, D., C. Chen, H. Yan, T. Liu, H. Yan, and J. Yuan. 2021. "Mortality risk after radioiodine therapy for hyperthyroidism: a systematic review and meta-analysis." *Endocrine Practice* 27 (4): 362–369. doi: 10.1016/j.eprac.2020.10.018.

68. Yu, C. Y., O. Saeed, A. S. Goldberg, S. Farooq, R. Fazelzad, D. P. Goldstein, et al. 2018. "A systematic review and meta-analysis of subsequent malignant neoplasm risk after radioactive iodine treatment of thyroid cancer." *Thyroid.* 28 (12): 1662–1673. doi: 10.1089/thy.2018.0244.
69. Peacock, J. G., M. N. Clemenshaw, and K. P. Banks. 2019. "Safety of the use of radioactive iodine in patients with hyperthyroidism." *JAMA Internal Medicine* 179 (12): 1737–1738. doi: 10.1001/jamainternmed.2019.5117.
70. Grady, E. E., K. Zukotynski, and B. S. Greenspan. 2019. "Safety of the use of radioactive iodine in patients with hyperthyroidism." *JAMA Internal Medicine* 179 (12): 1738–1739. doi: 10.1001/jamainternmed.2019.5120.
71. Toft, D. J. 2019. "Radioactive iodine therapy for hyperthyroidism is associated with increased solid cancer mortality." *Clinical Thyroidology* 31 (8): 326–329.
72. Zhang, X., G. Shan, Q. Liu, and Y. Lin. 2019. "Regarding the manuscript entitled 'Association of radioactive iodine treatment with cancer mortality in patients with hyperthyroidism'." *European Journal of Nuclear Medicine and Molecular Imaging* 46 (12): 2410–2411. doi: 10.1007/s00259-019-04522-1.
73. Greenspan, B. S., J. A. Siegel, A. Hassan, and E. B. Silberstein. 2019. "There is no association of radioactive iodine treatment with cancer mortality in patients with hyperthyroidism." *Journal of Nuclear Medicine* 60 (11): 1500–1501. doi: 10.2967/jnumed.119.235929.
74. Iakovou, I., E. Giannoula, V. Chatzipavlidou, and C. Sachpekidis. 2020. "Associating radioiodine therapy in hyperthyroidism with cancer mortality: robust or random results of a statistical analysis?" *Hellenic Journal of Nuclear Medicine* 23 (1): 94–95. doi: 10.1967/s002449912018.
75. Biondi, B. 2021. "Radioactive iodine treatment in hyperthyroidism and cancer mortality – a still controversial issue." *JAMA Network Open* 4 (9): e2126361. doi: 10.1001/jamanetworkopen.2021.26361.
76. Korevaar, T. I. M. 2020. "Is there a risk of cancer following radioactive iodine therapy for hyperthyroidism?" *Clinical Thyroidology* 32 (2): 58–61. 10.1089/ct.2020;32.58-61.
77. Dobyns, B. M., G. E. Sheline, J. B. Workman, E. A. Tompkins, W. M. McConahey, and D. V. Becker. 1974. "Malignant and benign neoplasms of the thyroid in patients treated for hyperthyroidism: a report of the cooperative thyrotoxicosis therapy follow-up study." *The Journal of Clinical Endocrinology & Metabolism* 38 (6): 976–998. doi: 10.1210/jcem-38-6-976.
78. Melo, D. R., A. B. Brill, P. Zanzonico, P. Vicini, B. Moroz, D. Kwon, et al. 2015. "Organ dose estimates for hyperthyroid patients treated with (131)I: an update of the thyrotoxicosis follow-up study." *Radiation Research* 184 (6): 595–610. doi: 10.1667/RR14160.1.
79. Zanzonico, P. B., D. V. Becker, A. B. Brill, O. Tsen, A. Strauss, J. R. Hurley, et al. 1989. "Extrathyroidal absorbed doses in radioiodine treatment of hyperthyroidism - based analysis of 468 patients." *Journal of Nuclear Medicine* 30:833. (As referenced in [8])
80. Boice, J. D., Jr., D. Preston, F. G. Davis, and R. R. Monson. 1991. "Frequent chest X-ray fluoroscopy and breast cancer incidence among tuberculosis patients in Massachusetts." *Radiation Research* 125 (2): 214–222.
81. Preston, D. L., A. Mattsson, E. Holmberg, R. Shore, N. G. Hildreth, and J. D. Boice, Jr. 2002. "Radiation effects on breast cancer risk: a pooled analysis of eight cohorts." *Radiation Research* 158 (2): 220–235. doi: 10.1667/0033-7587(2002)158[0220:reobcr]2.0.co;2.
82. Boice, J. D., Jr., E. B. Harvey, M. Blettner, M. Stovall, and J. T. Flannery. 1992. "Cancer in the contralateral breast after radiotherapy for breast cancer." *The New England Journal of Medicine* 326 (12): 781–785. doi: 10.1056/NEJM199203193261201.
83. Stovall, M., S. A. Smith, B. M. Langholz, J. D. Boice, Jr., R. E. Shore, M. Andersson, et al. 2008. "Dose to the contralateral breast from radiotherapy and risk of second primary breast cancer in the WECARE study." *International Journal of Radiation Oncology, Biology, Physics* 72 (4): 1021–1030. doi: 10.1016/j.ijrobp.2008.02.040.
84. Søgaard, M., D. K. Farkas, V. Ehrenstein, J. O. Jørgensen, O. M. Dekkers, and H. T. Sørensen. 2016. "Hypothyroidism and hyperthyroidism and breast cancer risk: a nationwide cohort study." *European Journal of Endocrinology* 174 (4): 409-414. doi: 10.1530/EJE-15-0989.
85. Journy, N. M. Y., M. O. Bernier, M. M. Doody, B. H. Alexander, M. S. Linet, and C. M. Kitahara. 2017. "Hyperthyroidism, hypothyroidism, and cause-specific mortality in a large cohort of women." *Thyroid* 27 (8): 1001–1010. doi: 10.1089/thy.2017.0063.
86. Tran, T. V., C. M. Kitahara, L. Leenhardt, F. de Vathaire, M. C. Boutron-Ruault, and N. Journy. 2022. "The effect of thyroid dysfunction on breast cancer risk: an updated meta-analysis." *Endocrine-Related Cancer* 30 (1): e220155. doi: 10.1530/ERC-22-0155.
87. Laugesen, K., J. F. Ludvigsson, M. Schmidt, M. Gissler, U. A. Valdimarsdottir, A. Lunde, et al. 2021. "Nordic Health Registry-based research: a review of health care systems and key registries." *Clinical Epidemiology* 13: 533–554. doi: 10.2147/CLEP.S314959.

88. Ludvigsson, J. F., E. Andersson, A. Ekbom, M. Feychting, J. L. Kim, C. Reuterwall, et al. 2011. "External review and validation of the Swedish national inpatient register." *BMC Public Health* 11: 450. doi: 10.1186/1471-2458-11-450.

89. Bakken, I. J., A. M. S. Ariansen, G. P. Knudsen, L. I. Johansen, and S. E. Vollset. 2020. "The Norwegian Patient Registry and the Norwegian Registry for Primary Health Care: research potential of two nationwide health-care registries." *Scandinavian Journal of Public Health* 48 (1): 49–55. doi: 10.1177/1403494819859737.

90. Schmidt, M., S. A. Schmidt, J. L. Sandegaard, V. Ehrenstein, L. Pedersen, and H. T. Sørensen. 2015. "The Danish National Patient Registry: a review of content, data quality, and research potential." *Clinical Epidemiology* 7: 449–490. doi: 10.2147/CLEP.S91125.

91. Rector, T. S., S. L. Wickstrom, M. Shah, N. Thomas Greenlee, P. Rheault, J. Rogowski, et al. 2004. "Specificity and sensitivity of claims-based algorithms for identifying members of Medicare+Choice health plans that have chronic medical conditions." *Health Service Research* 39 (6 Pt 1): 1839–1857. doi: 10.1111/j.1475-6773.2004.00321.x.

92. Centers for Medicare and Medicaid Services. Chronic Conditions among Medicare Beneficiaries, Chartbook, 2012 Edition. Baltimore, MD. 2012.

93. Seib, C. D., T. Meng, R. M. Cisco, D. T. Lin, E. A. McAninch, J. Chen, et al. 2023. "Risk of permanent hypoparathyroidism requiring calcitriol therapy in a population-based cohort of adults older than 65 undergoing total thyroidectomy for Graves' disease." *Thyroid* 33 (2): 223–229. doi: 10.1089/thy.2022.0140.

94. National Academy of Sciences. 1988. *Health Risks of Radon and Other Internally Deposited Alpha-Emitters (BEIR IV Report)*. Washington, DC: National Academy Press.

95. van Kaick, G., A. Karaoglou, and A. M. Kellerer, eds. 1995. *Health Effects of Internally Deposited Radionuclides: Emphasis on Radium and Thorium*. Singapore: World Scientific. 10.1142/2526.

96. Martinez, N. E., D. W. Jokisch, L. T. Dauer, K. F. Eckerman, R. E. Goans, J. D. Brockman, et al. 2022. "Radium dial workers: back to the future." *International Journal of Radiation Biology* 98 (4): 750–768. doi: 10.1080/09553002.2021.1917785.

97. Susser, M. 1991. "What is a cause and how do we know one? A grammar for pragmatic epidemiology." *American Journal of Epidemiology* 133 (7): 635–648. doi: 10.1093/oxfordjournals.aje.a115939.

98. International Agency for Research on Cancer. 2012. *IARC Monographs on the Evaluation of Carcinogenic Risks to Humans*. Vol 100D. *Radiation*. Lyon, France: IARC.

99. Fürst, C. J., M. Lundell, L. E. Holm, and C. Silfverswärd. 1988. "Cancer incidence after radiotherapy for skin hemangioma: a retrospective cohort study in Sweden." *Journal of the National Cancer Institute* 80 (17): 1387–1392. doi: 10.1093/jnci/80.17.1387.

100. Lundell, M., A. Mattsson, P. Karlsson, E. Holmberg, A. Gustafsson, and L. E. Holm. 1999. "Breast cancer risk after radiotherapy in infancy: a pooled analysis of two Swedish cohorts of 17,202 infants." *Radiation Research* 151 (5): 626–632.

101. Valent, P., B. Groner, U. Schumacher, G. Superti-Furga, M. Busslinger, R. Kralovics, et al. 2016. "Paul Ehrlich (1854-1915) and his contributions to the foundation and birth of translational medicine." *Journal of Innate Immunity* 8 (2): 111–120. doi: 10.1159/000443526.

102. American Thyroid Association Taskforce on Radioiodine Safety, J. C. Sisson, J. Freitas, I. R. McDougall, L. T. Dauer, J. R. Hurley, et al. 2011 "Radiation safety in the treatment of patients with thyroid diseases by radioiodine 131I: practice recommendation of the American Thyroid Association." *Thyroid* 21 (4): 335–346. doi: 10.1089/thy.2010.0403

103. Shaha, A. R, and R. M. Tuttle. 2022. "Nuances in the surgical management of thyroid cancer." *Indian Journal of Surgical Oncology* 13(1): 1–6. doi: 10.1007/s13193-021-01362-0.

104. do Prado Padovani, R., S. V. Chablani, and R. M. Tuttle. 2022. "Radioactive iodine therapy: multiple faces of the same polyhedron." *Archives of Endocrinology and Metabolism* 63: 393–406. doi: 10.20945/2359-3997000000461.

105. Tennvall, J., and B. Brans. 2007. "EANM procedure guideline for 32P phosphate treatment of myeloproliferative diseases." *European Journal of Nuclear Medicine and Molecular Imaging* 34 (8): 1324–1327. doi: 10.1007/s00259-007-0407-4.

106. Tennvall, J., M. Fischer, A. Bischof Delaloye, E. Bombardieri, L. Bodei, F. Giammarile, et al. 2007. "EANM procedure guideline of radio-immunotherapy for B-cell lymphoma with 90Y-radiolabeled ibritumomab tiuxetan (Zevalin)." *European Journal of Nuclear Medicine and Molecular Imaging* 34 (4): 616–622. doi: 10.1007/s00259-007-0372-y.

107. Pandit-Taskar, N., S. M. Larson, and J. A. Carrasquillo. 2014. "Bone-seeking radiopharmaceuticals for treatment of osseous metastases. Part 1: alpha therapy with 223Ra-dichloride." *Journal of Nuclear Medicine* 55 (2): 268–274. doi: 10.2967/jnumed.112.112482.

108. Chittenden, S. J., C. Hindorf, C. C. Parker, V. J. Lewington, B. E. Pratt, B. Johnson, et al. 2015. "A phase-1, open-label study of the biodistribution, pharmacokinetics, and dosimetry of 223Ra-dichloride in patients with hormone-refractory prostate cancer and skeletal metastases." *Journal of Nuclear Medicine* 56 (9): 1304–1309. doi: 10.2967/jnumed.115.157123.
109. George, S. L., N. Falzone, S. Chittenden, S. J. Kirk, D. Lancaster, S. J. Vaidya, et al. 2016. "Individualized 131I-mIBG therapy in the management of refractory and relapsed neuroblastoma." *Nuclear Medicine Communications* 37 (5): 466–472. doi: 10.1097/MNM.0000000000000470.
110. Bodei, L., J. Mueller-Brand, R. P. Baum, M. E. Pavel, D. Hörsch, M. S. O'Dorisio, et al. 2013. "The joint IAEA, EANM, and SNMMI practical guidance on peptide receptor radionuclide therapy (PRRNT) in neuroendocrine tumours." *European Journal of Nuclear Medicine and Molecular Imaging* 40 (5): 800–816. doi: 10.1007/s00259-012-2330-6.
111. Rahbar, K., H. Ahmadzadehfar, C. Kratochwil, U. Haberkorn, M. Schäfers, M. Essler, et al. 2017. "German multicenter study investigating 177Lu-PSMA-617 radioligand therapy in advanced prostate cancer patients." *Journal of Nuclear Medicine* 58 (1): 85–90. doi: 10.2967/jnumed.116.183194.
112. Kratochwil, C., F. Bruchertseifer, F. L. Giesel, M. Weis, F. A. Verburg, F. Mottaghy, et al. 2016. "225Ac-PSMA-617 for PSMAtargeted alpha-radiation therapy of metastatic castration-resistant prostate cancer." *Journal of Nuclear Medicine* 57 (12): 1941–1944. doi:10.2967/jnumed.116.178673.
113. Jurcic, J. G., and T. L. Rosenblat. 2014. "Targeted alpha-particle immunotherapy for acute myeloid leukemia." *American Society of Clinical Oncology Educational Book* 34, e126–e131. doi: 10.14694/EdBook_AM.2014.34.e126.
114. Larson, S. M., J. A. Carrasquillo, N-K. Cheung, and O. W. Press. 2015. "Radioimmunotherapy of human tumours." *Nature Reviews Cancer* 15 (6): 347–360. doi: 10.1038/nrc3925.
115. Hanaoka, K., M. Hosono, Y. Tatsumi, K. Ishii, S-W. Im, N. Tsuchiya, et al. 2015. "Heterogeneity of intratumoral 111Inibritumomab tiuxetan and 18F-FDG distribution in association with therapeutic response in radioimmunotherapy for B-cell non-Hodgkin's lymphoma." *EJNMI Research* 5: 10. doi: 10.1186/s13550-015-0093-3.
116. Ansell, B. M., A. Crook, J. R. Mallard, and E. G. Bywaters. 1963. "Evaluation of intra-articular colloidal gold Au 198 in the treatment of persistent knee effusions." *Annals of Rheumatic Diseases* 22 (6): 435–439. doi: 10.1136/ard.22.6.435.
117. Knut, L. 2015. "Radiosynovectomy in the therapeutic management of arthritis." *World Journal of Nuclear Medicine* 14 (1): 10–15. doi:10.4103/1450-1147.150509.
118. Giammarile, F., L. Bodei, C. Chiesa, G. Flug, F. Forrer, F. Kraeber-Bodere, et al. 2011. "EANM procedure guideline for the treatment of liver cancer and liver metastases with intra-arterial radioactive compounds." *European Journal of Nuclear Medicine and Molecular Imaging* 38 (7): 1393–1406. doi: 10.1007/s00259-011-1812-2.
119. Gomes Marin, J. R., R. F. Nunes, A. M. Coutinho, E. C. Zaniboni, L. B. Costa, F. G. Barbosa, et al. 2020. "Theranostics in nuclear medicine: emerging and re-emerging integrated imaging and therapies in the era of precision oncology." *Radiographics* 40 (6):1715–1740. doi: 10.1148/rg.2020200021.
120. Funkhouser, J. 2002. "Reinventing pharma: the theranostic revolution." *Current Drug Discovery* 2: 17–19.
121. Holland, J. P., M. J. Williamson, and L. S. Lewis. 2010. "Unconventional nuclides for radiopharmaceuticals." *Molecular Imaging* 9 (1): 1–20.
122. Williamson, J. J., and L. T. Dauer. 2014. "Activity thresholds for patient instruction and release for positron emission tomography radionuclides." *Health Physics* 106 (3): 341–352. doi: 10.1097/HP.0b013e31829efbc4.
123. Crisan, G., N. S. Moldovean-Cioroianu, D. Timaru, G. Andries, C. Cainap, and V. Chis. 2022. "Radiopharmaceuticals for PET and SPECT imaging: a literature review over the last decade." *International Journal of Molecular Science* 23 (9): 5023. doi: 10.3390/ijms23095023.
124. Steenhuysen, J. 2023. "US removes coverage curb on PET scans for Alzheimer's patients." Reuters October 13, 2023.
125. National Council on Radiation Protection and Measurements. 2006. *Management of Radionuclide Therapy Patients.* NCRP Report No. 155. Bethesda: NCRP.
126. Boice, J. D., Jr., L. T. Dauer, K. R. Kase, F. A. Mettler, Jr., and R. J. Vetter. 2020. "Evolution of radiation protection for medical workers." *British Journal of Radiology* 93 (1112): 20200282. 10.1259/bjr.20200282.

10 Adverse Effects of Radionuclide Therapy

Grace Kong, Raghava Kashyap, and Rodney J. Hicks

10.1 INTRODUCTION

Although there is much hype about the "emerging" field of theranostics, the therapeutic use of radionuclides preceded the advent of imaging by many decades. Soon after Marie Curie isolated radium, it was recognized that radiation can damage cells and could be used to treat cancer [1], resulting in medicinal uses of radioactivity in the promotion of health in the early 20th century [2]. However, subsequent recognition that radium dial painters died prematurely, particularly from sarcomas of the jaw, has resulted in research into its mechanisms in the modern era [3]. Localization to bone, reflecting physicochemical similarity to calcium, was a key to the toxicity of radium-226 (^{226}Ra), but also fundamental to the use of ^{223}Ra in metastatic prostate cancer [4].

The invention of the first cyclotron by Ernest Lawrence in 1930 [5] and the Joliot Curies' creation of radionuclides through bombardment of non-radioactive materials with alpha particles in 1934 [6] led to the synthesis of novel therapeutic agents. These included radioactive iodine (RAI). This was first used by Dr Saul Hertz to treat hyperthyroidism in 1941 [7]. Hertz, together with physicist Arthur Roberts, performed detailed dosimetry studies that helped define effective therapeutic activities based on thyroid volume. He also noted the development of late hypothyroidism in some patients [8]. Their partnership emblemized the convergence of clinical and physical sciences, which represents one of the fundamental strengths of nuclear medicine.

Dr Sam Seidlin first used RAI for thyroid cancer treatment at the Montefiore Hospital in the 1940s [9,10] but also reported one of the first cases of myeloid leukemia associated with RAI [11], highlighting that with benefits come potential risks. Other therapeutic radionuclides developed at this time included phosphorus-32 for hematological malignancies [12] and strontium-89 (^{89}SrCl) for prostate cancer bone pain palliation [13,14]. Since then, there has been significant development, advancement in understanding of radionuclide therapy targeting different tumor types, with many now incorporated into clinical guidelines. Importantly, many patients treated successfully were heavily pre-treated and had advanced disease. In this context, physiological reserves of patients were likely already compromised by the combination of malignant tissue infiltration and the toxic effects of prior treatments. Accordingly, any adverse effects from radionuclide therapy, including acute or long-term ones (Figure 10.1), must be weighed against the benefits derived in the duration or quality of life and an open mind must be applied when considering causality.

10.2 ACUTE TOXICITIES

Adverse effects occurring within hours to days following radionuclide therapy are grouped under acute toxicities. The causes of acute effects can be anticipated with an understanding of the effects of radiation on the sites of tumor and physiological uptake, and the pharmacological effects of the carrier used for the isotope or medications co-administered with the therapy. The factors that influence severity of radiation-induced damage include the activity of radionuclide administered, the type of particle and the energy of the emitted radiation and the percentage of administered activity taken up and retained in the individual organs, which influences radiation dose.

DOI: 10.1201/9781003250913-12

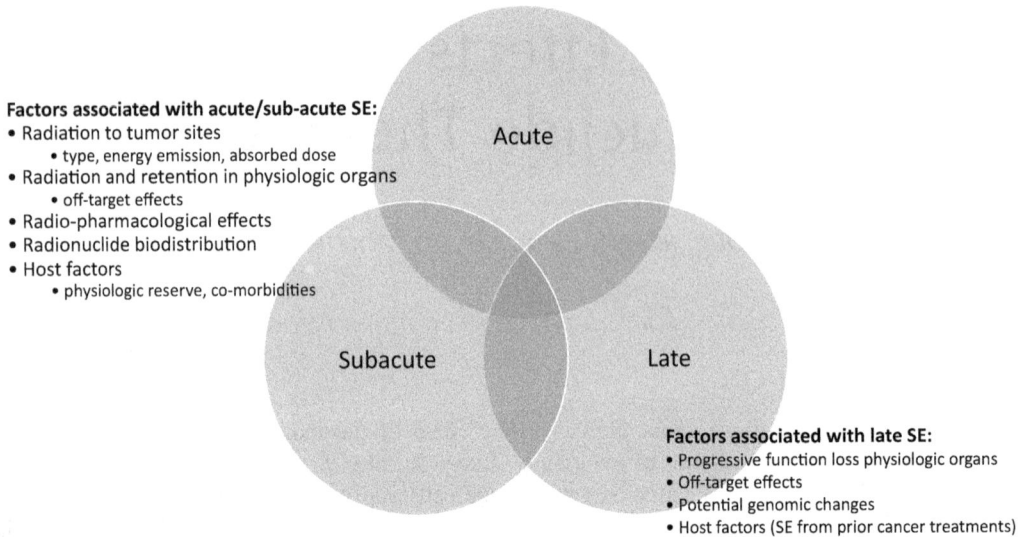

Factors associated with acute/sub-acute SE:
- Radiation to tumor sites
  - type, energy emission, absorbed dose
- Radiation and retention in physiologic organs
  - off-target effects
- Radio-pharmacological effects
- Radionuclide biodistribution
- Host factors
  - physiologic reserve, co-morbidities

Acute

Subacute

Late

Factors associated with late SE:
- Progressive function loss physiologic organs
- Off-target effects
- Potential genomic changes
- Host factors (SE from prior cancer treatments)

FIGURE 10.1 Late effects from radionuclide therapy. Side effects (SE) associated with radionuclide therapy can be classified as early (within hours of administration), subacute (occurring days to weeks later) or late (months to years after exposure). Some are discrete and limited to a particular period while some may overlap or persist across these intervals.

10.2.1 Adverse Effects Related to Cumulative Activity of Radionuclide

As an immediate effect of radiation-induced damage, edema and inflammation can occur in the tumor sites resulting in mechanical symptoms or signs. Lesions in bones can precipitate pain, which is often described as a "flare" phenomenon [15]. This occurs especially with bone-seeking radiopharmaceuticals used for pain palliation [16] but can also occur with lutetium-177 prostate specific membrane antigen (^{177}Lu-PSMA) therapy for prostate cancer, which commonly involves the skeleton. Pain flare may occur with capsular liver lesions, e.g., in the treatment of neuro-endocrine tumors (NET) [17].

A similar phenomenon is noticed in the treatment of hyperthyroidism with RAI. Pain and mild swelling of the thyroid is often noticed a few days following treatment. Importantly, radionuclide uptake in tumor sites in or adjacent to nervous system can result in pressure effects in the brain, or on the spinal cord and nerve roots. Tumor lysis is a potentially life-threatening acute adverse event following radionuclide therapy and is characterized by acute renal failure with hyperuricemia, hypocalcemia, hyperkalemia and metabolic acidosis [18]. It is a very rare toxicity of peptide receptor radionuclide therapy (PRRT) for NET [19].

10.2.2 Effects Related to Cumulative Activity in Normal Organs

Physiological uptake in organs results in "off-target" radiation delivery that may be dose-limiting or determine the dominant site of adverse effects related to the specific radionuclide therapy.

High physiologic uptake of RAI and ^{177}Lu-PSMA in the salivary and lacrimal glands can result in dryness of mouth and eyes. Prominent physiologic uptake of the upper gastrointestinal tract may also lead to nausea and vomiting with these therapies. Systemic radionuclide therapy is inevitably also associated with radiation exposure of bone marrow due to circulating radiotracer. An acute drop in hematological parameters is commonly encountered following radionuclide therapies and usually nadirs at around 3 weeks but is mostly transient. Platelets appear to be more susceptible among the three lineages to the acute effects of radionuclide therapy.

10.2.3 ADVERSE EFFECTS RELATED TO PHARMACEUTICAL PROPERTIES OF THE TRACER

Radionuclide therapy may contain a carrier molecule that has biological activity. Examples include meta-iodo-benzyl-guanidine (MIBG), which can result in degranulation of the adrenergic cells. When administered for therapeutic purposes to catecholamine-secreting tumors, the amount of carrier administered is relatively higher compared to diagnostic procedures and together with radiation effects may result in acute symptoms of excess adrenergic activity such as tachycardia, hypertension and palpitations [20]. When severe, hypertensive crisis can occur, and may be life-threatening [21]. This can also occur with PRRT of such tumors [22]. In NET, PRRT can also result in precipitation of carcinoid crisis [23–25], which manifests as sweating, intense flushing, tachycardia and diarrhea and vomiting. Less commonly, hormonal release from other functioning NET can also cause acute effects. For instance, hyperinsulinemia leading to profound hypoglycemia can occur following PRRT of insulinoma and may be life-threatening [26]. High-risk patients should be identified and provided with optimal medical therapy and monitoring for specific hormone syndromes. One of the most common acute side effects of PRRT is nausea and vomiting related to the use of renoprotective amino acids. This can be effectively prevented by premedication with anti-emetic medications [27].

10.3 SUBACUTE TOXICITIES

Subacute toxicities manifest from days to weeks after radionuclide therapy administration, usually related to radiation delivered to tumors, but also to off-target exposure. The specific toxicity profile will depend on the type of therapy and its biodistribution and retention.

10.3.1 PRRT FOR NET

PRRT is generally well tolerated. Fatigue following treatment is common and may last for a few weeks. Temporary, mild hair loss (generally grade 1) has been reported in 60% of patients after[177]Lu-DOTA-peptide therapy [27]. Patients with significant hormone-secretory symptoms may experience a temporary flare usually for a few days but is occasionally slightly more prolonged. Acute and subacute side effects are usually most severe after the first cycle [26]. Dose-limiting organs for PRRT are the kidneys and bone marrow. Subacute grade 3 or 4 hematological toxicities have been reported in up to 11% of patients [28]. Nadir usually occurs 4–6 weeks after therapy, but toxicity is generally mild and reversable within a few weeks [29].

10.3.2 ^{131}I MIBG FOR PHEOCHROMOCYTOMA AND PARAGANGLIOMA (PPGL)

For patients with functional disease, anti-hypertensive therapy typically requires alpha-adrenergic and beta-blockade to prevent acute hypertensive crisis and subacute clinical sequelae such as cerebrovascular hemorrhage. MIBG therapy is limited by hematological toxicity [20]. In a single-arm phase II trial, 68 adult PPGL patients were treated with up to two cycles of high specific activity ^{131}I-MIBG. The most common side effects were myelosuppression, nausea/vomiting and fatigue. Of significance, 72% of patients experienced ≥grade 3 hematotoxicity (41% thrombocytopenia, 41% leukopenia, 38% neutropenia and 21% anemia) and 25% required hematologic support. Other severe adverse events included pulmonary embolism in 3% (2/68). Nephrotoxicity was not reported in this trial [30].

10.3.3 [177]LU-PSMA FOR PROSTATE

Recently published prospective clinical trials have provided information on adverse effects of ^{177}Lu-PSMA-617 based on the phase III VISION trial [31] and phase II TheraP trial [32]. Fatigue, dry mouth and nausea were the most common subacute adverse events but were mainly of grade 1 or 2 severity. In the TheraP trial, Grade 3–4 adverse events occurred in 32 (33%) of 98 men in the ^{177}Lu-PSMA-617 group versus 45 (53%) of 85 men in the cabazitaxel group. However, grade 3–4 thrombocytopenia was more common with ^{177}Lu-PSMA-617 than with cabazitaxel (11% versus 0%), while grade 3–4 neutropenia was less common (4% versus 13%), with no episodes of febrile neutropenia (0% versus 8%) [32].

10.3.4 ^{131}I for Thyroid Cancer

Potential uncommon subacute side effects include dysgeusia (taste dysfunction) resulting from damage of the small mucous salivary glands in the vicinity of the taste buds and is usually a temporary side effect of ^{131}I therapy but may last for several weeks post-treatment [33].

10.3.5 ^{131}I Rituximab (Mabthera) for Lymphoma

The high expression of CD20 on B-lymphocytes makes this an attractive target for the treatment of both follicular and diffuse large B-cell lymphoma; this treatment has good evidence of efficacy [34]. Subacute toxicity is principally hematologic, but generally well tolerated. A phase II multicenter study with ^{131}I rituximab showed grade 4 thrombocytopenia occurring in 4% and grade 4 neutropenia in 16% of patients [34]. The median time to platelet nadir was 6 weeks, 7 weeks for neutrophils and 8 weeks for hemoglobin. Platelet nadirs were lower in patients with > 25% bone marrow involvement. In a study with 142 patients, the median time to platelet nadir was 5 weeks, 7 weeks for neutrophils and 5 weeks for hemoglobin, but no patient was hospitalized with infection, required intravenous antibiotics or had bleeding complications [34].

10.3.6 Bone-Seeking Radiopharmaceuticals (^{89}Sr, ^{153}Sm, ^{223}Ra)

Hematological toxicity of ^{89}SrCl is generally temporary and predominantly consists of mild myelosuppression [35]. The nadir usually occurs between the 12 and 16 weeks, showing resolution in the next six weeks, but depends significantly on the skeletal tumor extent and bone marrow reserve. For samarium-153 lexidronam pentasodium (^{153}Sm–EDTMP, Quadramet), bone marrow toxicity is mild in most patients. The platelet and white blood cell counts usually nadir in 3–5 weeks, recovering in 6–8 weeks after therapy [36]. Patients with severe grades of myelotoxicity usually had predisposing underlying conditions, including prior chemotherapy, extensive external beam radiotherapy (EBRT) or malignant bone marrow involvement [35]. Given the substantially shorter range of ^{223}Ra in tissues, hematological toxicity is expected to be less in comparison with β$^-$ emitters. Mild reversible myelosuppression occurs with a nadir in 2–4 weeks, usually resolving in 6 weeks after administration [35]. Diarrhea, nausea and vomiting may occur in ≥ 10% of cases [37].

10.4 LATE TOXICITIES

Late radiation effects are those that manifest months to years after treatment and that relate to either a progressive loss of function in a tissue or organ or are initiated by a genomic change that facilitates malignant transformation of irradiated cells .

The former effects are generally only seen at high cumulative radiation doses and are therefore relatively predictable, whereas the latter tend to occur as rare random events. Those that are dose-dependent are described as deterministic, while those that occur by chance are termed stochastic effects.

Most late effects from radionuclide therapies reflect off-target radiation exposure in areas with non-specific uptake or where normal cells also express the target. Radiation is passively delivered to bone marrow stem cells during blood circulation prior to uptake or excretion of the radiopharmaceutical. Therefore, rapid uptake by the tumor can reduce radiation exposure, whereas slow blood clearance due to low renal excretion may increase marrow exposure. Irradiation can also occur as a bystander effect due to radiopharmeceutical uptake or free radionuclide in bone lesions. Bystander effects are related to the type and energy of the particulate emissions.

Many of the current recommendations of radiation dose limits to normal tissues are based on extrapolation from data obtained from EBRT and ignore the fundamental differences that exist in the biological effects of internal particulate irradiation which include spatial heterogeneity of radiation dose, a much lower dose rate, the impact of the microenvironment and the varying biological effects of beta, alpha and Auger or conversion electron particles as well as host factors such as age [38]. Although the tools for measuring radiation dose to tumor and normal tissues are improving, much of what is considered dosimetry in terms of quantitative SPECT/CT [39] at multiple time points following therapy is, in fact, dose verification. While this may help to define dose–response relationships and safe dose limits to normal tissues, optimized planning of radionuclide therapy to avoid late toxicity while delivering as much radiation as possible to the tumor will likely require personalized prospective dosimetry. Therapeutic pairs with longer half-life PET radionuclides, such as $^{64}Cu/^{67}Cu$ [40] or $^{124}I/^{131}I$ [41], will enable improved understanding of the biological effects of radionuclide therapy and allow more accurate prescription prior to treatment. This will likely be important for selected patients with either impaired clearance of activity (e.g., renal failure) or with a very high tumor burden, who might need lower administered activity to avoid off-target toxicity or a higher administered activity to realize therapeutic benefit, respectively. The concept of "sink effect" is now being considered in the dosing of biological molecules that are effected by what is termed target-mediated drug distribution [42]. This is particularly relevant to the pharmacokinetics and biodistribution of agents with a high affinity for a specific target such as antibodies.

It is important to note that toxicities occur on the background radionuclide therapy that was delivered to patients often with metastatic disease and poor prognosis, with multiple lines of prior cancer treatment, some of which are independently known to be associated with cumulative and long-term toxicities, including induction of secondary malignancy. The generally low rates of severe late effects must be balanced against therapeutic benefits. The most important known late effects of the main types of radionuclide therapy in current use are detailed below.

10.4.1 Late Toxicities Related to PRRT

There have been a large number of studies documenting the efficacy and toxicity of PRRT [27]. The dominant concerns relate to therapy-related myeloid neoplasia (t-MN), presenting primarily as myelodysplastic syndrome (t-MDS), or subsequent or denovo acute myeloid leukemia (t-AML) [43], and long-term damage to the kidneys [44], which receive irradiation due to reabsorption of the radiopeptide by the megalin–cubilin transport system in the proximal convoluted tubules despite renoprotective amino acid solutions [45].

Of major concern for patients and clinicians is the risk of t-MN, which has been noted in most studies with adequate follow-up. A multicenter analysis in 807 patients using either ^{177}Lu or ^{90}Y agents reported a rate of just over 3% [46]. In a long-term follow-up of 1,631 patients receiving PRRT at the Bad Berka facility in Germany, there were 23 cases of t-MDS and 7 of t-AML, representing an overall t-MN rate of 1.8% with a median time to development of 43 months [47]. Another study identified 25 cases of t-MN among 521 patients (4.8%) treated with ^{177}Lu-DOT-ATATE PRRT with a median latency of 26 months [48], but this included patients treated with concurrent radiosensitizing chemotherapy (peptide receptor chemoradionuclide therapy (PRCRT)). A small series from France identified that prior alkylating treatments may be contributing in some patients [49]. This association was also suggested by a small prospective trial of 37 patients PRCRT with capecitabine and temozolomide in which the rate of MDS/AML was 8% [50]. The same group reported a cohort of 104 patients treated on various trials of PRCRT or PRRT with everolimus with a 6.7% incidence of t-MN [51]. They noted long overall survival across these trials. The exact cause or predictive factors are yet unknown, and underlying pre-existing biological or genetic susceptibility remains a possibility.

Concerns about the long-term risk of renal failure were initially raised in patients treated with ^{90}Y-DOTATOC without use of renoprotection [52]. In a recent systematic review that included 34 studies of over 5,000 patients followed for between 12 and 191 months, grade 3 or 4 renal impairment occurred in only <3% with these cases being primarily associated with ^{90}Y PRRT used alone or in combination with ^{177}Lu-based PRRT [53]. The occurrence of severe nephrotoxicity appears to be a rare event with ^{177}Lu-based PRRT [54,55].

Despite high uptake of PRRT agents in endocrine organs like the pituitary and adrenal medulla due to expression of somatostatin receptors, at least with ^{177}Lu-based peptides, late effects appear to be minimal and speak to the differential radiosensitivity of non-cycling cells compared to actively growing tumor cells [56].

10.4.2   MIBG for PPGL

There is some evidence of late toxicity in adults treated with ^{131}I-MIBG but this appears less frequent than in children treated with this agent for neuroblastoma, possibly reflecting the greater risks of radiation at younger ages. Second malignancies reported in neuroblastoma patients include leukemias and some soft tissue sarcomas [57]. Confounding causality factors in children include extensive prior chemotherapy and the use of radiotherapy to residual masses or as conditioning for bone marrow transplantation. For adult PPGL, a prospective single-arm phase II trial of high-specific-activity MIBG therapy involving 68 patients [58] showed a t-MDS rate of 4%, and leukemia of 3%, which are similar to the rates of t-MN following PRRT. No patients developed renal impairment on this trial. Despite the use of potassium iodide to block thyroid uptake of free ^{131}I, hypothyroidism is a recognized complication of MIBG therapy in both adults [59] and children [60]. This is readily corrected but ongoing monitoring is required.

10.4.3   PSMA for Prostate Cancer

Despite several prospective trials with impressive response rates when assessed biochemically [61–63], long-term follow-up of ^{177}Lu-PSMA has been relatively limited due to the modest overall survival of patients despite objective benefits. In longer-term follow-up of an extended cohort treated in a prospective phase II trial [64], early low-grade salivary toxicity had resolved in surviving patients and the mean reduction in glomerular filtration rate (GFR) was 11.7 mL/min in the 28 of 50 trial patients who had ^{51}Cr EDTA assessment. This appears higher than seen with PRRT and given that the median overall survival in this trial was only 13.3 months, the possibility of further later deterioration in renal function cannot be excluded. Of note, the mechanism of localization of PSMA ligands and somatostatin analogs differs and renoprotective amino acid infusions are not generally used for PSMA therapy. No MDS has been reported in these trials so far. A retrospective analysis of 145 patients found late grade 3–4 hematological toxicity in 18 (12%) patients, primarily anemia [65], but this is a common finding with advanced prostate cancer.

There is increasing interest in the use of alpha-emitting PSMA ligands to enhance response rates, or to treat resistance to ^{177}Lu-PSMA therapy. The higher radiobiological effects of alpha than beta particles may also have higher toxicity. A recent report of 26 patients treated with ^{225}Ac-PSMA showed more than one third had grade 3–4 hematological toxicity and 6 patients stopped treatment due to severe xerostomia [66]. Prior systemic treatments and advanced disease may have impacted marrow toxicity, but the relatively short survival of these patients may also underestimate its impact on the kidneys and duodenum if used earlier in the disease course or in patients with a higher likelihood of extended survival.

10.4.4 ^{131}I FOR THYROID CANCER

Radiation from the A-bomb in Japan was found to increase the risk of thyroid cancer only in individuals less than 20 years of age [67] but was not recapitulated in a large Swedish trial [68]. The Chernobyl accident exposed children and adolescents to relatively high levels of RAI and suggested that while there was a dose relationship to later development of thyroid cancer, this was heavily influenced by host and environmental factors with an individual or family history of thyroid disease and a low-iodine diet prior to exposure significantly increasing risk, whereas iodine supplementation after exposure decreased it. Late thyroid cancers were not observed in a study looking at the long-term outcomes of 215 children treated for differentiated thyroid cancer. Overall, of 15 patients who developed a second malignancy between 30 and 50 years after treatment, 11 had received radiation as part of their treatment [69]. Similarly, a study involving over 10,000 subjects in Sweden did not find an excess of thyroid cancer in patients treated with RAI for hyperthyroidism but did identify a time-dependent increase in gastric cancer [70]. While the stomach does receive incidental radiation exposure after RAI, Graves' autoimmune disease associated with atrophic gastritis is also at risk of gastric cancer. Another study demonstrated secondary cancers of the colon, salivary glands, and sarcoma with a dose relationship only for bone sarcomas [71]. Late hepatobiliary excretion of free RAI exposes the bowel to radiation and the salivary glands also concentrate RAI, so stochastic effects could explain the rare development of these cancers. The presence of bone metastases is an adverse prognostic indicator in thyroid cancer but there is evidence that RAI has a significant impact on disease control with >50% achieving a complete response with low short-term toxicity [72], emphasizing the need to balance concerns about uncommon late effects with important outcome benefits of this treatment.

There has been no evidence to suggest ovarian failure or impaired fertility in young females receiving RAI before 18 years of age [73]. Data from 10 thyroid cancer registries involving more than 6,000 women demonstrated no increase in the risk of breast cancer after RAI [74].

While uncommon, a slightly elevated risk of leukemia has been reported. Two cases were reported as part of the first series of thyroid cancer patients treated with RAI at the Montefiore Hospital (New York) in patients who received 13 and 20 therapeutic dosages (estimated activities of 53 and 64 GBq), respectively [9]. A Surveillance, Epidemiology and End-Results registry of >148,000 patients suggested an absolute risk difference of approximately 1 in 1,000 patients treated for 10 years [75]. Another study reported the median time to AML was 2.9 years, and that t-AML had a worse prognosis than de novo AML [76]. It is important to emphasize that the risk of secondary malignancies after RAI is overall exceptionally low. In each individual case, a risk-benefit analysis should be undertaken.

10.4.5 ^{131}I RITUXIMAB (MABTHERA) FOR LYMPHOMA

At a median follow-up of 23 months, there was a 5.5% rate of MDS with one progression to AML in a series of relapsed or refractory lymphoma patients treated with ^{131}I rituximab. Again, this must be balanced with the high objective response rate of 76% and poor prognosis of these patients without effective treatment [34]. Confounding factors were the prior use of chemotherapy and irradiation in many of these cases. There was a cumulative rate of hypothyroidism of 10%, likely reflecting RAI released from the labeled therapeutic agent. In a follow-up evaluation of patients who were retreated after relapse following a favorable prior response to ^{131}I Mabthera, an additional case of AML was recorded [77]. A subsequent trial in 16 patients reported hypothyroidism in 18% [78], but in this poor prognosis group, there was complete response in the lymphoma in all but one case at 3 months and sustained remission at a median of 44 months in 12 (75%) patients. Using a murine chimeric monoclonal antibody to CD20, tositumomab, radiolabeled with ^{131}I in a randomized control phase III trial comparing induction CHOP chemotherapy with and without radioimmunotherapy (RIT), there was a slightly higher rate of MDS/AML (3% versus 1%) but this was not statistically significant [79]. A phase III trial using a more myelotoxic chemotherapy with and without RIT reported a single case of MDS in each arm and the only case of AML occurred in the arm without radiation, an incidence of <1% in the RIT arm [80].

10.4.6 BONE-SEEKING RADIOPHARMACEUTICALS

The first agent to be tested for efficacy in relief of pain in a randomized control trial was ^{89}SrCl [14], but long-term toxicity was not reported. ^{153}Sm–EDTMP and ^{186}Re-HEDP [81] have proven effectiveness in controlling bone pain but limited toxicity beyond acute reductions in blood counts and a transient flare in symptoms have been observed. The limited survival of patients treated palliatively has constrained assessment of late effects. The newest agent ^{223}Ra, an alpha emitter, is delivered as multiple cycles of treatment and has been shown to prolong survival [82]. Longer-term follow-up revealed few persisting hematologic abnormalities and only 2 cases of AML were reported, both after 5–6 lines of treatment that may have contributed [83].

10.5 EXTRAVASATION

Inadvertent extravasation of radionuclide at the injection site into the subcutaneous space is a known complication of radionuclide therapy, albeit rare. This has, however, recently become an topic of significant interest in the United States where there has been a recommendation that extravasation becomes a reportable event to the regulatory authority [84].

While extravasation is a relatively common event with continuous IV infusions that are associated with cannulas sited for between hours and days, administration of radionuclides typically occurs within minutes of insertion of a secure line and demonstration of its patency. The infusion duration for both diagnostic and therapeutic radiopharmaceuticals is also typically short, and these procedures should be done under close medical supervision. These factors are likely to significantly reduce the likelihood of leakage into subcutaneous tissues, but the frequency of such events is currently unclear with most reports being anecdotal case reports. The lack of symptoms typically associated with small extravasations may introduce a reporting bias with cases associated with adverse outcomes arising from these episodes being more likely to be published than those without. Even with this caveat, most reports have not been associated with significant morbidity. For example, in a report of 2 cases receiving ^{223}Ra, a primarily alpha-emitting radionuclide, who developed unexplained edema in the arm used for infusion days to weeks after treatment, spontaneous resolution occurred without long-term effects [85]. Neither patient had evidence of extravasation acutely and, indeed, the authors of this study reported that their own post-treatment imaging of more than 180 patients treated with ^{223}Ra revealed no case of extravasation. These data were confirmed by real-time imaging of 15 ^{223}Ra infusions [86]. In the experience of the senior author (RJH) of thousands of therapeutic nuclear medicine procedures over the past 30 years, for which routine post-treatment imaging is performed at 24–48 hours, he has not observed any significant residual activity at the injection site, nor is he aware of development of a radionecrosis skin lesion as a late effect.

Although apparently uncommon, it is important to recognize that the deposition of a particle-emitting radionuclide into the subcutaneous tissues will both potentially limit its therapeutic effect by decreasing bioavailability to the tumor and deliver sufficient radiation to cause damage to the skin. Manifestations of this may include acute radiation changes such as erythema or desquamation,which can progress to ulceration over the area that can be difficult to heal. Most cases of poorly healing radionecrosis of skin have been associated with ^{90}Y, a relatively energetic beta emitter but even these appear to be rare, occurring in only 2 of 10 extravasation cases identified in a prior systematic review covering 8 publications [87]. The authors of this paper developed a complex protocol for management of suspected or proven extravasation that involved applying a cold compress to limit clearance until a surgical opinion could be obtained with a view to resection of the involved tissue but, thereafter, applying a warm compress to speed up lymphatic clearance if resection was not opted for. In our opinion, surgical excision seems excessive given the low rate of serious late effects.

As indicated above, prevention by insertion of a secure intravenous cannula and testing of its patency through flushing or drawing back of blood is much preferred in dealing with the consequences of extravasation. After an episode of extravasation of ^{131}I-MIBG, which was confirmed on post-treat scintigraphy, and that led to self-limiting erythema and desquamation, one group instituted a policy of confirming cannula patency by injecting a small activity of ^{99m}Tc pertechnetate prior to injection of the therapeutic radionuclide and later adapted their preventative measures to using probes over both arms to confirm free circulation of the therapeutic agent [88]. This paper assessed the radiation dose delivered to the dermis to be around 15 Gy with dependence on assumptions regarding the geometry of the extravasated dose and lymphatic clearance being required.

The subject of tissue clearance has recently been reviewed in some detail with evidence that the majority of currently used radionuclide therapies are relatively rapidly cleared via the lymphatic system and eventually localize in the tumor without significant late skin effects [89]. Warming of the extravasation site was recommended by the authors, although there is little direct evidence to support this suggestion. Infiltration of the skin with isotonic solutions and massage are other suggested maneuvers. The relatively rapid lymphatic clearance of ^{177}Lu-DOTATATE extravasation with mono-exponential curve fitting suggesting a tissue residence half-life of <80 minutes and subsequent accumulation at sites of known disease has been described [90]. The calculated dose to skin was around 10 Gy and not associated with adverse effects. Another case report of extravasation of ^{177}Lu-PSMA-617 treated extravasation with cooling rather than heating and also demonstrated clearance of subcutaneous tissues and accumulation in tumor sites on serial imaging within 20 hours of the extravasation event without reported late effects [91].

While lymphatic clearance of small molecules and beta-emitting radiopeptides appears to be of limited concern, larger biomolecules like monoclonal antibodies [92] and alpha-emitting radionuclides can cause late effects, including radionecrotic ulcers requiring skin grafting or late development of cutaneous malignancy [93]. Consequently, the European Association of Nuclear Medicine guideline on the use of ^{90}Y-ibritumomab tiuxetan (Zevalin) recommend local heating, massage and elevation of the site of extravasation [94].

In summary, much controversy exists about the frequency and significance of extravasation, but it appears to be either a very rare occurrence with good attention to infusion technique, or rarely associated with adverse consequences. In our opinion, if noted clinically or on imaging, probe measurements or imaging should be serially obtained to confirm clearance. While the benefits of heating and elevation remain uncertain [95], these are reasonable interventions to increase lymphatic flow. We would recommend that extravasation should be a reportable event if there is evidence of significant soft tissue retention beyond several hours, in which case a medical physicist should be engaged to estimate radiation dose to tissue [88], or if there is late development of a local complication.

REFERENCES

1. Blaufox, M.D., Becquerel and the discovery of radioactivity: early concepts. *Semin Nucl Med*, 1996. 26(3): pp. 145–154.
2. Blaufox, M.D., Radioactive artifacts: historical sources of modern radium contamination. *Semin Nucl Med*, 1988. 18(1): pp. 46–64.
3. Leenhouts, H.P. and M.J. Brugmans, An analysis of bone and head sinus cancers in radium dial painters using a two-mutation carcinogenesis model. *J Radiol Prot*, 2000. 20(2): pp. 169–188.
4. Parker, C. and O. Sartor, Radium-223 in prostate cancer. *N Engl J Med*, 2013. 369(17): pp. 1659–1660.
5. Saha, G.B., W.J. MacIntyre, and R.T. Go, Cyclotrons and positron emission tomography radiopharmaceuticals for clinical imaging. *Semin Nucl Med*, 1992. 22(3): pp. 150–161.

6. Joliot, F. and I. Curie, Artificial production of a new kind of radio-element. *Nature*, 1934. 133(3354): pp. 201–202.

7. Fahey, F.H., F.D. Grant, and J.H. Thrall, Saul Hertz, MD, and the birth of radionuclide therapy. *EJNMMI Phys*, 2017. 4(1): p. 15.

8. Hertz, S. and A. Roberts, Radioactive iodine in the study of thyroid physiology; the use of radioactive iodine therapy in hyperthyroidism. *J Am Med Assoc*, 1946. 131: pp. 81–86.

9. Siegel, E., The beginnings of radioiodine therapy of metastatic thyroid carcinoma: a memoir of Samuel M. Seidlin, M. D. (1895–1955) and his celebrated patient. *Cancer Biother Radiopharm*, 1999. 14(2): pp. 71–79.

10. Seidlin, S.M., L.D. Marinelli, and E. Oshry, Radioactive iodine therapy; effect on functioning metastases of adenocarcinoma of the thyroid. *J Am Med Assoc*, 1946. 132(14): pp. 838–847.

11. Seidlin, S.M., et al., Acute myeloid leukemia following prolonged iodine-131 therapy for metastatic thyroid carcinoma. *Science*, 1956. 123(3201): pp. 800–801.

12. Steinkamp, R.C., J.H. Lawrence, and J.L. Born, Long term experiences with the use of P-32 in the treatment of chronic lymphocytic leukemia. *J Nucl Med*, 1963. 4: pp. 92–105.

13. Pecher, C., Biological investigations with radioactive calcium and strontium. Preliminary report on the use of radioactive strontium in the treatment of metastatic bone cancer. *Univ Calif Pub Pharmacol*, 1942. 11: pp. 117–139.

14. Lewington, V.J., et al., A prospective, randomised double-blind crossover study to examine the efficacy of strontium-89 in pain palliation in patients with advanced prostate cancer metastatic to bone. *Eur J Cancer*, 1991. 27(8): pp. 954–958.

15. Pandit-Taskar, N., M. Batraki, and C.R. Divgi, Radiopharmaceutical therapy for palliation of bone pain from osseous metastases. J Nucl Med. 2004. 45(8): pp. 1358–1365.

16. Pollen, J.J., K.F. Witztum, and W.L. Ashburn, The flare phenomenon on radionuclide bone scan in metastatic prostate cancer. *AJR Am J Roentgenol*, 1984. 142(4): pp. 773–776.

17. Salner, A.L., et al., Lutetium Lu-177 dotatate flare reaction. *Adv Radiat Oncol*, 2021. 6(1): p. 100623.

18. Mirrakhimov, A.E., et al., Tumor lysis syndrome: A clinical review. *World J Crit Care Med*, 2015. 4(2): pp. 130–138.

19. Huang, K., W. Brenner, and V. Prasad, Tumor lysis syndrome: a rare but serious complication of radioligand therapies. *J Nucl Med*, 2019. 60(6): pp. 752–755.

20. Gonias, S., et al., Phase II study of high-dose [131I]metaiodobenzylguanidine therapy for patients with metastatic pheochromocytoma and paraganglioma. *J Clin Oncol*, 2009. 27(25): pp. 4162–4168.

21. Makis, W., K. McCann, and A.J. McEwan, The challenges of treating paraganglioma patients with (177)Lu-DOTATATE PRRT: catecholamine crises, tumor lysis syndrome and the need for modification of treatment protocols. *Nucl Med Mol Imaging*, 2015. 49(3): pp. 223–230.

22. Kong, G., et al., Efficacy of peptide receptor radionuclide therapy for functional metastatic paraganglioma and pheochromocytoma. *J Clin Endocrinol Metab*, 2017. 102(9): pp. 3278–3287.

23. Yadav, S.K., et al., Lutetium therapy-induced carcinoid crisis: a case report and review of literature. *J Cancer Res Ther*, 2020. 16(Supplement): pp. S206–S208.

24. Davi, M.V., et al., Carcinoid crisis induced by receptor radionuclide therapy with 90Y-DOTATOC in a case of liver metastases from bronchial neuroendocrine tumor (atypical carcinoid). *J Endocrinol Invest*, 2006. 29(6): pp. 563–567.

25. de Keizer, B., et al., Hormonal crises following receptor radionuclide therapy with the radiolabeled somatostatin analogue [177Lu-DOTA0,Tyr3]octreotate. *Eur J Nucl Med Mol Imaging*, 2008. 35(4): pp. 749–755.

26. Del Olmo-Garcia, M.I., et al., Prevention and management of hormonal crisis during theragnosis with LU-DOTA-TATE in neuroendocrine tumors. A systematic review and approach proposal. *J Clin Med*, 2020. 9(7): p. 2203.

27. Hicks, R.J., et al., ENETS consensus guidelines for the standards of care in neuroendocrine neoplasia: peptide receptor radionuclide therapy with radiolabeled somatostatin analogues. *Neuroendocrinology*, 2017. 105(3): pp. 295–309.

28. Bergsma, H., et al., Subacute haematotoxicity after PRRT with (177)Lu-DOTA-octreotate: prognostic factors, incidence and course. *Eur J Nucl Med Mol Imaging*, 2016. 43(3): pp. 453–463.

29. Frilling, A., et al., Recommendations for management of patients with neuroendocrine liver metastases. *Lancet Oncol*, 2014. 15(1): pp. e8–e21.

30. Pryma, D.A., et al., Efficacy and safety of high-specific-activity (131)I-MIBG therapy in patients with advanced pheochromocytoma or paraganglioma. *J Nucl Med*, 2019. 60(5): pp. 623–630.

31. Sartor, O., et al., Lutetium-177-PSMA-617 for metastatic castration-resistant prostate cancer. *N Engl J Med*, 2021. 385(12): pp. 1091–1103.
32. Hofman, M.S., et al., [(177)Lu]Lu-PSMA-617 versus cabazitaxel in patients with metastatic castration-resistant prostate cancer (TheraP): a randomised, open-label, phase 2 trial. *Lancet*, 2021. 397(10276): pp. 797–804.
33. Avram, A.M., et al., Management of differentiated thyroid cancer: The standard of care. J Nucl Med, 2022. 63(2): pp. 189–195.
34. Leahy, M.F., et al., Multicenter phase II clinical study of iodine-131-rituximab radioimmunotherapy in relapsed or refractory indolent non-Hodgkin's lymphoma. *J Clin Oncol*, 2006. 24(27): pp. 4418–4425.
35. Manafi-Farid, R., et al., Targeted palliative radionuclide therapy for metastatic bone pain. *J Clin Med*, 2020. 9(8): p. 2622.
36. Bodei, L., et al., EANM procedure guideline for treatment of refractory metastatic bone pain. *Eur J Nucl Med Mol Imaging*, 2008. 35(10): pp. 1934–1940.
37. Florimonte, L., L. Dellavedova, and L.S. Maffioli, Radium-223 dichloride in clinical practice: a review. *Eur J Nucl Med Mol Imaging*, 2016. 43(10): pp. 1896–1909.
38. Wahl, R.L., et al., Normal-tissue tolerance to radiopharmaceutical therapies, the knowns and the unknowns. *J Nucl Med*, 2021. 62(Suppl 3): pp. 23S–35S.
39. Jackson, P.A., et al., An automated voxelized dosimetry tool for radionuclide therapy based on serial quantitative SPECT/CT imaging. *Med Phys*, 2013. 40(11): p. 112503.
40. Hicks, R.J., et al., Cu-SARTATE PET imaging of patients with neuroendocrine tumors demonstrates high tumor uptake and retention, potentially allowing prospective dosimetry for peptide receptor radionuclide therapy. *J Nucl Med*, 2019. 60(6): pp. 777–785.
41. Kuker, R., M. Sztejnberg, and S. Gulec, I-124 imaging and dosimetry. *Mol Imaging Radionucl Ther*, 2017. 26(Suppl 1): pp. 66–73.
42. Mager, D.E., Target-mediated drug disposition and dynamics. *Biochem Pharmacol*, 2006. 72(1): pp. 1–10.
43. Bodei, L., et al., Myeloid neoplasms after chemotherapy and PRRT: myth and reality. *Endocr Relat Cancer*, 2016. 23(8): pp. C1–C7.
44. Bodei, L., et al., Long-term evaluation of renal toxicity after peptide receptor radionuclide therapy with 90Y-DOTATOC and 177Lu-DOTATATE: the role of associated risk factors. *Eur J Nucl Med Mol Imaging*, 2008. 35(10): pp. 1847–1856.
45. Rolleman, E.J., et al., Kidney protection during peptide receptor radionuclide therapy with somatostatin analogues. *Eur J Nucl Med Mol Imaging*, 2010. 37(5): pp. 1018–1031.
46. Bodei, L., et al., Long-term tolerability of PRRT in 807 patients with neuroendocrine tumours: the value and limitations of clinical factors. *Eur J Nucl Med Mol Imaging*, 2015. 42(1): pp. 5–19.
47. Chantadisai, M., H.R. Kulkarni, and R.P. Baum, Therapy-related myeloid neoplasm after peptide receptor radionuclide therapy (PRRT) in 1631 patients from our 20 years of experiences: prognostic parameters and overall survival. *Eur J Nucl Med Mol Imaging*, 2021. 48(5): pp. 1390–1398.
48. Goncalves, I., et al., Characteristics and outcomes of therapy-related myeloid neoplasms after peptide receptor radionuclide/chemoradionuclide therapy (PRRT/PRCRT) for metastatic neuroendocrine neoplasia: a single-institution series. *Eur J Nucl Med Mol Imaging*, 2019. 46(9): pp. 1902–1910.
49. Brieau, B., et al., High risk of myelodysplastic syndrome and acute myeloid leukemia after 177Lu-octreotate PRRT in NET patients heavily pretreated with alkylating chemotherapy.*Endocr Relat Cancer*, 2016. 23(5): pp. L17–L23.
50. Kesavan, M., et al., Long-term hematologic toxicity of 177Lu-octreotate-capecitabine-temozolomide therapy of GEPNET. *Endocr Relat Cancer*, 2021. 28(7): pp. 521–527.
51. Kennedy, K.R., et al., Long-term survival and toxicity in patients with neuroendocrine tumors treated with ¹⁷⁷Lu- octreotate peptide radionuclide therapy. *Cancer*, 2022. 128(11): pp. 2182–2192.
52. Cybulla, M., S.M. Weiner, and A. Otte, End-stage renal disease after treatment with 90Y-DOTATOC. *Eur J Nucl Med*, 2001. 28(10): pp. 1552–1554.
53. Stolniceanu, C.R., et al., Nephrotoxicity/renal failure after therapy with 90Yttrium- and 177Lutetium-radiolabeled somatostatin analogs in different types of neuroendocrine tumors: a systematic review. *Nucl Med Commun*, 2020. 41(7): pp. 601–617.
54. Sabet, A., et al., Accurate assessment of long-term nephrotoxicity after peptide receptor radionuclide therapy with (177)Lu-octreotate. *Eur J Nucl Med Mol Imaging*, 2014. 41(3): pp. 505–510.
55. Kashyap, R., et al., Rapid blood clearance and lack of long-term renal toxicity of 177Lu-DOTATATE enables shortening of renoprotective amino acid infusion. *Eur J Nucl Med Mol Imaging*, 2013. 40(12): pp. 1853–1860.

56. Elston, M.S., et al., Pituitary function following peptide receptor radionuclide therapy for neuroendocrine tumours. *Cancer Med*, 2021. 10(23): pp. 8405–8411.
57. Garaventa, A., et al., Second malignancies in children with neuroblastoma after combined treatment with 131I-metaiodobenzylguanidine. *Cancer*, 2003. 97(5): pp. 1332–1338.
58. Pryma, D.A., et al., Efficacy and safety of high-specific-activity ^{131}I-MIBG therapy in patients with advanced pheochromocytoma or paraganglioma. J Nucl Med, 2019. 60(5): pp. 623–630.
59. Shapiro, B., et al., Radiopharmaceutical therapy of malignant pheochromocytoma with [131I]metaiodobenzylguanidine: results from ten years of experience. *J Nucl Biol Med,* 1991. 35(4): pp. 269–276.
60. van Santen, H.M., et al., High incidence of thyroid dysfunction despite prophylaxis with potassium iodide during (131)I-meta-iodobenzylguanidine treatment in children with neuroblastoma. *Cancer*, 2002. 94(7): pp. 2081–2089.
61. Hofman, M.S., et al., [177Lu]-PSMA-617 radionuclide treatment in patients with metastatic castration-resistant prostate cancer (LuPSMA trial): a single-centre, single-arm, phase 2 study. *Lancet Oncol*, 2018. 19(6): pp. 825–833.
62. Sartor, O., et al., Lutetium-177-PSMA-617 for Metastatic Castration-Resistant Prostate Cancer. *N Engl J Med*, 2021. 385(12): pp. 1091–1103.
63. Hofman, M.S., et al., [177 Lu]Lu-PSMA-617 versus cabazitaxel in patients with metastatic castration-resistant prostate cancer (TheraP): a randomised, open-label, phase 2 trial. *Lancet*, 2021. 397(10276): pp. 797–804.
64. Violet, J., et al., Long-term follow-up and outcomes of retreatment in an expanded 50-patient single-center phase II prospective trial of 177Lu-PSMA-617 theranostics in metastatic castration-resistant prostate cancer. *J Nucl Med*, 2020. 61(6): pp. 857–865.
65. Rahbar, K., et al., German multicenter study investigating 177Lu-PSMA-617 radioligand therapy in advanced prostate cancer patients. *J Nucl Med*, 2017. 58(1): pp. 85–90.
66. Feuerecker, B., et al., Activity and adverse events of actinium-225-PSMA-617 in advanced metastatic castration-resistant prostate cancer after failure of lutetium-177-PSMA. *Eur Urol*, 2021. 79(3): pp. 343–350.
67. Wood, J.W., et al., Thyroid carcinoma in atomic bomb survivors Hiroshima and Nagasaki, *Am J Epidemiol*, 1969. 89(1): pp. 4–14.
68. Hall, P. and L.E. Holm, Late consequences of radioiodine for diagnosis and therapy in Sweden. *Thyroid*, 1997. 7(2): pp. 205–208.
69. Hay, I.D., et al., Long-term outcome in 215 children and adolescents with papillary thyroid cancer treated during 1940 through 2008. *World J Surg*, 2010. 34(6): pp. 1192–1202.
70. Holm, L.E., et al., Cancer risk after iodine-131 therapy for hyperthyroidism. *J Natl Cancer Inst*, 1991. 83(15): pp. 1072–1077.
71. Rubino, C., et al., Second primary malignancies in thyroid cancer patients. *Br J Cancer*, 2003. 89(9): pp. 1638–1644.
72. Petrich, T., et al., Outcome after radioiodine therapy in 107 patients with differentiated thyroid carcinoma and initial bone metastases: side-effects and influence of age. *Eur J Nucl Med*, 2001. 28(2): pp. 203–208.
73. Nies, M., et al., Long-term effects of radioiodine treatment on female fertility in survivors of childhood differentiated thyroid carcinoma. *Thyroid*, 2020. 30(8): pp. 1169–1176.
74. Reiners, C., et al., Breast cancer after treatment of differentiated thyroid cancer with radioiodine in young females: what we know and how to investigate open questions. Review of the literature and results of a multi-registry survey. *Front Endocrinol (Lausanne)*, 2020. 11: p. 381.
75. Molenaar, R.J., et al., Risk of hematologic malignancies after radioiodine treatment of well-differentiated thyroid cancer. *J Clin Oncol*, 2018. 36(18): pp. 1831–1839.
76. Oluwasanjo, A., et al., Therapy-related acute myeloid leukemia following radioactive iodine treatment for thyroid cancer. *Cancer Causes Control*, 2016. 27(1): pp. 143–146.
77. Bishton, M.J., et al., Repeat treatment with iodine-131-rituximab is safe and effective in patients with relapsed indolent B-cell non-Hodgkin's lymphoma who had previously responded to iodine-131-rituximab. *Ann Oncol*, 2008. 19(9): pp. 1629–1633.
78. Kruger, P.C., J.P. Cooney, and J.H. Turner, Iodine-131 rituximab radioimmunotherapy with BEAM conditioning and autologous stem cell transplant salvage therapy for relapsed/refractory aggressive non-Hodgkin lymphoma. *Cancer Biother Radiopharm*, 2012. 27(9): pp. 552–560.

79. Press, O.W., et al., Phase III randomized intergroup trial of CHOP plus rituximab compared with CHOP chemotherapy plus (131)iodine-tositumomab for previously untreated follicular non-Hodgkin lymphoma: SWOG S0016. *J Clin Oncol*, 2013. 31(3): pp. 314–320.

80. Vose, J.M., et al., Phase III randomized study of rituximab/carmustine, etoposide, cytarabine, and melphalan (BEAM) compared with iodine-131 tositumomab/BEAM with autologous hematopoietic cell transplantation for relapsed diffuse large B-cell lymphoma: results from the BMT CTN 0401 trial. *J Clin Oncol*, 2013. 31(13): pp. 1662–1668.

81. Paes, F.M. and A.N. Serafini, Systemic metabolic radiopharmaceutical therapy in the treatment of metastatic bone pain. *Semin Nucl Med*, 2010. 40(2): pp. 89–104.

82. Parker, C., et al., Alpha emitter radium-223 and survival in metastatic prostate cancer. *N Engl J Med*, 2013. 369(3): pp. 213–223.

83. Jacene, H., et al., Hematologic toxicity from radium-223 therapy for bone metastases in castration-resistant prostate cancer: risk factors and practical considerations. *Clin Genitourin Cancer*, 2018. 16(4): pp. e919–e926.

84. Goans, R.E., A forum on extravasation in nuclear medicine. *Health Phys*, 2022. 122(4): p. 518.

85. Frantellizzi, V., et al., Analysis of unusual adverse effects after radium-223 dichloride administration. *Curr Radiopharm*, 2020. 13(2): pp. 159–163.

86. Wright, C.L., et al., Real-time scintigraphic assessment of intravenous radium-223 administration for quality control. *Biomed Res Int*, 2015. 2015: p. 324708.

87. van der Pol, J., et al., Consequences of radiopharmaceutical extravasation and therapeutic interventions: a systematic review. *Eur J Nucl Med Mol Imaging*, 2017. 44(7): pp. 1234–1243.

88. Bonta, D.V., R.K. Halkar, and N. Alazraki, Extravasation of a therapeutic dose of 131I-metaiodobenzylguanidine: prevention, dosimetry, and mitigation. *J Nucl Med*, 2011. 52(9): pp. 1418–1422.

89. Arveschoug, A.K., et al., Extravasation of [^{177}Lu]Lu-DOTATOC: case report and discussion. *EJNMMI Res*, 2020. 10(1): p. 68.

90. Maucherat, B., et al., Effective management of 177Lu-DOTA0-Tyr3-octreotate extravasation. *Clin Nucl Med*, 2021. 46(2): pp. 144–145.

91. Schlenkhoff, C.D., M. Essler, and H. Ahmadzadehfar, Possible treatment approach to an extravasation of 177Lu-PSMA-617. *Clin Nucl Med*, 2017. 42(8): pp. 639–640.

92. Williams, G., et al., Extravazation of therapeutic yttrium-90-ibritumomab tiuxetan (zevalin): a case report. *Cancer Biother Radiopharm*, 2006. 21(2): pp. 101–105.

93. Benjegerdes, K.E., S.C. Brown, and C.D. Housewright, Focal cutaneous squamous cell carcinoma following radium-223 extravasation. *Proc (Bayl Univ Med Cent)*, 2017. 30(1): pp. 78–79.

94. Tennvall, J., et al., EANM procedure guideline for radio-immunotherapy for B-cell lymphoma with 90Y-radiolabelled ibritumomab tiuxetan (Zevalin). *Eur J Nucl Med Mol Imaging*, 2007. 34(4): pp. 616–622.

95. Martin, C.J., et al., Guidance on prevention of unintended and accidental radiation exposures in nuclear medicine. *J Radiol Prot*, 2019. 39(3): pp. 665–695.

Part 3

Radiation Chemistry and Physics

11 Radionuclide Production

Gokce Engudar, Valery Radchenko, and Thomas J. Ruth

11.1 INTRODUCTION

As described in an earlier chapter, the concept of theranostics involves coupling, or pairing, diagnostic radiotracers labeled with radionuclides suitable for imaging with the same or similar radiotracer labeled with radionuclides that can deliver a therapeutic dose of radiation to the target area. The concept for theranostic pairs is shown in Figure 11.1. In the ideal case, theranostic isotope pairs are composed of isotopes of the same element. For example, $^{123/124}$I and ^{131}I [1] would be ideal as long as the targeting compound to which the radionuclides are attached can be used for both imaging and therapy. The terbium isotope series (^{149,152,155,161}Tb) [2] would be another situation where imaging and therapy complexes would be the same as that of $^{61/64}$Cu and ^{67}Cu [3,4]. In the case of element-equivalent theranostic pairs, there is no doubt that the biodistribution of both diagnostic and therapeutic complexes is identical due to the chemical equivalence of both radiotracers. In some instances, a single radioisotope can be used for both imaging and therapy. Examples include ^{131}I, ^{177}Lu and ^{67}Cu, all of which decay via both photon- and particle-emitting pathways (Figure 11.1).

In the event that suitable isotopes of the same element are not available, the next best pairing approach is to use isotope pairs from the same chemical family. Examples of this approach include using ^{99m}Tc for imaging and either ^{186}Re or ^{188}Re as the therapeutic isotope [5]. Because they are in the same chemical family, similar binding motifs can be used. However, the same chemical properties do not guarantee the same in vivo behavior due to small differences in oxidation states, potential and atomic/ionic size. An extreme pairing example include the use of ^{18}F and ^{211}At. Even though they are considered halogens, their respective chemical properties could not be more extreme with astatine having seven oxidation states including At$^+$ [6,7].

Regardless of the radionuclide pairs, their production and application need to consider the following concepts:

Half-life, decay mode/branching ratios, chemical purity, radioisotopic and radiochemical purity, specific and molar activity, chemical binding and feasibility of production and distribution at clinical quantities.

In many respects, these topics seem self-evident, but it is important to appreciate the underlying issues so that the development of new approaches to diagnose and treatment move forward in a realistic manner.

- Half-life – a balance of length to allow for radiopharmaceutical synthesis, distribution logistics and patient dose.
- Decay mode/branching ratio – prevalence of preferred decay for diagnostic/therapeutic application.
- Chemical purity – the need for chemical purity is based on the fact that very small quantities of materials are used, and any excess chemicals can lower the efficiency with which the delivery system can operate.

DOI: 10.1201/9781003250913-14

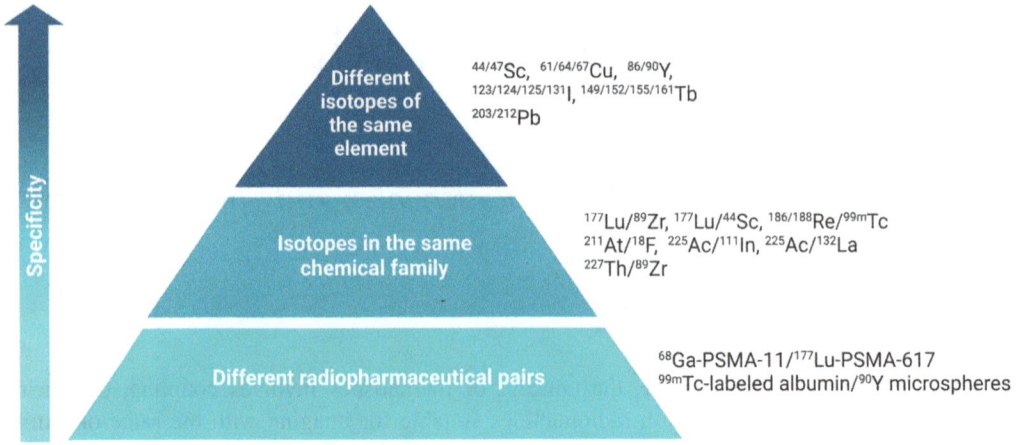

FIGURE 11.1 Concept for theranostic pairs – therapeutic and diagnostic radionuclides.

- Radioisotopic and radiochemical purity – for both imaging and therapy- it is important that there are no extraneous isotopes or other radionuclidic species that can interfere with the ability to identify the site of disease and to ensure that the optimal radiation dose is delivered to that site.
- Specific and molar activity – the quantity of radioactivity per mass of element can impact the ability to combine the radioactive isotope to the appropriate molecule(s) as well as deliver sufficient radioactivity for imaging and/or the cell killing power to the site [8].
- Chemical binding – understanding the nature of the chemical interaction between isotope, binding motif and targeting compound is very important.
- Feasibility of production and distribution at clinical quantities – there are a number of exciting radionuclides that have been identified by their physical characteristics as potential candidates for use in therapy. While these entities should be explored, the possibility of producing sufficient quantities on a routine basis should be included in the decision process. This includes availability of starting materials and post-processing, including radiochemical yields of the final products.

11.2 PRODUCTION

For the most part, radionuclides suitable for imaging are "proton" rich and decay via positron emission or electron capture. There are a few cases where the imageable photon occurs within the metastable sate of an radionuclide, as famously demonstrated by ^{99m}Tc [9].

Typically, the production of these radionuclides occurs via proton-induced reactions such as (p,n), (p,2n), (p,pn) or (p,α). These reactions are typically performed at lower proton energies, <20 MeV [10].

As of 2023, the most widely used radionuclides for imaging are ^{99m}Tc [9,11] and ^{18}F [12], with emerging community interests in ^{68}Ga [13,14] and ^{89}Zr [15] and perhaps ^{64}Cu [16,17] and ^{123}I [18,19]. While ^{99m}Tc and ^{68}Ga can be produced from, ^{99}Mo/^{99m}Tc and ^{68}Ge/^{68}Ga generators, respectively, ^{68}Ga is becoming a companion diagnostic for some therapeutic nuclides such as ^{177}Lu and ^{225}Ac. With the increasing demand for ^{68}Ga, there are efforts underway to implement direct production via the ^{68}Zn (p,n)^{68}Ga reaction [20,21]. While ^{99m}Tc has also been produced at TBq quantities using the ^{100}Mo (p,2n) transformation, and is still the most widely used radionuclide in nuclear medicine, it has not been widely used with a therapeutic entity. Further representations for proposed imaging radionuclides are presented in Table 11.1 along with the relevant routes of production.

TABLE 11.1

Imaging Radionuclides

Radionuclide	Half-Life	Decay Mode	Emission Energy (keV)	Production Method[*]	Reaction	Ref
^{18}F	109.8 min	β^+ (97%) EC (3%)	$E_{\beta^+\,max} = 633$ $E_{\beta^+\,mean} = 250$	accelerator	$^{18}O(p,n)\ ^{18}F$ $(H_2{}^{18}O,\ ^{18}O_2\ targets)$	[22]
^{44}Sc	3.97 h	β^+ (94%) EC (6%)	$E_{\beta^+\,max} = 1474$ $E_{\beta^+\,mean} = 632$ $E_\gamma = 1157$	accelerator $^{44}Ti/^{44}Sc$ generator	$^{nat}Ca(p,xn)\ ^{44}Sc\ (^{44m/47}Sc)$ $^{44}Ca(p,n)\ ^{44}Sc$ (E < 18 MeV) $^{44}Ca(d,2n)\ ^{44}Sc$ $^{45}Sc(p,2n)\ ^{44}Ti$ $^{44}Ti/^{44}Sc$ generator $^{51}V(p,2p6n)\ ^{44}Ti$ $^{54}Fe(p,^{11}B)\ ^{44}Ti$	[23, 24]
^{61}Cu	3.35 h	β^+ (62%) EC (38%)	$E_{\beta^+\,max} = 1159$ $E_{\beta^+\,mean} = 500$ (61%) $E_\gamma = 283$ (13%), 656 (10%)	accelerator	$^{61}Ni(p,n)\ ^{61}Cu$ (E = 19 MeV) $^{64}Zn(p,\alpha)\ ^{61}Cu$ $^{62}Ni(p,2n)\ ^{61}Cu$ $^{60}Ni(d,n)\ ^{61}Cu$ $^{58}Ni(\alpha,p)\ ^{61}Cu$ $^{59}Co(\alpha,2n)\ ^{61}Cu$	[17, 25]
^{64}Cu	12.7 h	β^+ (18%) EC (44%) β^- (38%)	$E_{\beta^+\,max} = 653$ $E_{\beta^+\,mean} = 278$ $E_{\beta^-\,mean} = 191$ (38%)	neutron source and accelerator	$^{64}Zn(n,p)\ ^{64}Cu$ $^{63}Cu(n,\gamma)\ ^{64}Cu$ $^{64}Ni(p,n)\ ^{64}Cu$ (E = 5–20 MeV) $^{64}Ni(d,2n)\ ^{64}Cu$ (E = 19 MeV) $^{nat}Zn(p,xn)\ ^{64}Cu$	[17, 22]
^{68}Ga	67.7 min	β^+ (89%) EC (11%)	$E_{\beta^+\,max} = 1899$ $E_{\beta^+\,mean} = 830$	accelerator $^{68}Ge/^{68}Ga$ generator	$^{68}Zn(p,n)\ ^{68}Ga$ (E = 12 MeV) $^{69}Ga(p,2n)\ ^{68}Ge$ (E = 23 MeV) $^{65}Cu(\alpha,n)\ ^{68}Ga$ $^{68}Ge/^{68}Ga$ generator $^{nat}Ga(p,xn)\ ^{68}Ge$	[26, 27]

(Continued)

TABLE 11.1 (Continued)
Imaging Radionuclides

Radionuclide	Half-Life	Decay Mode	Emission Energy (keV)	Production Method*	Reaction	Ref
					^{71}Ga(p,4n) ^{68}Ge ^{66}Zn(α,2n) ^{68}Ge	
^{86}Y	14.7 h	β^+ (32%) EC (68%)	$E_{\beta^+ max} = 1481$ $E_{\beta^+ mean} = 664$ $E_\gamma = 443$ (17%), 627 (33%)	accelerator	^{86}Sr(p,n) ^{86}Y ^{86}Sr(d,2n) ^{86}Y ^{88}Sr(p,3n) ^{86}Y ^{89}Sr(p,4n) ^{86}Zr ^{nat}Rb(^{3}He,xn) ^{86}Y ^{85}Rb(α,3n) ^{86}Y ^{90}Zr(p,αn) ^{86}Y ^{nat}Zr(p,x) ^{86}Y	[28]
^{89}Zr	78.4 h	β^+ (23%) EC (77%)	$E_{\beta^+ max} = 902$ $E_{\beta^+ mean} = 396$	accelerator	^{89}Y(p,n) ^{89}Zr (E = 13 - 19 MeV) ^{89}Y(d,2n) ^{89}Zr (E = 5.6 MeV)	[15, 29]
^{99m}Tc	6.0 h	EC (98%)	$E_\gamma = 140$	neutron source, accelerator and ^{99}Mo/^{99m}Tc generator	^{235}U(n,f) (6.07%) ^{99}Mo ^{98}Mo(n,γ) ^{99}Mo ^{100}Mo(γ,n) ^{99}Mo ^{96}Zr(α,n) ^{99}Mo ^{102}Ru(n,α) ^{99}Mo ^{99}Mo/^{99m}Tc generator ^{100}Mo(p,2n) ^{99m}Tc	[30]
^{111}In	2.8 days	EC (100%)	$E_\gamma = 171$ (91%), 245 (94%)	accelerator	^{113}Cd(p,3n) ^{111}In ^{112}Cd(p,2n) ^{111}In ^{111}Cd(p,n) ^{111}In ^{111}Cd(d,2n) ^{111}In ^{110}Cd(d,n) ^{111}In ^{109}Ag(^{4}He,2n) ^{111}In Sb spallation	[31]

	Half-life	Decay mode	Energy (keV)	Production method	Production reactions	Ref.
^{123}I	13.2 h	EC (97%)	E_γ = 159 (83%)	accelerator	^{123}Te(p,n) ^{123}I ^{124}Te(p,2n) ^{123}I ^{127}I(p,5n) ^{123}Xe (EC, β^+, 2.1 h) ^{123}I ^{124}Xe(p,2n) ^{123}Cs ^{123}Xe ^{123}I ^{124}Xe(p,pn) ^{123}Xe ^{123}I ^{124}Xe(p,2p) ^{123}I ^{124}Xe(p,x) ^{123}I	[27,32]
^{124}I	4.2 days	β^+ (23%) EC (77%)	$E_{\beta^+, max}$ = 2135 (11%), 1532 (11%) $E_{\beta^+, mean}$ = 819 E_γ = 603 (63%)	accelerator	^{124}Te(p,n) ^{124}I (E = 5–20 MeV) ^{124}Te(d,2n) ^{124}I (E = 5–20 MeV) ^{125}Te(p,2n) ^{124}I (E = 15–30 MeV)	[33]
^{152}Tb	17.5 h	β^+ (18%) EC	$E_{\beta^+, mean}$ = 1140 E_γ = 344 (57%)	accelerator	^{nat}Nd(^{12}C,xn) ^{152}Dy ^{152}Tb ^{155}Gd(p,4n) ^{152}Tb high-energy proton spallation of Ta	[2,34]
^{155}Tb	5.32 days	EC	E_γ = 87 (32%), 105 (25%)	accelerator	^{155}Tb by ISOL facility (ISAC) at TRIUMF ^{155}Gd(p,n) ^{155}Tb ^{154}Gd(d,n) ^{155}Tb ^{159}Tb(p,x) (E > 50 MeV) ^{159}Tb(p,5n) ^{155}Dy (ε, 9.9 h) ^{155}Tb ^{nat}Gd(d,nx) ^{152,155}Tb	[35–37]
^{203}Pb	51.9 h	EC	E_γ = 279 (81%),	accelerator	^{203}Tl(p,n) ^{203}Pb	[38]

* Production method: Accelerator refers to cyclotrons that are capable of accelerating protons, deuterons and alpha particles to produce radionuclides via (p,n), (p,pn), (p,xn), (p,α), (d,n), (α,n) and (^{3}He, n) reactions, and linear accelerators (linacs) that can be used to produce radionuclides via (γ,n) reaction. Neutron source refers to reactors and a number of new approaches using electron linear accelerators (e-linacs) or other devices that are capable of producing neutrons, to produce radionuclides via (n,γ) and (n,α) reactions.

The production of β^- radionuclides is typically performed via (n,γ) reactions or fission [39] (Table 11.2). The challenges with this approach are associated with the low specific activity (SA) inherent with having target and product being the same element (e.g., ^{176}Lu $(n,\gamma)^{177}$Lu).

Auger electron emitters are often proton-rich nuclei, while alpha emitters are generally of high mass and are often derived from naturally occurring elements [40] (Table 11.3). One of the main advantages in using Auger electron-emitting radionuclides for targeted radionuclide therapy are that the many potent candidates can be produced with low- to medium-energy cyclotrons, ^{103}Pd, ^{111}In, ^{119}Sb, $^{197m/g}$Hg [40].

For alpha emitters, proton-induced spallation or fission of these heavy elements is commonly used to produce alpha-emitting radionuclides [41] (Table 11.4).

With fission of spallation reaction, the chemical extraction of other radionuclides from this chemical mix provides access to a number of imaging and therapeutic radionuclides [42].

11.2.1 GENERAL APPROACHES TO BE CONSIDERED IN RADIONUCLIDE PRODUCTION

The production of radionuclides requires careful consideration of several aspects that begin with (i) the selection of an appropriate irradiation approach (proton, electron/gamma, neutron) and (ii) preparation of the corresponding target material; this is followed by (iii) deciding on a target extraction and radionuclidic purification strategy, and concludes with (iv) an assessment of the quality (e.g., radiochemical purity, SA) of the radionuclide of interest [26,43].

11.2.1.1 Irradiation Approach and Target Material Selection – Cross Sections

Nuclear cross section refers to the probability of a particular reaction occurring as a function of the bombarding particle using the reaction routes described below. An analysis of the cross section will provide both the threshold energy for the desired reaction. and the energy at which the maximum yield is achieved. Complete cross-sectional data will also include the energies where other competing reactions occur. These competing reactions can impact radionuclidic and radio-chemical purity, SA, and yield.

11.2.1.2 Targetry

Once the reaction pathway is selected, the next step is to design the chemical and physical form of the target material to be used. Considerations include the ease associated with the chemistry for extracting the desired product from the target matrix and the thermal properties of the target matrix since all reactions will involve the transfer of kinetic/thermal energy during the irradiation process. The target material can be in any of the physical forms, while recognizing the density of the material can impact the yield as well as the chemistry employed for isolating the desired product.

11.2.1.3 Target Isotopic Enrichment

Most target materials involve the use of isotopically enriched elements. Ideally, the desired element should be 100% enriched for the isotope needed. While there are a few elements that exist as only one isotopic form (e.g., ^{209}Bi, ^{127}I, ^{89}Y) that have been used as target materials, the enrichment process is never quantitative, and thus, the isotopic mixture will be variable. In addition, the greater the enrichment required, the more expensive the target material. Also, the non-desired isotopes can be a source of radionuclidic impurities. The source of many enriched isotopes is from legacy enrichment processes and is in limited supply. In the planning process for producing a particular radionuclide, the requirement for enriched target material, its availability and the possibility to recover and reuse the target must be considered. A recent example of significance is the enrichment of ^{176}Yb for the production of ^{177}Lu without carrier Lu.

TABLE 11.2

Beta-Particle-Emitting Therapeutic Radionuclides [32,46,47]

Radionuclide	Half-Life	Decay Mode	Emission Energy (keV)	γ-Ray Emission (Eγ, keV)	Production Method*	Reaction	Ref
^{90}Y	2.7 days	β⁻ (100%)	$E_{\beta^- \text{ max}} = 2280$ $E_{\beta^- \text{ mean}} = 935$	-	neutron source and ^{90}Sr/^{90}Y generator	^{89}Y(n,γ) ^{90}Y ^{90}Zr(n,p) ^{90}Y ^{90}Sr/^{90}Y generator	[48]
^{131}I	8.02 days	β⁻ (89%) EC (81%)	$E_{\beta^- \text{ max}} = 606$ $E_{\beta^- \text{ mean}} = 192$	364 (82%)	neutron source	^{235}U(n,f) (2.89%) ^{130}Te(n,γ) ^{131g}Te (β⁻, 25.0 min)	[49]
^{177}Lu	6.65 days	β⁻ (100%) EC (11%)	$E_{\beta^- \text{ max}} = 497$ (79%) $E_{\beta^- \text{ mean}} = 133.6$	113 (6.4%) 209 (11%)	neutron source and accelerator	^{176}Lu(n,γ) ^{177}Lu ^{176}Yb(n,γ) ^{177}Yb (β⁻, 1.9 h) ^{176}Yb(d,p) ^{177}Lu and high-energy proton irradiation of Hf and Ta	[50]
^{47}Sc	3.35 days	β⁻ (100%) EC (68%)	$E_{\beta^- \text{ max}} = 600$ (32%) $E_{\beta^- \text{ mean}} = 162$	159 (68%)	neutron source and accelerator	^{46}Ca(n,γ) ^{47}Ca (β⁻, 4.54 d) ^{47}Sc (E_n = 0.025 eV) ^{47}Ti(n,p) ^{47}Sc (E_n > 1 MeV) ^{48}Ti(p,2p) ^{47}Sc ^{48}Ti(γ,p) ^{47}Sc (E_{photon} = 60 MeV) ^{48}Ca(γ,n) ^{47}Ca ^{47}Sc (E_{photon} = 40 MeV)	[34,51]
^{67}Cu	2.58 days	β⁻ (100%)	$E_{\beta^- \text{ max}} = 562$ $E_{\beta^- \text{ mean}} = 141$	93 (16%) 185 (49%)	neutron source and accelerator	^{67}Zn(n,p) ^{67}Cu ^{68}Zn(p,2p) ^{67}Cu (E > 50 MeV) ^{70}Zn(p,α) ^{67}Cu (E = 12–21 MeV) ^{70}Zn(d,nα) ^{67}Cu ^{64}Ni(α,p) ^{67}Cu ^{68}Zn(γ,p) ^{67}Cu	[22,30,34,52]

(Continued)

TABLE 11.2 (Continued)

Beta-Particle-Emitting Therapeutic Radionuclides [32,46,47]

Radionuclide	Half-Life	Decay Mode	Emission Energy (keV)	γ-Ray Emission (Eγ, keV)	Production Method*	Reaction	Ref
^{89}Sr	50.5 days	β⁻ (100%)	$E_{\beta\text{-max}}$ = 1501		neutron source	^{88}Sr(n,γ) ^{89}Sr	[53]
^{161}Tb	6.89 days	β⁻ (100%) EC (10%)	$E_{\beta\text{-max}}$ = 593 $E_{\beta\text{-mean}}$ = 154	26 (23%) 49 (17%) 75 (10%)	neutron source and accelerator	^{160}Gd(n,γ) ^{161}Gd (β⁻, 3.66 min) ^{161}Tb ^{160}Gd(d,x) ^{161}Tb ^{nat}Gd(d,nx) ^{161}Tb	[54]
^{166}Ho	26.83 h	β⁻	$E_{\beta\text{-max}}$ = 1855 (49.9%) 1774 (48.8%) $E_{\beta\text{-mean}}$ = 667	81 (6.4%)	neutron source and ^{166}Dy/^{166}Ho generator	^{165}Ho(n,γ) ^{166}Ho ^{164}Dy(n,γ) ^{165}Dy (β⁻, 2.33 h) ^{165}Dy(n,γ) ^{166}Dy (β⁻, 81.5 h) ^{166}Dy/^{166}Ho generator	[55]
^{188}Re	16.9 h	β⁻	$E_{\beta\text{-max}}$ = 2118 (72%) $E_{\beta\text{-mean}}$ = 784	155 (15%)	neutron source and ^{188}W/^{188}Re generator	^{188}W/^{188}Re generator ^{187}Re(n,γ) ^{188}Re ^{186}W(n,γ) ^{187}W(n,γ) ^{188}W ^{188}Re	[27,48]
^{212}Pb	10.64 h	β⁻ (100%)	$E_{\beta\text{-max}}$ = 570 $E_{\beta\text{-mean}}$ = 100 E_{α} = 8736	239 (44%)	^{224}Ra/^{212}Pb generator	^{224}Ra/^{212}Pb generator	[38]

* Production method: Accelerator refers to cyclotrons that are capable of accelerating protons, deuterons and alpha particles to produce radionuclides via (p,n), (p,pn), (p,xn), (p,α), (d,n), (α,n) and (³He, n) reactions, and linacs that can be used to produce radionuclides via (γ, n) reaction. Neutron source refers to reactors and a number of new approaches using e-linacs or other devices that are capable of producing neutrons to produce radionuclides via (n,γ) and (n,α) reactions.

TABLE 11.3

Auger Electron-Emitting Therapeutic Radionuclides [40]

Radionuclide	Half-Life	Decay Mode	Emission Energy (E$_{Auger, max}$, keV)	γ-Ray Emission (E$_\gamma$, keV)	Production Method*	Reaction	Ref
^{125}I	59.4 days	EC (100%)	23 (E$_{Auger, max}$), 19	35	neutron source	^{124}Xe(n,γ) ^{125}Xe (β⁻, 16.9 h)	[32]
^{111}In	2.8 days	EC (100%)	19 (E$_{Auger, max}$), 7	171 (91%) 245 (94%)	accelerator	^{113}Cd(p,3n) ^{111}In ^{112}Cd(p,2n) ^{111}In ^{111}Cd(p,n) ^{111}In ^{111}Cd(d,2n) ^{111}In ^{110}Cd(d,n) ^{111}In ^{109}Ag(^{4}He,2n) ^{111}In Sb spallation	[32]
^{149}Tb	4.12 h	EC (76%) α (16.7%) β⁺ (7%)	35	165 (26%) 352 (29%) 388 (18%) 652 (16%)	accelerator	high-energy proton induced spallation of Ta ^{152}Gd(p,4n) ^{149}Tb ^{nat}Gd(p,x) ^{149}Tb ^{151}Eu(^{3}He,5n) ^{149}Tb (E = 70–40 MeV) ^{152}Gd(α,7n) ^{149}Dy(ε) ^{149}Tb (E > 100 MeV) ^{nat}Ta(p,x) ^{149}Tb ^{nat}Nd(^{12}C,xn) ^{149}Dy(ε) ^{149}Tb ^{141}Pr(^{12}C,4n) ^{149}Tb	[2,35]
^{197g}Hg	64.14 h	EC	13.4	70	accelerator	^{197}Au(p,n) ^{197}Hg (E = 13 MeV)	[32]
^{103m}Rh	56 min	IT	38	38	^{103}Pd/^{103m}Rh generator	^{103}Pd/^{103m}Rh generator	[32]
^{103}Pd	17 days	EC (100%)	44	16	accelerator	^{103}Rh(p,n) ^{103}Pd (E = 5–15 MeV)	[32]
^{119}Sb	38 hours	EC	26	23	accelerator	^{119}Sn(p,n) ^{119}Sb	[56]

(Continued)

TABLE 11.3 (Continued)

Auger Electron-Emitting Therapeutic Radionuclides [40]

Radionuclide	Half-Life	Decay Mode	Emission Energy (E Auger, keV)	γ-Ray Emission (Eγ, keV)	Production Method*	Reaction	Ref
^{135}La	19.93 hours	β^+, EC	6.9	36	accelerator	^{nat}Ba(p,x) ^{13x}La (E = 12–70 MeV)	[57]
^{155}Tb	5.32 days	EC	16.8	87 (32%) 105 (25%)	accelerator	^{155}Tb by ISOL facility (ISAC) at TRIUMF ^{155}Gd(p,n) ^{155}Tb ^{154}Gd(d,n) ^{155}Tb ^{159}Tb(p,x) (E > 50 MeV) ^{159}Tb(p,5n) ^{155}Dy (ε, 9.9 h) ^{155}Tb ^{nat}Gd(d,nx) ^{152,155}Tb	[35–37]
^{161}Tb	6.89 days	β^- (100%) EC (10%)	29.3	26 (23%) 49 (17%) 75 (10%)	neutron source and accelerator	^{160}Gd(n,γ) ^{161}Gd (β^-, 3.66 min) ^{160}Gd(d,x) ^{161}Tb ^{nat}Gd(d,nx) ^{161}Tb	[54]

* Production method: Accelerator refers to cyclotrons that are capable of accelerating protons, deuterons and alpha particles to produce radionuclides via (p,n), (p,pn), (p,xn), (p,α), (d,n), (α,n) and (^{3}He, n) reactions, and linacs that can be used to produce radionuclides via (γ, n) reaction. Neutron source refers to reactors and a number of new approaches using e-linacs or other devices that are capable of producing neutrons to produce radionuclides via (n,γ) and (n,α) reactions.

TABLE 11.4
Alpha-Particle-Emitting Therapeutic Radionuclides [65,66]

Radionuclide	Half-Life	Decay Mode	Emission Energy ($E\alpha$, keV)	γ-Ray Emission ($E\gamma$, keV)	Production Method*	Reaction	Ref
211At	7.21 h	α (41.8%) EC (58.2%)	5870 (41.8%) 7450 (58.1%)	77 (12%) 79 (21%) 687 (0.3%) 569 (0.5%) 898 (0.6%)	accelerator	high-energy proton induced Th spallation (E = 160–660 MeV) 232Th(p,xn) 211Rn 238U(p,x) 211Rn 209Bi(7Li,5n) 211Rn 209Bi(6Li,4n) 211Rn 211Rn/211At generator 209Bi(α,2n) 211At (E = 20–28 MeV)	[6,67–69]
213Bi	45.61 min	α (2.2%) β⁻ (97.8%)	5875 (2.2%) 8376 (97.8%)	440 (25.9%)	225Ac generator	225Ac generator	[70]
223Ra	11.43 days	α (100%)	5540 (9.0%) 5607 (25.2%) 5716 (51.6%) 5747 (9.0%)	122 (1.2%) 144 (3.3%) 154 (5.7%) 269 (13.9%) 324 (4.0%) 338 (2.8%) 445 (1.3%)	neutron source	226Ra(n,γ) 227Ra(β⁻, 42.2 m) 227Ac(β⁻, 21.8 y) 227Th(β⁻, 18.7 d) 227Th/223Ra generator	[65]
224Ra	3.63 days	α (100%)	5449 (5.0%) 5685 (94.9%)	241 (4%)		232Th decay 232U decay 226Ra(xn,γ) 227/228Ra	[65]
225Ac	9.9 days	α (100%)	5732 (8.0%) 5791 (8.6%) 5793 (18.1%) 5830 (50.7%)	154 (0.2%) 157 (0.3%) 188 (0.5%) 440 (26%) 217 (11%)	neutron source and accelerator	228Ra(n,γ) 229Th 229Th/225Ac generator 226Ra(p,2n) 225Ac (E = 15–30 MeV) (226Ra, $T_{1/2}$ = 1600 a) high-energy proton-induced Th spallation 232Th(p,x) 225Ac	[65]

(Continued)

TABLE 11.4 (Continued)
Alpha-Particle-Emitting Therapeutic Radionuclides [65,66]

Radionuclide	Half-Life	Decay Mode	Emission Energy (Eα, keV)	γ-Ray Emission (Eγ, keV)	Production Method*	Reaction	Ref
						^{226}Ra(γ,n) ^{225}Ra ^{226}Ra(n,2n) ^{225}Ra ^{226}Ra(n,3d) ^{225}Ac	
^{227}Th	18.7 days	α (100%)	5709 (8.3%) 5713 (5.0%) 5757 (20.4%) 5978 (23.5%) 6038 (24.2%)	236 (12.9%) 256 (7.0%) 286 (1.7%) 290 (1.9%) 300 (2.2%) 330 (2.9%)		^{227}Ac decay ^{235}U decay	[65]
^{226}Th	30.57 min	α (100%)	6234 (22.8%) 6337 (75.5%)	111 (3.3%) 131 (0.3%) 242 (0.9%)		^{230}U decay	[65]
^{149}Tb	4.12 h	EC (76%) α (16.7%) β^+ (7%)	3967 (16.7%)	165 (26% %) 352 (29%) 388 (18%) 652 (16%)	accelerator	high-energy proton-induced spallation of Ta ^{152}Gd(p,4n) ^{149}Tb ^{nat}Gd(p,x) ^{149}Tb ^{151}Eu(^{3}He,5n) ^{149}Tb (E = 70–40 MeV) ^{152}Gd(α,7n) ^{149}Dy(ε) ^{149}Tb (E > 100 MeV) ^{nat}Ta(p,x) ^{149}Tb ^{nat}Nd(^{12}C,xn) ^{149}Dy(ε) ^{149}Tb ^{141}Pr(^{12}C,4n) ^{149}Tb	[2,35]

* Production method: Accelerator refers to cyclotrons that are capable of accelerating protons, deuterons and alpha particles to produce radionuclides via (p,n), (p,pn), (p,xn), (p,α), (d,n), (α,n) and (^{3}He, n) reactions, and linacs that can be used to produce radionuclides via (γ, n) reaction. Neutron source refers to reactors and a number of new approaches using e-linacs or other devices that are capable of producing neutrons to produce radionuclides via (n,γ) and (n,α) reactions.

11.2.1.4 Irradiation Parameters

Equation 11.1 for representing the production radionuclides is defined as

$$A = \phi \sigma n \, (1 - e^{-\lambda t}) \tag{11.1}$$

where

A = quantity (activity) of produced radionuclide
ϕ = flux, particles per cm^2/s
σ = formation cross section in barn (10^{-24} cm^2)
n = number of target atoms
$n = W*K/A_w \, 6.02 \times 10^{23}$
W = weight of target material
K = natural abundance of target element
A_w = atomic weight
$(1 - e^{-\lambda t})$ refers to saturation factor which accounts for the fact that the produced radionuclide is decaying at its own rate (λ), as it is being produced.
λ = decay constant given by $0.693/t_{1/2}$ (s^{-1})
t = duration of irradiation (s)

The conditions of the irradiation include the energy of the incoming particle and the energy at which the bombarding particle exits the matrix [44]. This represents the energy deposited in the matrix and will have implications in which nuclear transformations take place. In addition to nuclear considerations, consideration of physical factors such as heat transfer and dissipation will be required. At this stage, the issue of volatile radionuclides must be considered since this represents a potential major safety issue.

Figure 11.2 illustrates the typical reaction routes at low energies (<30 MeV for bombarding particle).

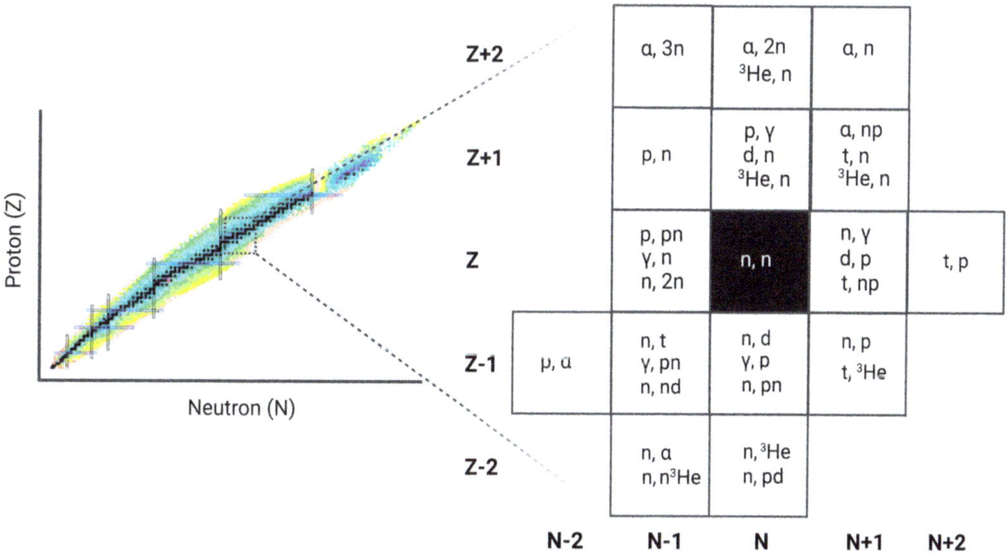

		N-2	N-1	N	N+1	N+2
Z+2		α, 3n	α, 2n / ³He, n	α, n		
Z+1		p, n	p, γ / d, n / ³He, n	α, np / t, n / ³He, n		
Z		p, pn / γ, n / n, 2n	n, n	n, γ / d, p / t, np	t, p	
Z-1	p, α	n, t / γ, pn / n, nd	n, d / γ, p / n, pn	n, p / t, ³He		
Z-2		n, α / n, n³He	n, ³He / n, pd			

FIGURE 11.2 General production approaches based on targets and source irradiation with neutrons, protons, deuterons, alphas, gammas and other nuclear particles. The use of the Chart of Nuclides can aid in establishing pathways including potential side products.

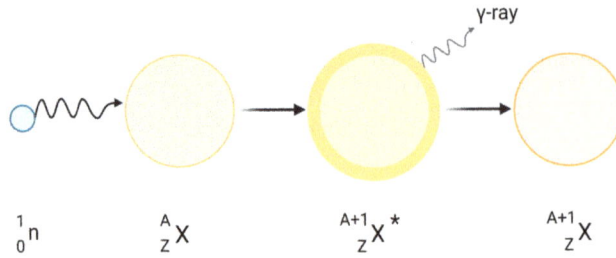

FIGURE 11.3   Production of radionuclides (e.g., ^{99}Mo, ^{177}Lu) by neutron capture. See also Figure 11.2

11.3   PRODUCTION VIA NEUTRON CAPTURE

Reactors are the primary source of neutrons with fluxes ranging from 10^{13} to 10^{15} n/s/cm^2. These neutrons are used to produce radionuclides on the neutron-rich side of stability. Neutrons can also induce fission in heavy nuclei such as uranium. Reactions typically involve neutron absorption followed by the emission of γ-rays (Figure 11.3). If the energy of the neutron is sufficiently high, particles may be emitted such as extra neutrons or charged particles such as protons or α-particles.

The most commonly used reactor-produced radionuclides are ^{99}Mo, ^{131}I, ^{89}Sr, ^{153}Sm and ^{177}Lu where the first two are products of fission in ^{235}U and the latter neutron capture (^{88}Sr(n,γ)^{89}Sr, ^{152}Sm(n,γ)^{153}Sm and ^{176}Lu(n,γ)^{177}Lu; ^{176}Yb(n,γ)^{177}Yb followed by decay to ^{177}Lu).

It should be noted that ^{99}Mo can also be produced via neutron capture of ^{98}Mo; however, this product is of low SA because of the two Mo isotopes in the target/product mix. A commercial version of this process exists [45]. See Tables 11.2 and 11.4 for beta-particle-emitting and alpha-particle-emitting therapeutic radionuclides produced by neutron irradiation, respectively.

11.4   CYCLOTRON-PRODUCED RADIONUCLIDES

From Figure 11.2, it can be seen that the typical bombarding particles produced by cyclotrons are protons, deuterons and alpha particles.

Table 11.1 provides the most common radionuclides used in imaging that are produced via accelerators. Typical reactions involve bombarding targets with protons in the energy range of 10–30 MeV to induce (p,n), (p,α) or (p,2n) reactions. By examining the excitation functions for the production of the desired radionuclide, the optimal energy window can be chosen, while keeping in mind the yield as well as the potential to produce undesired isotopes or other contaminating radionuclides.

Other radionuclides may require higher energies to induce (p,xn) reactions. In some cases, the use of very high energies (>200 MeV) may be used to induce what is called a spallation reaction which entails many particles being released from the reaction mix. In this case, the selective chemistry and/or half-lives can be used to isolate the desired species. In some cases, isotope mass-separators have been used (see below).

11.5   RADIONUCLIDES PRODUCED VIA DIFFERENT METHODS

11.5.1   PHOTONUCLEAR

While the concept of using photons to initiate nuclear reactions has been explored for a very long time, it is only recently when high-powered electron machines have become available, that it is now possible to explore the use of bremsstrahlung radiation to produce radionuclides of interest.

When electrons are slowed in passing through materials, the resulting bremsstrahlung radiation is emitted in a continuous spectrum with photons of low energy having the highest flux and dropping off exponentially, asymptotically reaching the energy of the initial energy of the electron beam [58]. The resonant energy for emission of a neutron from the target material is approximately 16 MeV [59]. Thus, electron beams of 40 MeV or so are required in order to generate a photon beam that has sufficient flux in the resonate region making use of the (γ,n) reaction [60].

This reaction can be viewed as the inverse of the (n,γ) reaction. In both cases, the product is of the same element as the target and is thus of low SA. Radionuclides of interest to the medical community that have been proposed for production via photons include $^{100}Mo(\gamma,n)^{99}Mo$ and ^{226}Ra $(\gamma,n)^{225}Ra \rightarrow ^{225}Ac$ [61,62]. Table 11.4 provides the production routes for alpha-particle-emitting radionuclide, ^{225}Ac.

At higher energies, it is possible to initiate the emission of a proton (γ,p) [63]. ^{67}Cu has been proposed as a good candidate for being produced via the $^{68}Zn(\gamma,p)^{67}Cu$ reaction [64] (Table 11.2).

11.5.2 ALPHA PARTICLES

During the 1960s and 1970s, nuclear physicists used multi-particle cyclotrons for research. These cyclotrons could accelerate protons, deuterons, $^{3}He^{++}$ and $^{4}He^{++}$ (alpha) particles [71]. As a result, a number of routes for producing radionuclides of medical interest were explored.

For a period, the $^{20}Ne(d,a)^{18}F$ reaction was the primary source for ^{18}F-F_2 [72]. The other important radionuclide, ^{211}At, is still produced using alpha particles via the $^{209}Bi(\alpha,2n)^{211}At$ reaction [73] (Table 11.4). Another tracer used extensively throughout this period was the ^{14}N $(d,n)^{15}O$ reaction [74]. Even with the concerted effort to move to proton only cyclotrons, the simplicity of using natural nitrogen with deuterons resulted in building small accelerators for the sole purpose of generating ^{15}O in its various forms (O_2, CO and CO_2) [75].

11.5.3 MASS SEPARATION ISOL, OFF-LINE

Most of the isotopically enriched non-gaseous target materials were produced via mass separators of the calutron type [76]. With the need for higher SAs and higher radionuclidic purity, a number of high energy accelerator facilities have used on-line isotope separators capable of selecting radioisotopes of extraordinary purity. These separators are connected to the target, usually irradiated with high energy protons (500 MeV to 1 GeV or more) [77,78]. The resulting mix of isotopes is passed through an ionizing field and then through a high magnetic field separating the electrically charged ions by mass.

High-energy physics accelerators using radioactive ion beams (RIBs) as probes in nuclear and particle physics research have made use of ion separators to produce these RIBs. These same facilities have used these separated beams to isolate radioisotopes that have potential for use in medicine [79]. See the press release for CERN's medical isotope program in Switzerland [78] and for TRIUMF in Canada [80]. These programs, which enable to produce rare and exotic radionuclides successfully, suggested that radioisotope separators could be used to isolate the desired radioisotope from the mixture of unwanted radioisotopes obtained from the production process [81] (Figure 11.4). As of 2023, there are no dedicated off-line isotope separators.

11.6 RADIONUCLIDE GENERATORS (PARENT/DAUGHTER PAIRS FOR BOTH DIAGNOSTIC AND THERAPEUTIC RADIONUCLIDES)

During radioactive decay, the resultant nuclide can be radioactive. If this pair has sufficiently different half-lives, they can form what is known as a generator. Typically, the parent radionuclide

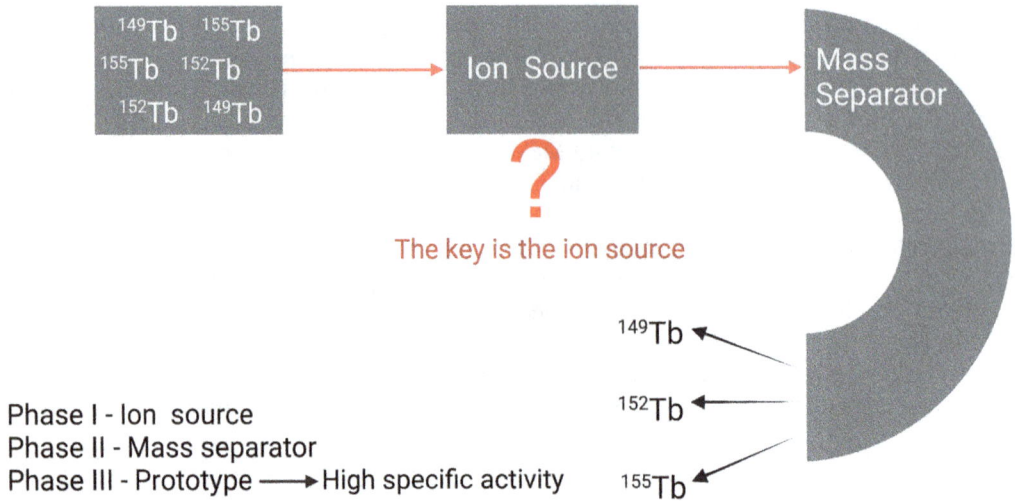

FIGURE 11.4 Schematic principle for an electromagnetic isotope separator. The key to the efficient separation is the ion source capable of high output.

has a longer half-life than the product daughter radionuclide. In this way, the parent can be produced at one location and moved to the site where the decay product (daughter) can be extracted and isolated from the mix. Generators are produced by using an ion column (stationary phase) on which the parent adheres and will allow the daughter to be removed by adding an elution solvent (mobile phase).

Because only one radioactive species is eluted from the mix, this product will be of high SA. The cost of these generators is typically cheaper than having to produce the desired radionuclide on site for each use. Also depending upon the half-lives of the pair, the product can be eluted on demand depending upon the in-growth of the eluted daughter.

The equations for determining the decay and growth of the isotopic pair are beyond the scope of this chapter but can be found in [48].

Table 11.5 illustrates the parent/daughter pairs actively used in nuclear medicine.

11.7   RADIOCHEMISTRY

Although it is beyond the scope of this chapter to provide details as to how to separate and isolate the various radionuclides of interest from the various production targets, there are a number of issues that need to be kept in mind in assessing the feasibility of creating a source for these tracers.

The actual chemical or physical separation approaches will make use of the difference in chemical properties and/or physical characteristics for achieving the separation. Traditionally, the chemical approaches have used solvent extraction, precipitation and column chromatography. The physical approaches have made use of thermochromatographic properties.

In selecting the optimal approach, the requirements for Good Manufacturing Practices (GMP) must be kept in mind as well as the reproducible, safe handling procedures. Remote or automated processes would help in these efforts.

Keeping the tracer principle in mind, the isolated radionuclide should be of the highest possible SA and radiochemically pure. While the goal is to have no-carrier-added isotopes, this is difficult to achieve if the desired radionuclide is produced from an isotope of the product.

TABLE 11.5

Radionuclide Generators

Generator System	Source of Parent	Production Method* (Parent)	Half-Life (p/d)	Decay Mode (Daughter)	Application	Ref
^{44}Ti/^{44}Sc	^{45}Sc(p,2n) ^{44}Ti proton induced V or Cr spallation	accelerator	58.9 a/3.97 h	β^+ (94%)	PET imaging	[82]
^{68}Ge/^{68}Ga	^{66}Ga(p,2n) ^{68}Ge ^{nat}Zn(α,xn) ^{68}Ge proton induced Rb, Br or As spallation	accelerator	270.8 d/67.7 min	β^+ (89%)	PET imaging	[48]
^{99}Mo/^{99m}Tc	^{235}U(n,f) ^{99}Mo ^{98}Mo(n,γ) ^{99}Mo	neutron source	65.9 h/6 h	IT	SPECT imaging	[30]
^{81}Rb/^{81m}Kr	^{80}Kr(d,n) ^{81}Rb	accelerator	4.6 h/13 s	IT	SPECT imaging	[82]
^{82}Sr/^{82}Rb	^{85}Rb(p,4n) ^{82}Sr ^{82}Kr(^{3}He,3n) ^{82}Sr proton induced Rb, Mo or Y spallation	accelerator	25.6 d/1.27 min	β^+ (95%)	PET imaging	[48]
^{90}Sr/^{90}Y	^{235}U(n,f) ^{90}Sr	neutron source	28.5 a/2.67 d	β^- (100%)	Beta-particle therapy	[48]
^{103}Pd/^{103m}Rh	^{130}Rh(p,n) ^{103}Pd	accelerator	17 d/56.1 min	IT	Auger-therapy	[32]
^{211}Rn/ ^{211}At	^{209}Bi(^{7}Li,5n) ^{211}Rn	accelerator	14.6 h/7.21 h	α	Alpha-particle therapy	[6,67–69]
^{212}Pb/^{212}Bi	^{224}Ra decay ^{228}Th decay		10.6 h/60.5 min	α	Alpha-particle therapy	[38]
^{225}Ac/^{213}Bi	^{232}Th(p,x) ^{225}Ac ^{226}Ra(p,2n) ^{225}Ac	accelerator	9.9 d/45.6 min	α	Alpha-particle therapy	[83]
^{227}Ac/^{227}Th/^{223}Ra	^{235}U decay ^{226}Ra(n, γ) ^{227}Ra(β^-, 42 min) ^{227}Ac	neutron source	21.8 d/11.4 d	α	Alpha-particle therapy	[65]

* Production method: Accelerator refers to cyclotrons that are capable of accelerating protons, deuterons and alpha particles to produce radionuclides via (p,n), (p,pn), (p,xn), (p,α), (d,n), (α,n) and (^{3}He, n) reactions, and linacs that can be used to produce radionuclides via (γ, n) reaction. Neutron source refers to reactors and a number of new approaches using e-linacs or other devices that are capable of producing neutrons to produce radionuclides via (n,γ) and (n,α) reactions.

11.8   CONCLUSION

While the production of theranostic pairs using isotopes of the same element is possible, as seen from the production parameters, and even for radionuclides from the same chemical family, the most widely used pairs presently include ^{18}F, ^{68}Ga or ^{99m}Tc for imaging and ^{177}Lu for therapy. This is partly due to the availability of ^{18}F, ^{68}Ga or ^{99m}Tc and the fact that ^{177}Lu-PSMA agents have the approval of the Food and Drug Administration of the United Sates.

While the use of radionuclides for therapy such as ^{89}Sr, ^{90}Y and ^{153}Sm will continue to play a significant role in cancer treatment, there are no reported studies using imaging isotopes in conjunction with these products in the manner discussed in this chapter.

The possibility of using alpha emitters such as ^{211}At and ^{225}Ac will depend upon the widespread production and availability of these radionuclides. These particular radionuclides do not have natural isotopic or chemical imaging pairs; thus, the imaging will depend upon the ease with which an imaging radionuclide can be incorporated into the targeting agent [46,84].

Based on the wide array of possibilities for both imaging and dose-delivering radionuclides, the field of theranostics is well positioned to make a significant impact on healthcare.

ACKNOWLEDGMENTS

This review is supported by a Canadian Cancer Society Research Institute Innovation Grant to Gokce Engudar and the US National Institute of Health (NIH 1R01EB029259-01) and NSERC Discovery Grant RGPIN-2018–04997 to Valery Radchenko. TRIUMF received funding via a contribution agreement with the National Research Council of Canada.

The authors greatly appreciate Dr. Paul Schaffer's review of the manuscript.

REFERENCES

1. Iwano S, Kato K, Nihashi T, Ito S, Tachi Y, Naganawa S. Comparisons of I-123 diagnostic and I-131 post-treatment scans for detecting residual thyroid tissue and metastases of differentiated thyroid cancer. *Ann Nucl Med.* 2009;23(9):777–782.
2. Naskar N, Lahiri S. Theranostic terbium radioisotopes: challenges in production for clinical application. *Front Med (Lausanne).* 2021;8:675014.
3. Mou L, Martini P, Pupillo G, Cieszykowska I, Cutler CS, Mikolajczak R. (67)Cu production capabilities: a mini review. *Molecules.* 2022;27(5):1501.
4. Pupillo G, Mou L, Martini P, Pasquali M, Boschi A, Cicoria G, et al. Production of 67Cu by enriched 70Zn targets: first measurements of formation cross sections of 67Cu, 64Cu, 67Ga, 66Ga, 69mZn and 65Zn in interactions of 70Zn with protons above 45 MeV. *Radiochimica Acta.* 2020;108(8):593–602.
5. Eary JF, Durack L, Williams D, Vanderheyden JL. Considerations for imaging Re-188 and Re-186 isotopes. *Clin Nucl Med.* 1990;15(12):911–916.
6. Zalutsky MR, Pruszynski M. Astatine-211: production and availability. *Curr Radiopharm.* 2011;4(3):177–185.
7. Ruth TJ, Dombsky M, D`auria JM, Ward TE. *Radiochemistry of Astatine.* Oak Ridge, United States: United States Department of Energy; 1988. Contract No. NAS-NS-3064.
8. Coenen HH, Gee AD, Adam M, Antoni G, Cutler CS, Fujibayashi Y, et al. Consensus nomenclature rules for radiopharmaceutical chemistry – setting the record straight. *Nucl Med Biol.* 2017;55:v–xi.
9. Kane SM, Davis DD. Technetium-99m. April 2023. Available from: https://www.ncbi.nlm.nih.gov/books/NBK559013/.
10. Herman M, Capote R, Carlson BV, Oblozinsky P, Sin M, Trkov A, et al. EMPIRE: nuclear reaction model code system for data evaluation. *Nucl Data Sheets.* 2007;108(12):2655–2715.
11. Jurisson SS, Lydon JD. Potential technetium small molecule radiopharmaceuticals. *Chem Rev.* 1999;99(9):2205–2218.
12. Jacobson O, Kiesewetter DO, Chen X. Fluorine-18 radiochemistry, labeling strategies and synthetic routes. *Bioconjug Chem.* 2015;26(1):1–18.

13. Bartholoma MD, Louie AS, Valliant JF, Zubieta J. Technetium and gallium derived radio-pharmaceuticals: comparing and contrasting the chemistry of two important radiometals for the molecular imaging era. *Chem Rev*. 2010;110(5):2903–2920.

14. Rosch F, Baum RP. Generator-based PET radiopharmaceuticals for molecular imaging of tumours: on the way to THERANOSTICS. *Dalton Trans*. 2011;40(23):6104–6111.

15. Holland JP, Sheh Y, Lewis JS. Standardized methods for the production of high specific-activity zirconium-89. *Nucl Med Biol*. 2009;36(7):729–739.

16. Hao G, Singh AN, Liu W, Sun X. PET with non-standard nuclides. *Curr Top Med Chem*. 2010;10(11):1096–1112.

17. Williams HA, Robinson S, Julyan P, Zweit J, Hastings D. A comparison of PET imaging characteristics of various copper radioisotopes. *Eur J Nucl Med Mol Imaging*. 2005;32(12):1473–1480.

18. Matthay KK, Shulkin B, Ladenstein R, Michon J, Giammarile F, Lewington V, et al. Criteria for evaluation of disease extent by (123)I-metaiodobenzylguanidine scans in neuroblastoma: a report for the International Neuroblastoma Risk Group (INRG) Task Force. *Br J Cancer*. 2010;102(9):1319–1326.

19. Parisi MT, Eslamy H, Park JR, Shulkin BL, Yanik GA. (1)(3)(1)I-Metaiodobenzylguanidine theranostics in neuroblastoma: historical perspectives; practical applications. *Semin Nucl Med*. 2016;46(3):184–202.

20. Alves F, Bertrand S, DeGrado T, Gagnon K, Guerin B, Hoehr C, Pandey M, Tremblay S *Gallium-68 Cyclotron Production*. Vienna: International Atomic Energy Agency; 2019. Contract No. IAEA-TECDOC-1863.

21. McElvany KD, Hopkins KT, Hanrahan TJ, Moore HAJ, Welch MJ. Comparison of Ge-68/Ga-68 generator systems for radiopharmaceutical production. *J Label Compd Radiopharm*. 1982;19(11-12):1419–1420.

22. Qaim SM. Cyclotron production of medical radionuclides. In: Vertes A, Nagy S, Klencsar Z, Lovas RG, Rosch F, editors. *Handbook of Nuclear Chemistry*, Springer,New York, NY; 2011. pp. 1903–1933.

23. Kurakina ES, Wharton L, Hoehr C, Orvig C, Magomedbekov EP, Filosofov D, et al. Improved separation scheme for (44)Sc produced by irradiation of (nat)Ca targets with 12.8 MeV protons. *Nucl Med Biol*. 2022;104–105:22–27.

24. Filosofov DV, Loktionova NS, Rosch F. A 44Ti/44Sc radionuclide generator for potential application of 44Sc-based PET-radiopharmaceuticals. *Radiochim Acta*. 2010;98:149–156.

25. Qaim SM. Theranostic radionuclides: recent advances in production methodologies. *J Radioanal Nucl Chem*. 2019;322:1257–1266.

26. Talip Z, Favaretto C, Geistlich S, Meulen NPV. A step-by-step guide for the novel radiometal production for medical applications: case studies with (68)Ga, (44)Sc, (177)Lu and (161)Tb. *Molecules*. 2020;25(4):966.

27. Qaim SM. Nuclear data for production and medical application of radionuclides: present status and future needs. *Nucl Med Biol*. 2017;44:31–49.

28. Rosch F, Herzog H, Qaim SM. The beginning and development of the theranostic approach in nuclear medicine, as exemplified by the radionuclide pair (86)Y and (90)Y. *Pharmaceuticals (Basel)*. 2017;10(2).

29. Severin GW, Engle JW, Barnhart TE, Nickles RJ. 89Zr radiochemistry for positron emission tomography. *Med Chem*. 2011;7(5):389–394.

30. Mirzadeh S, Mausner LF, Garland MA. Reactor-produced medical radionuclides. In: Vertes A, Nagy S, Klencsar Z, Lovas RG, Rosch F, editors. *Handbook of Nuclear Chemistry*: Springer, New York, NY; 2011:1857

31. Kurakına ES, Velichkov AI, Karaivanov DV, Marinova AP, Marinov GM, Radchenko V, et al. Production of 111In and radioisotopes of Te and Sn from an antimony target irradiated with high-energy protons. *Radiochemistry*. 2020;62:393–399.

32. Ruth TJ, Pate BD, Robertson R, Porter JK. Radionuclide production for the biosciences. *Nucl Med Biol*. 1989;16(4):323–336.

33. Braghirolli AM, Waissmann W, da Silva JB, dos Santos GR. Production of iodine-124 and its applications in nuclear medicine. *Appl Radiat Isot*. 2014;90:138–148.

34. Qaim SM, Scholten B, Neumaier B. New developments in the production of theranostic pairs of radionuclides. *J Radioanal Nucl Chem*. 2018;318:1493–1509.

35. Muller C, Zhernosekov K, Koster U, Johnston K, Dorrer H, Hohn A, et al. A unique matched quadruplet of terbium radioisotopes for PET and SPECT and for alpha- and beta-radionuclide therapy: an in vivo proof-of-concept study with a new receptor-targeted folate derivative. *J Nucl Med*. 2012;53(12):1951–1959.

36. Muller C, Fischer E, Behe M, Koster U, Dorrer H, Reber J, et al. Future prospects for SPECT imaging using the radiolanthanide terbium-155 - production and preclinical evaluation in tumor-bearing mice. *Nucl Med Biol*. 2014;41 Suppl:e58–e65.

37. Fiaccabrino DE, Kunz P, Radchenko V. Potential for production of medical radionuclides with on-line isotope separation at the ISAC facility at TRIUMF and particular discussion of the examples of (165) Er and (155)Tb. *Nucl Med Biol*. 2021;94-95:81–91.

38. McNeil BL, Robertson AKH, Fu W, Yang H, Hoehr C, Ramogida CF, et al. Production, purification, and radiolabeling of the (203)Pb/(212)Pb theranostic pair. *EJNMMI Radiopharm Chem*. 2021;6(1):6.

39. Akaboshi M, Alberto R, Ananthakrishnan M, Aungurarat G, Beets AL, Bhagwat AM, Brihaye C et al. Manual for reactor produced radioisotopes. Vienna, Austria: International Atomic Energy Agency; 2003. Contract No. IAEA-TECDOC-1340.

40. Filosofov D, Kurakina E, Radchenko V. Potent candidates for targeted auger therapy: production and radiochemical considerations. *Nucl Med Biol*. 2021;94-95:1–19.

41. Radchenko V, Morgenstern A, Jalilian AR, Ramogida CF, Cutler C, Duchemin C, et al. Production and supply of alpha-particle-emitting radionuclides for targeted alpha-therapy. *J Nucl Med*. 2021;62(11):1495–1503.

42. Mastren T, Radchenko V, Owens A, Copping R, Boll R, Griswold JR, et al. Simultaneous separation of actinium and radium isotopes from a proton irradiated thorium matrix. *Sci Rep*. 2017;7(1):8216.

43. Radchenko V, Baimukhanova A, Filosofov D. Radiochemical aspects in modern radiopharmaceutical trends: a practical guide. *Solvent Extr Ion Exch*. 2021;39(7):714–744.

44. Friedlander G, Kennedy JW, Macias ES, Miller JM. Nuclear and radiochemistry. 3rd edition United States 1981.

45. Harvey J. NorthStar: The new producer and distributor of Mo-99, Mo-99 Stakeholders Meeting, Chicago IL, 2019. Available from: https://mo99.ne.anl.gov/2019stakeholders/pdfs/2.3_Harvey.pdf.

46. Miller C, Rousseau J, Ramogida CF, Celler A, Rahmim A, Uribe CF. Implications of physics, chemistry and biology for dosimetry calculations using theranostic pairs. *Theranostics*. 2022;12(1):232–259.

47. Kostelnik TI, Orvig C. Radioactive main group and rare earth metals for imaging and therapy. *Chem Rev*. 2019;119(2):902–956.

48. Filosofov DV, Garland M, John KD, Knapp FF, Kuznetsov R, Mausner L, Mirzadeh S et al. Production of long lived parent radionuclides for generators:68Ga, 82Sr, 90Sr and 188W. Vienna, Austria: International Atomic Energy Agency; 2010. Contract No. STI/PUB/1436.

49. Gourani M, Nabardi B, Farahani H. *Technology of iodine-131 production and its application*. Kazakhstan: IAEA; 2005. Available from: https://inis.iaea.org/search/search.aspx?orig_q= RN:38022907.

50. Banerjee S, Pillai MR, Knapp FF. Lutetium-177 therapeutic radiopharmaceuticals: linking chemistry, radiochemistry, and practical applications. *Chem Rev*. 2015;115(8):2934–2974.

51. Domnanich KA, Muller C, Benesova M, Dressler R, Haller S, Koster U, et al. (47)Sc as useful beta (-)-emitter for the radiotheragnostic paradigm: a comparative study of feasible production routes. *EJNMMI Radiopharm Chem*. 2017;2(1):5.

52. Hao G, Mastren T, Silvers W, Hassan G, Oz OK, Sun X. Copper-67 radioimmunotheranostics for simultaneous immunotherapy and immuno-SPECT. *Sci Rep*. 2021;11(1):3622.

53. Lever SZ, Lydon JD, Cutler CS, Jurisson SS. Radioactive metals in imaging and therapy. In: McCleverty JA, Meyer TJ, editors. *Comprehensive Coordination Chemistry II*. Elsevier, Pergamon; Oxford, United Kingdom. 2003. pp. 883–911.

54. Gracheva N, Muller C, Talip Z, Heinitz S, Koster U, Zeevaart JR, et al. Production and characterization of no-carrier-added (161)Tb as an alternative to the clinically-applied (177)Lu for radionuclide therapy. *EJNMMI Radiopharm Chem*. 2019;4(1):12.

55. Vosoughi S, Shirvani-Arani S, Bahrami-Samani A, Salek N, Jalilian A. Production of no-carrier-added Ho-166 for targeted therapy purposes. *Iran J Nucl Med*. 2017;25(Suppl 1):15–20.

56. Thisgaard H, Jensen M. Production of the Auger emitter 119Sb for targeted radionuclide therapy using a small PET-cyclotron. *Appl Radiat Isot*. 2009;67(1):34–38.

57. Aluicio-Sarduy E, Hernandez R, Olson AP, Barnhart TE, Cai W, Ellison PA, et al. Production and in vivo PET/CT imaging of the theranostic pair (132/135)La. *Sci Rep*. 2019;9(1):10658.

58. Yeung J, Schultz K. bremsstrahlung radiation 2011, May 2022.

59. Chemerisov S. Accelerator-based production of Mo-99: photonuclear approach, Argonne National Laboratory, Knoxville, TN; 2018. Available from: https://mo99.ne.anl.gov/2018/pdfs/presentations/ S11-P2.pdf.

60. Ruth TJ. The shortage of technetium-99m and possible solutions. *Annu Rev Nucl Sci*. 2020;70:77–94.

61. Galea R, Ross C, Wells RG. Reduce, reuse and recycle: a green solution to Canada's medical isotope shortage. *Appl Radiat Isot*. 2014;87:148–151.

62. Maslov OD, Sabel'nikov AV, Dmitriev SN. Preparation of 225Ac by 226Ra(γ, n) photonuclear reaction on an electron accelerator, MT-25 microtron. *Radiochemistry*. 2006;48:195–197.

63. Kanazawa M, Homma S, Koike M, Murata Y, Okuno H, Soga F, et al. (γ,p), (γ,pn), and (γ,pp) reactions on light nuclei in the Delta (1232) resonance region. *Phys Rev C*. 1987;35(5):1828.

64. Yagi M, Kondo K. Preparation of carrier-free 67Cu by the 68Zn (γ,p) reaction. *Int J Appl Radiat Isot*. 1978;29(12):757–759.

65. Ferrier MG, Radchenko V, Wilbur DS. Radiochemical aspects of alpha emitting radionuclides for medical application. *Radiochim Acta*. 2019;107(9-11):1065–1085.

66. Wilbur DS. The radiopharmaceutical chemistry of alpha-emitting radionuclides. In: Lewis JS, Windhorst AD, Zeglis BM editors. *Radiopharmaceutical Chemistry [Internet]*. Switzerland: Springer. 2019. 409–424.

67. Meyer G-J, Lambrecht RM. Excitation function for the 209Bi(7Li, 5n)211Rn nuclear reaction. *Int J Appl Radiat Isot*. 1980;31(6):351–355.

68. Feng Y, Zalutsky MR. Production, purification and availability of (211)At: near term steps towards global access. *Nucl Med Biol*. 2021;100-101:12–23.

69. Crawford JR, Yang H, Kunz P, Wilbur DS, Schaffer P, Ruth TJ. Development of a preclinical (211) Rn/(211)At generator system for targeted alpha therapy research with (211)At. *Nucl Med Biol*. 2017;48:31–35.

70. Ahenkorah S, Cassells I, Deroose CM, Cardinaels T, Burgoyne AR, Bormans G, et al. Bismuth-213 for targeted radionuclide therapy: from atom to bedside. *Pharmaceutics*. 2021;13(5).

71. Mackenzie GH, Schmor PW, Schneider HR. Cyclotrons. In: Achanta G, De Luca M, Ng TK, Parkinson P, Seidel P, editors. Encyclopedia of Applied Physics. Wiley-VCH. Verlag GmbH & Co. 2009.

72. Casella V, Ido T, Wolf AP, Fowler JS, MacGegor RR, Ruth TJ. Anhydrous F-18 labeled elemental fluorine for radiopharmaceutical preparation. *J Nucl Med*. 1980;21(8):750–757.

73. Mortenzi S, Bonardi M, Groppi F, Zona C, Persico E, Menapace E, et al. Cyclotron production of 211At/211gPo by 209Bi(α,2n) reaction. *J Radioanal Nucl Chem*. 2008;276:843–847.

74. Evans W, Green T, Middleton R. An investigation of the reaction 14N(d,n)15O at 8 MeV deuteron energy. *Proc Phys Soc A*. 2002;66(1):108.

75. DeGrazia J. Short-lived radioactive gases for clinical use. *Med Phys*. 1981;8(5):723.

76. Donev JMKC. Energy Education – Calutron [Online] 2017.Available from: https://energyeducation. ca/encyclopedia/Calutron.

77. Hoehr C, Benard F, Buckley K, Crawford J, Gottberg A, Hanemayeer V, et al. Medical isotope production at TRIUMF – from imaging to treatment. *Phys Procedia*. 2017;90:200–208.

78. Schaeffer A. ISOLDE to produce isotopes for medical research, CERN; 2012 [Available from: https:// home.cern/news/news/experiments/isolde-produce-isotopes-medical-research.

79. Beyer GJ, Ruth TJ. The role of the electromagnetic separators in the production of radiotracers for biomedical research and nuclear medical application. *Nucl Instrum Methods Phys Res B*. 2003;204:694–700.

80. Hoehr C. Medical isotope production at TRIUMF – from imaging to treatment: Triumf; 2017. Available from: https://www.triumf.ca/sites/default/files/2016%20TARA-Hoehr.pdf.

81. D`Auria JM, Keller R, Ladouceur K, Lapi SE, Ruth TJ, Schmor P. An alternate approach to the production of radioisotopes for nuclear medicine applications. *Rev Sci Instrum*. 2013;84:034705.

82. Rosch F, Knapp FF. Radionuclide generators. 2011. In: Vertes A, Nagy S, Klencsár Z, Rezso GL, Rosch F, editors. *Handbook of Nuclear Chemistry [Internet]*. Springer Science Business Media. New York, NY. 1935–1976.

83. Ermolaev S, Skasyrskaya A, Vasiliev A. A radionuclide generator of high-purity Bi-213 for instant labeling. *Pharmaceutics*. 2021;13(6):914.

84. Bailey TA, Mocko V, Shield KM, An DD, Akin AC, Birnbaum ER, et al. Developing the (134)Ce and (134)La pair as companion positron emission tomography diagnostic isotopes for (225)Ac and (227)Th radiotherapeutics. *Nat Chem*. 2021;13(3):284–289.

12 Radioactivity Measurement and Traceability

Andrew Robinson

12.1 INTRODUCTION

Measurement traceability to primary standards of radioactivity underpins all clinical administrations of radiopharmaceuticals and is a critical component in ensuring their safe and effective clinical use in nuclear medicine diagnostics and therapies. Traceable calibration of radioactivity measurements provides confidence in the measurement results for clinical users, harmonization of measurements across sites, and is often needed to fulfill regulatory requirements [1–3].

Metrological traceability is defined as a "property of a measurement result whereby the result can be related to a reference through a documented unbroken chain of calibrations, each contributing to the measurement uncertainty" [4]. Traceability is *only* achieved with comprehensive documentation of the calibration chain, calibration against an appropriate measurement standard, and with an accompanying assessment of uncertainty in the measurement result [2]. The most common chains for establishing traceability for radioactivity measurements are shown in Figure 12.1. The Bureau International des Poids et Mesures (BIPM) provides the highest reference point for these measurements, with interactions at a national level with National Metrology Institutes (NMIs) or a Designated Institute (hereafter included in discussion of NMIs) to ensure equivalence. NMIs are responsible for establishing primary standards for specific radionuclides and for extending traceability, through links with secondary laboratories, to end-users. These routes vary between countries and in the case when a country does not have a dedicated NMI, then the primary standard from an NMI in another country may be recognized.

When considering radiotheranostic applications, multiple traceable calibration standards are required for both diagnostic tracers and therapeutic agents. In addition, activity quantification from quantitative imaging (from SPECT or PET) requires appropriate traceable calibration [5].

12.2 PRIMARY STANDARDS OF RADIOACTIVITY

A primary standard measurement of radioactivity aims to perform a direct measurement of nuclear transitions occurring per unit time for a specific radionuclide [6]. These measurements are based on the detection of emitted radiation and should depend on absolute measurement and not on other standards. The measurement should be traceable to the SI (typically for units of mass, time, frequency, and length). There are a variety of primary measurement techniques, the choice of which will depend on the specific decay scheme of the radionuclide of interest [6]. Although primary standardizations are designed in such a way that their result is independent of nuclear decay data, all standardization techniques will have a direct or indirect dependence on knowledge of the decay scheme and half-life of the radionuclide and corrections may be required for any impurities present. [7]. Consequently, care must be taken to choose sources of nuclear decay data which have been evaluated with metrology best practices, including uncertainty evaluation such as the Decay Data Evaluation Project (DDEP) [8].

DOI: 10.1201/9781003250913-15

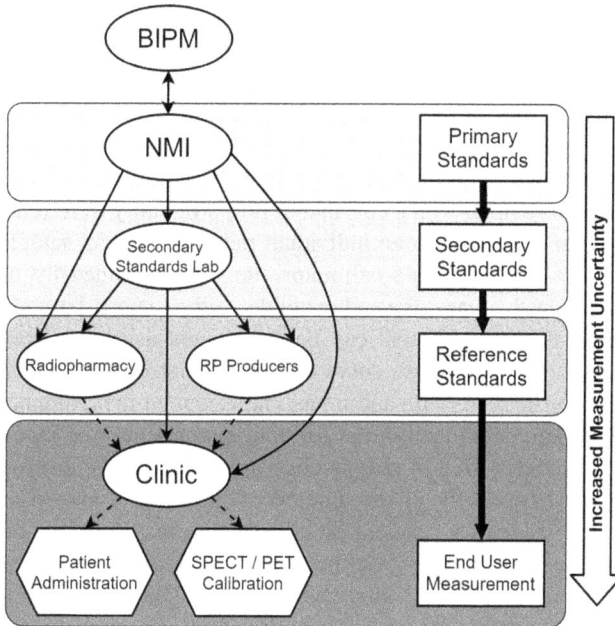

FIGURE 12.1 Traceability chain for radioactivity measurements in clinical nuclear medicine. Solid arrows indicate direct traceability links and dashed arrows indicate potential secondary routes. The measurement standards commonly provided by each organization are also indicated. In general, the measurement uncertainty will increase down the chain toward end-user measurements. (BIPM, Bureau International des Poids et Mesures; NMI, National Metrology Institute (or Designated Institute); RP, Radiopharmaceutical; SPECT, single-photon computed emission tomography; PET, positron emission tomography).

12.2.1 INTERNATIONAL EQUIVALENCE

The wide variety of techniques that can be used to realize a primary standard for radioactivity [6] enables NMIs to compare results against other institutions, increasing the confidence in the results. The radioactive nature of the samples being standardized presents a unique challenge for international comparisons, requiring samples to be received simultaneously across multiple countries with differing regulations and geographies. This can be further complicated when the isotope of interest has a short (< 1 day) half-life. The BIPM plays a key role both in the organization of these comparisons and with the provision of the Système International de Référence (SIR) [9]. This system, based on a simple and stable measurement system (well-type ionization chamber), allows NMIs to submit samples for comparison outside of a comparison exercise – removing many of the scheduling complexities. For short-lived radionuclides (e.g. ^{18}F with a half-life of just 1.82890 (23) hours [10]), an alternative traveling system, based on a sodium iodide well-type crystal, has been developed (SIRTI – SIR Traveling Instrument [11]). This system allows measurements performed with the instrument at different international sites to be directly compared. The system was used to perform an international comparison of ^{18}F, which included measurements from NMIs across Europe, North America, Australia, and South Africa [12].

12.3 RADIONUCLIDE CALIBRATORS

The principal instrument used for measurements of radioactivity for clinical applications is the radionuclide calibrator (alternatively referred to as a (radionuclide) "dose calibrator" – a practice which should be avoided to prevent any confusion with units based upon the energy absorbed per unit mass of irradiated material, especially in the context of radiotheranostics and dosimetry).

These instruments provide the most common route for dissemination of primary activity measurements into the clinic (in the form of secondary and reference standards, see Figure 12.1) [13,14]. A radionuclide calibrator consists of a well-type ionization chamber (filled with gas at a pressure of several atmospheres) with a potential difference applied, coupled to electronics to read out the current produced from the ionization of the gas by incident radiation from a radioactive sample placed in the chamber. The time-averaged ionization current will be proportional to the activity of the radionuclide sample, with a constant of proportionality (referred to as the *calibration factor* or *dial setting*) that is specific to an individual radionuclide and sample geometry [13].

Calibration factors for a radionuclide calibrator can be determined by measurement with a primary standard source; in this case, the radionuclide calibrator can be considered a secondary standard. Alternatively, calibration factors can be determined using a range of traceable radionuclide standards and an energy-response curve can be calculated, from which calibration factors for all radionuclides can be derived (with additional knowledge of the radionuclide decay scheme). This calibration methodology is typically used for field instruments (see Figure 12.1). The use of non-carrier-added radionuclides (free of radionuclide impurities) is preferable when making these transfer measurements. Alternatively, if the amount of impurity is known and appropriate corrections applied, a carrier-added (or "patient dose") solution may be used, provided the level of impurities is consistent across samples. Calibration factors for a specific radiopharmaceutical compound (e.g. radiolabeled peptides, microspheres, colloidal solutions) may also be established using this calibration methodology [13]. In this case, care must be taken to establish the same geometry and distribution of compound for subsequent measurements with a specific calibration factor. Standard uncertainty [15] for a well-calibrated field instrument can be expected to be in the region of ~2% for medium-energy gamma emitters (100 - 2000 keV), or ~5% for low-energy gamma emitters (< 100 keV) and pure beta emitters. It is important to note that calibration factors are determined for a standard volume in a particular container geometry and any deviation from this requires the determination of a new calibration factor (e.g. by cross-calibration with a secondary standard calibrator or traceable source) to maintain measurement traceability and accuracy [13].

12.3.1 NATIONAL COMPARISONS OF RADIONUCLIDE CALIBRATOR MEASUREMENTS

There have been a number of studies published that report the intercomparison results of activity measurements using radionuclide calibrators in different clinical centers [16–21]. These comparisons are typically coordinated by a country's NMI, with the most common comparison protocol involving test sources that are prepared in a common clinical geometry calibrated by the NMI against the national standard and subsequently shipped to the participating clinics. Comparison exercises can be essential for highlighting problems with the transfer of standards to clinical use. For example, the impact of an incorrect ^{68}Ga radionuclide calibration factor on quantitative PET imaging, leading to the underestimation of the Standardized Uptake Values by up to 23%, has been demonstrated in a multicenter clinical trial [19]. A key aspect of these comparisons is the continued involvement of clinical centers and the accompanying improvement in measurement capabilities. An example of this improvement is seen in the case of ^{123}I measurement capabilities in UK hospitals where an increase in the fraction of centers with measurements within 5% of the certificated value was reported from 28% in 1996 to 85% by 2015 [20]. In the Czech Republic, a similar improvement was demonstrated for ^{131}I, with 80% of the institutions within 10% of the calibrated value in 1991 and 100% of the institutions within the 10% limits in 2002 [16].

12.4 ACTIVITY MEASUREMENTS FOR RADIOTHERANOSTICS

For clinically established radiotheranostic combinations of isotopes, there is now an accompanying corpus of activity standards, intercomparison exercises, and evaluated nuclear data providing an excellent foundation for establishing traceability. In the case of the broadly established radioiodine nuclides, the therapeutic nuclide ^{131}I has to date had 18 NMIs and one other laboratory perform comparisons of ^{131}I activity measurements through BIPM [22], with a number of reported standardization and national intercomparisons [23–25] and evaluated nuclear data [26]. Similarly, for the diagnostic nuclide ^{123}I, three NMIs and two other laboratories have performed comparisons of ^{123}I activity [27] and evaluated nuclear data produced [10]. In the case of the positron-emitting radionuclide ^{124}I, although results of a BIPM comparison have not been published, a number of primary standardizations have been reported [28–31] along with evaluated nuclear data [32]. Recently, the radiotheranostic pairing of diagnostic ^{68}Ga PET and therapeutic ^{177}Lu has become increasingly common. As with the radioiodine nuclides, there is an accompanying strong foundation for establishing traceability for both nuclides [33–45] and the alternative ^{64}Cu diagnostic companion [12,46–50].

The increasing interest in the development of novel radiotheranostic approaches will introduce radionuclides into preclinical and clinical use for which there are not currently primary activity standards and for which the nuclear data may have significantly increased uncertainties. Development of the standards to support these isotopes is an extensive process due to the relative complexity of performing primary standard measurements, the need for intercomparisons between NMIs, and the requirements to establish traceability to end-users through appropriate secondary standards. It is therefore advantageous to have NMIs involvement as early as possible in the development of new radiotheranostic treatments to establish these standards [5]. This process is demonstrated in recent work establishing new standards and nuclear data to support the development of the quartet of terbium isotopes (^{149,152,155,161}Tb) for radiotheranostics [51]. The first activity standardization of ^{161}Tb was recently reported [52], along with new determinations of the half-life [53,54] and gamma emission intensities [55]. The availability to the radionuclide metrology community of relatively small quantities of these novel radionuclides from facilities such as CERN-MEDICIS [56] has accelerated the establishment of standards, allowing harmonization of measurements and results in any potential clinical trials.

12.5 CONCLUSION

This chapter has reviewed the principles of measurement traceability that underpin clinical administrations of radiopharmaceuticals and the calibration of associated measurement devices. The systems to ensure international equivalence between primary standards of radioactivity are well established, with robust international comparisons in place for common nuclear medicine radionuclides. There are multiple routes to establishing traceability for measurements in a nuclear medicine clinic, accommodating a range of geographical and regulatory differences. Regardless of the route, traceability will include comprehensive documentation of the calibration chain, calibration against an appropriate measurement standard, and provide an assessment of uncertainty in the measurement result. Ongoing engagement with NMIs, especially participation in intercomparison exercises of clinical measurements, can be highly effective in improving the accuracy of clinical activity measurements at participating sites.

Radiotheranostics requires traceable activity calibration for multiple radionuclides, often in the form of "matched" pairs of diagnostic and therapeutic radionuclides. In addition, the requirements for quantified imaging and accompanying absorbed dose calculations necessitate traceable calibration of SPECT and PET imaging and traceable nuclear decay data. For clinically established radiotheranostic combinations of isotopes, these activity standards and evaluated nuclear data are well established, providing a foundation for the harmonization of measurements across clinical sites. As new radiotheranostic approaches, and associated novel radionuclides, are introduced, there is a need for accompanying new activity standards and improved nuclear data to establish traceability and allow harmonization of measurements.

FUNDING ACKNOWLEDGMENT

This work was supported by the National Measurement System of the UK's Department for Business, Energy and Industrial Strategy.

REFERENCES

1. B. E. Zimmerman and S. Judge, "Traceability in nuclear medicine," *Metrologia*, vol. 44, no. 4, pp. S127–S132, Aug. 2007, doi: 10.1088/0026-1394/44/4/S16.
2. L. Karam, "Measurement traceability in medical physics," *J. Med. Phys.*, vol. 39, no. 1, p. 1, 2014, doi: 10.4103/0971-6203.125470.
3. INTERNATIONAL ATOMIC ENERGY AGENCY, *Quality Assurance for Radioactivity Measurement in Nuclear Medicine, Technical Reports Series No. 454,* IAEA, Vienna (2006)
4. BIPM, IEC, IFCC, ILAC, ISO, IUPAC, IUPAP, and OIML. International vocabulary of metrology — Basic and general concepts and associated terms (VIM). Joint Committee for Guides in Metrology, JCGM 200:2012. (3rd edition), https://www.bipm.org/documents/20126/2071204/JCGM_200_2012.pdf/f0e1ad45-d337-bbeb-53a6-15fe649d0ff1.
5. A. J. Fenwick, J. L. Wevrett, K. M. Ferreira, A. M. Denis-Bacelar, and A. P. Robinson, "Quantitative imaging, dosimetry and metrology; Where do National Metrology Institutes fit in?," *Appl. Radiat. Isot.*, vol. 134, pp. 74–78 2018, doi: 10.1016/j.apradiso.2017.11.014
6. S. Pommé, "Methods for primary standardization of activity," *Metrologia*, vol. 44, no. 4, pp. S17–S26, Aug. 2007, doi: 10.1088/0026-1394/44/4/S03.
7. S. M. Judge *et al.*, "100 Years of radionuclide metrology," *Appl. Radiat. Isot.*, vol. 87, pp. 27–31, 2014, doi: 10.1016/j.apradiso.2013.11.121.
8. "Decay Data Evaluation Project – Laboratoire National Henri Becquerel." http://www.lnhb.fr/ddep_wg/ (accessed May 18, 2022).
9. G. Ratel, "The Système International de Référence and its application in key comparisons," *Metrologia*, vol. 44, no. 4, pp. S7–S16, Aug. 2007, doi: 10.1088/0026-1394/44/4/S02.
10. M.-M. Bé *et al.*, *Table of Radionuclides*, vol. 1. Pavillon de Breteuil, F-92310 Sèvres, France: Bureau International des Poids et Mesures, 2004. [Online]. Available: http://www.bipm.org/utils/common/pdf/monographieRI/Monographie_BIPM-5_Tables_Vol1.pdf
11. Michotte C., Nonis M., Bobin C., Altzizoglou T., Sibbens G. "Rapport BIPM-2013/02: The SIRTI: a new tool developed at the BIPM for comparing activity measurements of short-lived radionuclides worldwide," p. 1–23 2013
12. C. Michotte, T. Dziel, A. Listkowska, T. Ziemek, Z. Tymiński, and I. D. Silva, "Activity measurements of the radionuclides ^{99m}Tc, ^{18}F and ^{64}Cu for the POLATOM, Poland, in the ongoing comparisons BIPM.RI (II)-K4 series and KCRV update in the corresponding BIPM.RI(II)-K1 comparison," *Metrologia*, vol. 59, no. 1A, pp. 06004, Jan. 2022, doi: 10.1088/0026-1394/59/1A/06004.
13. R. Gadd *et al.*, "NPL GPG 93: Protocol for Establishing and Maintaining the Calibration of Medical Radionuclide Calibrators and their Quality Control," 2006. [Online]. Available: https://eprintspublications.npl.co.uk/3661/
14. E. Nickoloff *et al.*, "The Selection, Use, Calibration, and Quality Assurance of Radionuclide Calibrators Used in Nuclear Medicine," AAPM, Jun. 2012. doi: 10.37206/137.
15. BIPM, IEC, IFCC, ILAC, ISO, IUPAC, IUPAP, and OIML, "Evaluation of measurement data — Guide to the expression of uncertainty in measurement." Joint Committee for Guides in Metrology, JCGM 100:2008, https://www.bipm.org/documents/20126/2071204/JCGM_100_2008_E.pdf/cb0ef43f-baa5-11cf-3f85-4dcd86f77bd6.
16. V. Olšovcová, "Activity measurements with radionuclide calibrators in the Czech Republic," *Appl. Radiat. Isot.*, vol. 60, no. 2–4, pp. 535–538, Feb. 2004, doi: 10.1016/j.apradiso.2003.11.072.
17. M. K. Schultz *et al.*, "A performance evaluation of 90Y dose-calibrator measurements in nuclear pharmacies and clinics in the United States," *Appl. Radiat. Isot.*, vol. 66, no. 2, pp. 252–260, Feb. 2008, doi: 10.1016/j.apradiso.2007.09.002.
18. K. Kossert *et al.*, "Comparison of 90Y activity measurements in nuclear medicine in Germany," *Appl. Radiat. Isot.*, vol. 109, pp. 247–249, 2016, doi: 10.1016/j.apradiso.2015.11.005.
19. D. L. Bailey *et al.*, "Accuracy of dose calibrators for 68Ga PET imaging: Unexpected findings in a multicenter clinical pretrial assessment," *J. Nucl. Med.*, vol. 59, no. 4, pp. 636–638, 2018, doi: 10.2967/jnumed.117.202861.

20. K. M. Ferreira and A. J. Fenwick, "123I intercomparison exercises: Assessment of measurement capabilities in UK hospitals," *Appl. Radiat. Isot.*, vol. 134, no. November 2017, pp. 108–111, 2018, doi: 10.1016/j.apradiso.2017.11.015.

21. C. Saldarriaga Vargas *et al.*, "An international multi-center investigation on the accuracy of radionuclide calibrators in nuclear medicine theragnostics," *EJNMMI Phys.*, vol. 7, no. 1, 2020, doi: 10.1186/s40658-020-00338-3.

22. C. Michotte *et al.*, "BIPM comparison BIPM.RI(II)-K1.I-131 of activity measurements of the radionuclide [131] I for the NMIJ (Japan), the NIST (USA) and the LNE-LNHB (France), with linked results for the APMP.RI(II)-K2.I-131 comparison," *Metrologia* , vol. 51, no. 4, , 2014, doi: 10.1088/0026-1394/51/1A/06003.

23. L. Joseph, R. Anuradha, R. Nathuram, V. V. Shaha, and M. C. Abani, "National intercomparisons of 131I radioactivity measurements in nuclear medicine centres in India," *Appl. Radiat. Isot.*, vol. 59, no. 5–6, pp. 359–362, Nov. 2003, doi: 10.1016/S0969-8043(03)00192-1.

24. B. E. Zimmerman, A. Meghzifene, and K. R. Shortt, "Establishing measurement traceability for national laboratories: Results of an IAEA comparison of 131I," *Appl. Radiat. Isot.*, vol. 66, no. 6–7, pp. 954–959, 2008, doi: 10.1016/j.apradiso.2008.02.067.

25. D. B. Kulkarni, R. Anuradha, P. J. Reddy, and L. Joseph, "Standardization of 131I: Implementation of CIEMAT/NIST method at BARC, India," *Appl. Radiat. Isot.*, vol. 69, no. 10, pp. 1512–1515, Oct. 2011, doi: 10.1016/j.apradiso.2011.06.004.

26. M.-M. Bé *et al.*, *Table of Radionuclides*, vol. 8. Pavillon de Breteuil, F-92310 Sèvres, France: Bureau International des Poids et Mesures, 2016. [Online]. Available: http://www.bipm.org/utils/common/pdf/monographieRI/Monographie_BIPM-5_Tables_Vol8.pdf

27. G. Ratel and C. Michotte, "BIPM comparison BIPM.RI(II)-K1.I-123 of activity measurements of the radionuclide [123] I and links for the 1983 EUROMET.RI(II)-K2.I-123 comparison," *Metrologia*, vol. 40, no. 1A, pp. 06022, Jan. 2003, doi: 10.1088/0026-1394/40/1A/06022.

28. D. H. Woods *et al.*, "The Standardization and Measurement of Decay Scheme Data of 124I," International Journal of Radiation Applications and Instrumentation. Part A. Applied Radiation and Isotopes, vol. 43, 4, p. 551-560, doi: 10.1016/0883-2889(92)90138-5.

29. A. Luca, M. Sahagia, M.-R. Ioan, A. Antohe, and B. L. Savu, "Experimental determination of some nuclear decay data in the decays of 177 Lu, 186 Re and 124 I," *Appl. Radiat. Isot.*, vol. 109, pp. 146–150, Mar. 2016, doi: 10.1016/j.apradiso.2015.11.072.

30. M. Sahagia, M.-R. Ioan, A. Antohe, A. Luca, and C. Ivan, "Measurement of 124I," *Appl. Radiat. Isot.*, vol. 109, pp. 349–353, Mar. 2016, doi: 10.1016/j.apradiso.2015.12.002.

31. D. E. Bergeron, J. T. Cessna, R. Fitzgerald, L. Pibida, and B. E. Zimmerman, "Standardization of I-124 by three liquid scintillation-based methods," *Appl. Radiat. Isot.*, vol. 154, p. 108849, Dec. 2019, doi: 10.1016/j.apradiso.2019.108849.

32. B. E. Zimmerman, "Decay data for the positron emission tomography imaging radionuclide 124I: A DDEP evaluation," *Appl. Radiat. Isot.*, vol. 134, pp. 433–438, Apr. 2018, doi: 10.1016/j.apradiso.2017.10.051.

33. B. E. Zimmerman, M. P. Unterweger, and J. W. Brodack, "The standardization of 177Lu by 4pb liquid scintillation spectrometry with 3H-standard efficiency tracing," *Appl. Radiat. Isot.*, vol. 54, no. 5, p. 623,-631, 2001, doi: 10.1016/S0969-8043(00)00316-X.

34. M.-M. Bé *et al.*, *Table of Radionuclides*, vol. 2. Pavillon de Breteuil, F-92310 Sèvres, France: Bureau International des Poids et Mesures, 2004. [Online]. Available: http://www.bipm.org/utils/common/pdf/monographieRI/Monographie_BIPM-5_Tables_Vol2.pdf

35. M. Capogni, M. L. Cozzella, P. De Felice, and A. Fazio, "Comparison between two absolute methods used for 177Lu activity measurements and its standardization," *Appl. Radiat. Isot.*, vol. 70, no. 9, pp. 2075–2080, Sep. 2012, doi: 10.1016/j.apradiso.2012.02.040.

36. K. Kossert, O. J. Nähle, O. Ott, and R. Dersch, "Activity determination and nuclear decay data of 177Lu," *Appl. Radiat. Isot.*, vol. 70, no. 9, pp. 2215–2221, Sep. 2012, doi: 10.1016/j.apradiso.2012.02.104.

37. B. E. Zimmerman *et al.*, "Results of an international comparison for the activity measurement of 177Lu," *Appl. Radiat. Isot.*, vol. 70, no. 9, pp. 1825–1830, 2012, doi: 10.1016/j.apradiso.2012.02.014.

38. M.-M. Bé *et al.*, *Table of Radionuclides*, vol. 7. Pavillon de Breteuil, F-92310 Sèvres, France: Bureau International des Poids et Mesures, 2013. [Online]. Available: http://www.bipm.org/utils/common/pdf/monographieRI/Monographie_BIPM-5_Tables_Vol7.pdf

39. C. Michotte *et al.*, "BIPM comparison BIPM.RI(II)-K1.Lu-177 of activity measurements of the radionuclide [177] Lu for the NPL (UK) and the IRMM (EU), with linked results for the comparison

CCRI(II)-K2.Lu-177," *Metrologia*, vol. 51, no. 1A, pp. 06002– 06002, Jan. 2014, doi: 10.1088/ 0026-1394/51/1A/06002.

40. P. Dryák, J. Sochorová, J. Šolc, and P. Auerbach, "Activity standardization, photon emission probabilities and half-life measurements of 177Lu," *Appl. Radiat. Isot.*, vol. 109, pp. 160–163, 2016, doi: 10.1016/j.apradiso.2015.11.059.

41. W. M. van Wyngaardt, M. L. Smith, T. W. Jackson, B. Howe, S. M. Tobin, and M. I. Reinhard, "Development of the Australian standard for germanium-68 by two liquid scintillation counting methods," *Appl. Radiat. Isot.*, vol. 134, pp. 79–84, Apr. 2018, doi: 10.1016/j.apradiso.2017.10.005.

42. J. T. Cessna *et al.*, "Results of an international comparison of activity measurements of 68Ge," *Appl. Radiat. Isot.*, vol. 134, pp. 385–390, Apr. 2018, doi: 10.1016/j.apradiso.2017.10.052.

43. C. Bobin, C. Thiam, and J. Bouchard, "Standardization of 68 Ge/ 68 Ga using the $4\pi\beta$–γ coincidence method based on Cherenkov counting," *Appl. Radiat. Isot.*, vol. 134, pp. 252–256, Apr. 2018, doi: 10.1016/j.apradiso.2017.06.044.

44. P. O. Verdecia, L. G. Rodríguez, R. A. S. Águila, Y. M. León, Y. J. Magaña, and P. Cassette, "68 Ga activity calibrations for nuclear medicine applications in Cuba," *Appl. Radiat. Isot.*, vol. 134, pp. 112–116, Apr. 2018, doi: 10.1016/j.apradiso.2017.11.010.

45. C. Michotte *et al.*, "BIPM comparison BIPM.RI(II)-K1.Ge-68 of activity measurements of the radionuclide [68]Ge for the LNMRI/IRD, NIST, NIM, IRA-METAS, LNE-LNHB and the TAEK, and the linked 2015 CCRI(II)-K2.Ge-68 comparison," *Metrologia*, vol. 57, no. 1A, pp. 06014, Jan. 2020, doi: 10.1088/0026-1394/57/1A/06014.

46. M. Capogni, P. De Felice, A. Fazio, F. Latini, and K. Abbas, "Development of a primary standard for calibration of 64Cu activity measurement systems," *Appl. Radiat. Isot.*, vol. 66, no. 6–7, pp. 948–953, Jun. 2008, doi: 10.1016/j.apradiso.2008.02.041.

47. C. Wanke, K. Kossert, O. J. Nähle, and O. Ott, "Activity standardization and decay data of 64Cu," *Appl. Radiat. Isot.*, vol. 68, no. 7–8, pp. 1297–1302, Jul. 2010, doi: 10.1016/j.apradiso.2010.01.005.

48. M. Sahagia, A. Luca, A. Antohe, and C. Ivan, "Standardization of 64Cu and 68Ga by the $4\pi(PC)\beta$-γ coincidence method and calibration of the ionization chamber," *Appl. Radiat. Isot.*, vol. 70, no. 9, pp. 2025–2030, Sep. 2012, doi: 10.1016/j.apradiso.2012.02.043.

49. D. E. Bergeron, J. T. Cessna, R. Fitzgerald, L. Pibida, and B. E. Zimmerman, "Standardization of 64Cu activity," *Appl. Radiat. Isot.*, vol. 139, pp. 266–273, Sep. 2018, doi: 10.1016/j.apradiso.2018.05.023.

50. M.-M. Bé *et al.*, *Table of Radionuclides*, vol. 6. Pavillon de Breteuil, F-92310 Sèvres, France: Bureau International des Poids et Mesures, 2011. [Online]. Available: http://www.bipm.org/utils/common/ pdf/monographieRI/Monographie_BIPM-5_Tables_Vol6.pdf

51. C. Müller *et al.*, "A unique matched quadruplet of terbium radioisotopes for PET and SPECT and for α- and β- radionuclide therapy: an in vivo proof-of-concept study with a new receptor-targeted folate derivative.," *J. Nucl. Med.*, vol. 53, no. 12, pp. 1951–1959, 2012, doi: 10.2967/jnumed.112.107540.

52. Y. Nedjadi *et al.*, "Activity standardisation of 161Tb," *Appl. Radiat. Isot.*, vol. 166, p. 109411, Dec. 2020, doi: 10.1016/j.apradiso.2020.109411.

53. M. T. Durán *et al.*, "Determination of 161Tb half-life by three measurement methods," *Appl. Radiat. Isot.*, vol. 159, p. 109085, May 2020, doi: 10.1016/j.apradiso.2020.109085.

54. S. M. Collins *et al.*, "Determination of the 161Tb half-life," *Appl. Radiat. Isot.*, vol. 182, p. 110140, Apr. 2022, doi: 10.1016/j.apradiso.2022.110140.

55. F. Juget *et al.*, "Determination of the gamma and X-ray emission intensities of terbium-161," *Appl. Radiat. Isot.*, vol. 174, p. 109770, Aug. 2021, doi: 10.1016/j.apradiso.2021.109770.

56. C. Duchemin *et al.*, "CERN-MEDICIS: A review since commissioning in 2017," *Front. Med.*, vol. 8, p. 693682, Jul. 2021, doi: 10.3389/fmed.2021.693682.

13 Instrumentation, Calibration, Quantitative Imaging, and Quality Control

Michael Ljungberg

13.1 INTRODUCTION

Imaging of theranostic radionuclides is based on measuring photons that are emitted following a decay of radionuclides that also emit charged particles that are used for patient therapy. The photons are emitted isotropically, and since some of the photons penetrate the patient, it is possible to detect them using a gamma camera, SPECT (single-photon emission computed tomography) and in some cases using PET (positron emission tomography). The photon emission is proportional to the activity; therefore, if the number of impinging photons detected is proportional to the number of decays in a certain volume of interest (VOI) in the image, the activity in that VOI can also be estimated. A quantitative accurate measurement of the activity distribution in vivo will be needed to estimate the total amount of energy emitted from the charged particles, which is important because the deposited energy is generally assumed to correlate with damage to the tissue (i.e., the treatment outcome). However, there are several physical factors and instrumentation-imposed limitations in such a measurement that will result in deterioration of the image and therefore need to be considered to accurately estimate the activity in a specific VOI from images. The purpose of this chapter is to briefly outline these factors.

13.2 INSTRUMENTATION

High-energy photons cannot be viewed directly with the naked eye. Therefore, we need a process that converts the relatively high energy that is transported by photons originating from radioactive decay and subsequently deposits it in a detector system with the purpose of generating a measurable signal. Over the years, the most common way of doing this has been to use a sodium iodide (NaI(Tl)) scintillation detector, where the NaI crystal is doped with a small amount of thallium (Tl). The principle behind scintillation detection is that when a high-energy photon interacts in the crystal, it releases electrons that gain kinetic energy so that they can further interact with other atomic electrons with a subsequential release of scintillation photons with wavelengths in the blue part of the visible spectrum. The process causes many light photons to be emitted during these excitations and de-excitations with an intensity that is proportional to the total deposited energy. This light is guided to a photomultiplier tube (PMT) that generates an electric signal proportional to the light intensity. Therefore, by measuring the electrical signal from a PMT, the energy of the impinging photons can indirectly be estimated from the energy deposited in the NaI(Tl) crystal. As a crystalline material, NaI(Tl) has been used in nuclear medicine scintillation cameras for many years. Although it has pros and cons, the use of NaI(Tl) has proven itself over many years and it has become the method of choice for nuclear medicine detectors.

DOI: 10.1201/9781003250913-16

13.2.1 Scintillation Cameras – NaI(Tl)

NaI(Tl) scintillation cameras are based on three fundamental parts, namely (a) a thin NaI(Tl) crystal with a large field-of-view (FOV), (b) a collimator to restrict the detection of photons based on their angular distribution, and (c) a grid of multiple PMTs that together form not only the energy signal but also provide an estimate of the position of impinging energy. The initial design was conceived by Hal O. Anger [1,2] and this design has remained the core of commercial cameras for over 50 years. The principle is that the collimator, which is made of a high-Z material (usually lead), only allows photons with certain direction angles to pass through it and interact in the NaI(Tl) crystal. The detected interaction locations will then be used to create 2D projection images. The most common collimator type is the parallel-hole collimator that consists of many holes parallel in direction to each other. The principle is that only photons passing through the holes will reach the detector and contribute to scintillation light and the measured signal. As many PMTs are used that each cover a specific part of the crystal, the position of the interaction locations for a certain incoming photon can then be determined by weighting the energy signal from surrounding PMT tubes with their PMT's absolute position (x,y) on the crystal (center-of-gravity calculation). The precision of this measurement is about 3–4 mm FWHM (Full-Width at Half Maximum) which is less than the size of the PMTs used. However, the system's spatial resolution is mainly dependent on the geometrical properties and the material of the collimator. To obtain a reasonable counting statistic (i.e., less noise), the hole diameter cannot be too small; alternatively, the hole-length cannot be too long, since both define the acceptance angle that determines if the photon can pass through the hole. Thus, to obtain high sensitivity (cps/MBq), the hole diameter should be large and the hole length short, while for high spatial resolution the opposite applies. Furthermore, if the distance from the source to the camera increases, geometrically there will be an increased possibility that a photon can pass through adjacent holes and interact at some distance away from the projection line which leads to reduced spatial resolution. Different types of collimators favoring either resolution or sensitivity are therefore available for a particular study. Theranostic radionuclides often emit photons of relatively high energies, so this also requires collimators with thicker hole walls to prevent septal penetration, which leads to poorer spatial resolution and potentially streak artifacts.

13.2.2 Solid-State Cameras – CZT

Even though NaI(Tl) has proven to be a very good and robust all-round scintillator for photon detection, use of this crystal has some limitations, namely, (a) the relatively poor energy resolution, (b) the long decay time for the scintillation light and (c) the need for relatively large number of PMTs. The recently increased use of solid-state CZT (cadmium zinc telluride) detectors has shown these to be a good alternative. This type of detector is based on direct collection of charges, created by secondary electrons released by interacting photons. By applying an electrical potential between a cathode and multiple small anodes, an image can be directly formed. The detector modules used in the latest commercial systems are usually in the form of 16×16 anodes (2.46×2.46 mm^2 pixels) with detectors of thicknesses 5–7.25 mm. The modules are thus very compact in size when compared to NaI(Tl) connected to PMTs, and this therefore enables a design with multi-detector camera systems. The first commercial clinical systems were dedicated cardiac cameras (D-SPECT by Spectrum Dynamics, Inc, and Discovery 530n by GE Healthcare). Full-sized CZT SPECT/CT systems (GE 870 CZT Pro) are available from GE Healthcare. Two new dedicated SPECT/CT CZT systems with multiple detectors are the Veriton system by Spectrum Dynamics, Inc, and the StarGuide SPECT/CT by GE Healthcare. Both systems have 12 detectors positioned around the patient and the whole detector package can rotate. In addition, each detector can swivel allowing the acquisition to focus on just a part inside the patient (e.g., the heart) or make it possible to cover the whole body. Since the projections are acquired simultaneously around the patient, dynamic SPECT recordings are possible. It will become apparent in the future whether this system will be useful for theranostic images because of potential problems in changing collimators. However, in principle, it should be possible to image the 113 keV photon with low-energy collimators in a ^{177}Lu decay if proper correction is made for the downscatter contribution from the 208 keV photons. It should also be mentioned here that hand-held CZT cameras, based on a single 16×16 detector module, are available [3,4].

The principle behind CZT detectors differs from that behind scintillation cameras in that electron/hole pairs are directly created from incoming photons. However, during the detection process, the electrons and holes can recombine so that the charge measured at detection will be less than expected. Furthermore, since multiple anodes are used in a CZT pixelized camera, the charge cloud can be shared between anodes, which also leads to reduced detected energy.

13.2.3   PET CAMERAS

PET systems use imaging radionuclides that emit positrons (the antiparticle of an electron, i.e., equivalent to an electron but with a positive charge) because the radionuclides have an excess of protons. When coming to rest, positrons cannot co-exist in proximity to electrons so electron–positron annihilation occurs, which creates two photons of 511 keV (the energy corresponding to two electron masses) because of energy conservation. As the conservation of momentum principle must also be observed, the two photons will be emitted in opposite directions.

A PET system consists of many small individual scintillation detectors that are symmetrically positioned in a 360-degree ring system. The principle behind PET imaging is that if two individual detectors each detect scintillation light from two photon interactions within a very narrow timing window, then these two detections are assumed to come from the same positron annihilation (a coincidence event). The positions of the two detectors will then define a line-of-response (LOR), that is an imaginary line along which the annihilation must have occurred. By rebinning the measured LORs into projection data as a function of LOR angle (sinograms), a transversal image of the locations of the annihilation can be obtained using some of the image reconstruction methods described in the next section.

It is only the coincidence events that are of interest in PET imaging. However, most detections occur as single events in one of the crystals. Since these events are not useful but still occupy the detector for some time, it is very important that the processing and decay time for a detector event be as low as possible. BGO (bismuth germanate) is a standard crystal material that has been used for many years due to its high effective atomic number and density. However, if faster crystals are used, it is possible to use Time-of-Flight (TOF) information, that is, to measure the time difference between detection of the two annihilation photons. Modern PET systems therefore use crystals that have much faster timing properties. Table 13.1 lists the properties of some crystal materials.

TABLE 13.1
Characteristics of Scintillation Crystals Used for PET

Scintillator	Composition	Density [g cm^{-3}]	Z_{eff}	Decay Time [ns]
BGO	$Bi_4Ge_3O_{12}$	7.1	75	300
NaI	NaI(Tl)	3.7	51	230
GSO	$Gd_2SiO_5(Ce)$	6.7	59	60
LSO	$Lu_2SiO_5(Ce)$	7.4	66	40
YAP	$YAlO_3(Ce)$	5.5	33.5	30
LPS	$Lu_2Si_2O_7(Ce)$	6.2	63.8	30
LUAP	$LuAlO_3(Ce)$	8.3	64.9	18

Source: Data compiled from Humm et al. [5].

The spatial resolution is limited by the number of possible LORs. One difficulty in making small detectors is the need for PMTs. However, the number of LORs can be increased by slicing the crystal into small compartments (tunnels). By using multiple PMTs for each detector and the same principle as used in the center-of-gravity calculation applied in scintillation cameras, a much larger number of LORs can be defined resulting in improved spatial resolution. Recent PET systems have also replaced scintillators with photon detection based on solid-state detectors, so-called Silicon PhotoMultiplier (SiPM) detectors, due to their better intrinsic timing properties and higher photon-detection efficiency [6].

13.2.4   HYBRID SYSTEMS (SPECT/CT AND PET/CT)

The interest in using hybrid system equipped with a CT (Computed Tomography) unit combined with a SPECT or PET detector has increased considerably and they are now a standard in many applications. A major focus of interest for the first designs was the facility of having a CT image as an aid for locating uptakes and attenuation correction. The GE Millenium[TM] hybrid SPECT/CT camera equipped with the HawkEye[TM] single-slice CT (GE Healthcare, Haifa, Israel) was the first commercially available SPECT/CT system and this system created CT images with a thickness of 10 mm. The spatial resolution was about 3.5 mm, the tube voltage was either 120 or 140 kV, and the tube current – exposure time product (measure of the total radiation produced over a set amount of time) was 2.5 mAs. A CT acquisition that matched the FOV for the SPECT cameras took approximately 10 minutes to complete. Due to the low resolution resulting from physiological movements, the system was not regarded as a diagnostic CT.

One of the most important applications for a combined SPECT and CT unit is the ability to fuse anatomical and morphological images because of the, in most cases, poor landmarks in a SPECT image. However, if a SPECT image is geometrically adjusted on the CT image and both are displayed together using dual-color table techniques, the location of a lesion becomes more evident. Prior to SPECT/CT, some manufacturers offered attenuation compensation methods based on simultaneous transmission imaging with a radioactive source such as ^{153}Gd line sources or ^{57}Co flood sources [7]. However, the poor spatial resolution and image quality, and crosstalk between emission and transmission photons, prohibited more diverse applications. The requirement for a faster and better method of obtaining attenuation maps and anatomical localization therefore led to the development of SPECT/CT hybrid systems.

The CT information is expressed in Hounsfield Units (HU), defined as: $1 \text{ HU} = 1000 \cdot (\mu-\mu_{water}) / (\mu_{water}-\mu_{air})$. It should be remembered that the HU values from a CT are obtained from a continuous energy spectrum of X-ray photons. This needs to be considered when converting an image of HU numbers to attenuation coefficient images for a fixed energy.

A CT image, registered to a SPECT image, is also very useful for volume segmentation due to its superior spatial resolution. However, when calculating activity and activity concentration using CT-based VOIs, there is a need for a correction for the spill-out and spill-in of counts. This can be made by applying partial volume corrections [7].

13.3   TOMOGRAPHIC RECONSTRUCTION

A major limitation in scintillation camera imaging is that the raw images are 2D projections and represent the distribution of events from photons incoming along projection lines. Thus, no information about from where on the line the photons were emitted from a decay can be determined. This also holds true for PET since LORs in one sense also represent projections. A single projection is therefore not sufficient to obtain the source depth. However, if it is assumed that the source distribution does not change during the acquisition time, by acquiring projections at different angles around the object, sufficient information can be obtained to mathematically reconstruct the activity distribution in 3D.

The two most important tomographic reconstruction methods that have been used clinically over the years are the filtered back projection (FBP) and model-based iterative reconstruction methods (ML-EM/OS-EM).

13.3.1   FILTERED BACK PROJECTION

As stated above, for scintillation camera imaging, the acquired image reflects the sum of counts (interactions) from photons traveling along a straight line (forward projection). Therefore, using a computer it is possible to reverse the process by backprojecting the measured data over an image matrix that represents an imaginary area. Since it is not known where the photons that generated the data come from, the measured data are often distributed evenly along the line over the area defined by an image matrix. This procedure is called direct back projection (DBP). It turns out that this method creates blurred images with low contrast because data are also backprojected in areas of no activity and even outside the object. This effect can, however, be compensated for by applying filtering of the raw data by a ramp filter that is constructed in such a way that it reduces the blurring to a large extent. The mathematical justification for using this filter is discussed elsewhere [8], but an important effect is that the nature of the ramp filter is a high-pass filter meaning that it will amplify the image noise (often a high-frequency component). Since noise usually appears in nuclear medicine projections, this leads to an even noisier reconstructed image. This noise amplification can, however, be suppressed partly by applying a second low-pass filter (for example, a Butterworth filter with a shape tailored by specific cut-off and order values). However, this additional low-pass filtering procedure generally also decreases the spatial resolution. Figure 13.1 shows the principles of the filtered back projection (FBP) reconstruction.

A FBP can mathematically be described by

$$f(x, y) = \int_{0}^{\pi} F^{-1}[\,|v|F\{p(r, \theta)\}\,]d\theta, \tag{13.1}$$

where F and F^{-1} represent the Fourier transform and inverse Fourier transform operations, respectively, and $r = x \cdot cos(\theta) + y \cdot sin(\theta)$. By (a) calculating the Fourier transform of the acquired projection data $p(r, \theta)$, (b) multiplying the result of this transformation with a ramp-shaped filter $|v|$ and (c) finally calculating the inverse Fourier transform, the result can then be back-projected to obtain an image of acceptable resolution.

As mentioned above, probably the most used method for reducing statistical image noise is to apply a low-pass filter that weights a specific pixel value based on the contents of its neighbors. The filtering can in principle be (a) applied in 2D on projection data prior to reconstruction, (b) applied as a post-reconstruction operation in 3D on the noisy reconstructed image or (c) applied as an additional multiplicative 1D filtering step within the FBP procedure by multiplying with a second low-pass filter function, $lp(v)$, as shown below:

$$f(x, y) = \int_{0}^{\pi} F^{-1}[lp(v)|v|F\{p(r, \theta)\}\,]d\theta. \tag{13.2}$$

An optimization procedure for a particular kind of study is thus to find the optimal impact of the filter that reduces the noise to an acceptable level while at the same time keeping as many as possible of the high frequencies that represent true information.

13.3.2   MODEL-BASED ITERATIVE RECONSTRUCTION

This category of reconstruction methods is today the method of choice for both SPECT and PET. It is based on a computer model of the imaging system and the patient geometry. From these, an

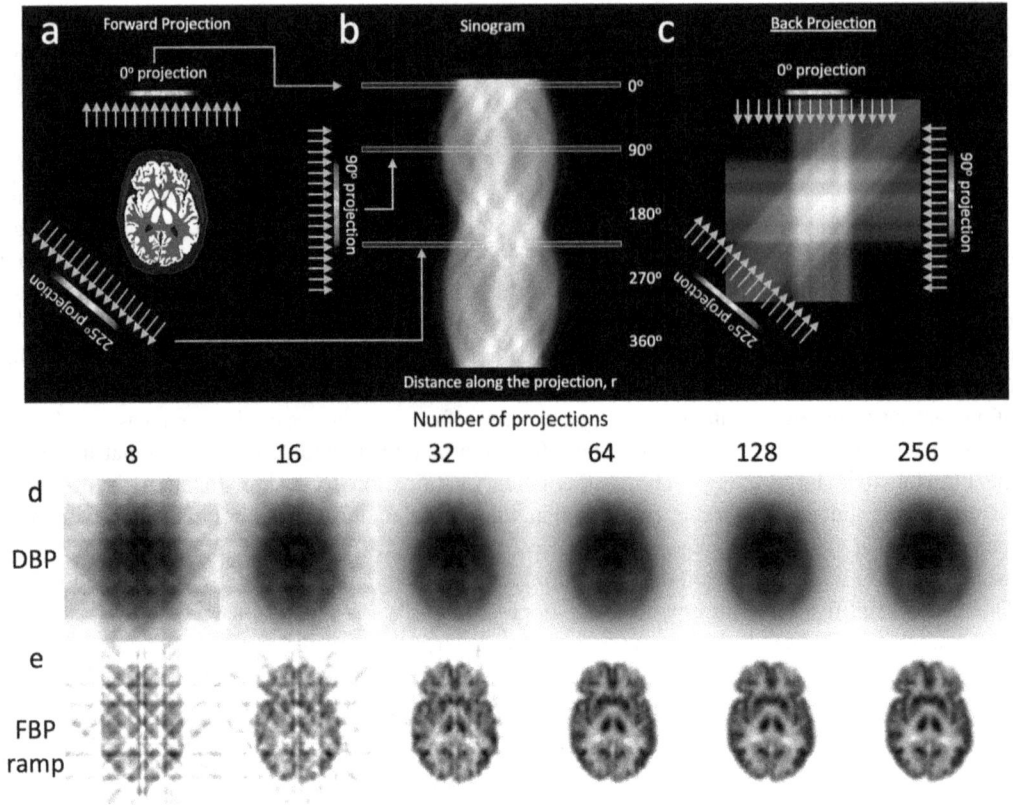

FIGURE 13.1 Three basic steps in the reconstruction of a tomographic image. (a) Photons emitted in parallel directions are passing though the collimator and generate a projection image. The camera is rotated to get different views of the same distribution. (b) The data acquired are reorganized into a sinogram. (c) The data are backprojected into the object domain to generate an estimated activity distribution. The middle row (d) shows images reconstructed from a different number of projections ranging from 8 to 256 using direct back projection (DBP. The poor image quality can here be seen clearly. The lower row (e) shows, for the same number of projection angles as for (d), reconstructed images but now from filtered back projection (FBP). The figure has been taken with permission from Ljungberg et al. in Chapter 16 [8].

estimate projection image is created using an initial estimate of the source distribution obtained using a forward-projection procedure. The estimated projections are then compared to measured projections and the difference between these two projections is then estimated and used to calculate an error image which can then be used to modify (or update) the initial image estimate. Most commercial systems use the maximum-likelihood expectation-maximization (ML-EM) algorithm, introduced by Shepp and Vardi [9], which is the ratio of the estimated projection to the measured projection that defines the difference between the two types of projections. Here, it is customary to start with an image in which all voxels have a constant value (uniform estimate), but it is also possible to start with an FBP image. One restriction is, however, that the starting value needs to be greater than zero. The ratios of the projections are then back-projected for all projection angles to form an error image that upon conclusion will be multiplied with the initial estimate to obtain an updated version (better estimate). The procedure iterates until the difference is small (i.e., for the ML-EM algorithm, the ratio converges to unity). Thus, the assumption here is that if the estimated and measured projections agree within some criteria, then the estimated images will reflect the unknown activity distribution in the object. Mathematically, the ML-EM algorithm can be expressed as follows:

$$f_i^{n+1} = \frac{f_i^n}{\sum_j a_{ij}} \sum_j a_{ij} \frac{p_j}{\left(\sum_k a_{kj} f_k^n\right)}, \tag{13.3}$$

where f^n and f^{n+1} are the current and new estimates, respectively, of the tomographic image at the ith voxel location, and p_j is the measured value at the jth pixel in the projection.

In an iterative reconstruction, the model that describes the emission and detection process that relates to the object activity distribution and forms the projection data is referred to as the system matrix (a_{ij} in Equation 13.3). This system matrix represents the probability that photons emitted from a voxel location in the object will be detected in a specific pixel in the projection. The system matrix accounts for the system geometry, but, in principle, also considers physical factors such as attenuation, scatter, and collimator effects. These factors can be incorporated into the system model by simply modifying the weighting of the matrix elements based on the probability of each occurrence.

One limitation of the ML-EM algorithm has been the slow convergence rate of the iteration to obtain a reliable solution. This is partly because data from all projection angles are used to form the error image (ratio) before it is used to update the estimate. Consequently, in the early days of its use, the reconstruction time was found to be too long for clinical use. However, Hudson and Larkin [10] proposed an alternative method, called ordered-subsets expectation-maximization (OS-EM), that is a method based very closely on the principles of ML-EM, but which differs in that the error image is created from data representing only a subset of projection angles. A typical number of projection angles in a subset can be 6–10 with the angles evenly distributed. This means that for each iteration (i.e., data from all projection angles having been processed), the image estimate will be updated equal to the number of subsets, n. A rule of thumb is therefore that the OS-EM procedure is n times faster than the ML-EM to obtain roughly the same image quality. Figure 13.2 shows a flow chart of the major parts of an OS-EM algorithm. Note that if n equals one, then OS-EM is equivalent to ML-EM.

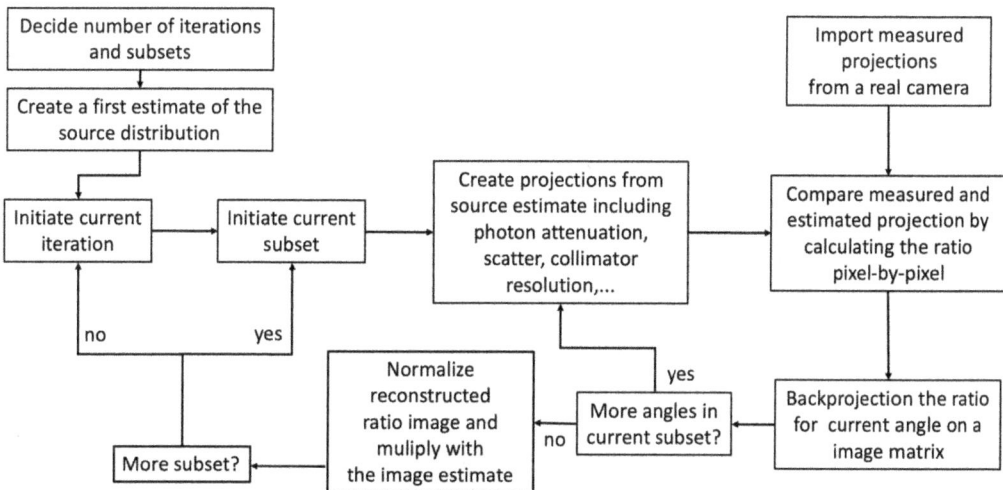

FIGURE 13.2 Main components of the ML-EM/OS-EM algorithms. After an arbitrary initial estimate of the source distribution, projections are calculated using a camera/patient model and the results are compared to measured projections. The projection ratio, voxel-by-voxel, are then calculated, back-projected, and used to update the source estimate until convergence is reached. Note that when only one subset of projection angle is used, the OS-EM algorithm is equivalent to the ML-EM algorithm.

It is very important to understand that the purpose of the iterative process is to modify the initial estimate so that the generated projections from this estimate subsequently compared to the measured projections. However, whether the final image will correctly represent the activity distribution will depend on how well the projection mimics the camera performance and the radiation transport through the computer model of the patient. For example, if the effect of attenuation is not included in the computer model, then the iterative method will indeed converge to a stable solution, but this solution will not match the activity distribution in the patient because the measured projection is affected by attenuation, but the estimated projection is not. Therefore, adding an accurate model of attenuation, including information on heterogeneities from a registered set of CT images, results in compensation for attenuation and thus a better estimate of the activity distribution. The same holds true for scatter contribution, collimator resolution, and other effects. Thus, a realistic projection model is essential for accurate tomographic reconstruction. The following section will discuss some of the major physical effects that may need to be implemented in the forward projection.

13.4 PROBLEMS RELATED TO QUANTITATIVE IMAGING

13.4.1 Photon Attenuation

Photon attenuation is a general term for physical interactions that could affect a photon traveling in a certain direction and prevent detection. These effects include (a) photon absorption where the energy of the photon is completely transferred to an orbital electron resulting in an ionization event, (b) Compton scattering when the photon only loses a part of its energy by interacting with an orbital electron but continues its onward travel with a change in direction, (c) coherent scattering where the photon changes direction without any loss of energy, and (d) the photon interacts with the atom and creates an electron–positron pair (only relevant for incoming photons with energies greater than 1.022 MeV). All these types of interaction can thus lead to a loss of detection within a main photopeak energy window, and the general effect will be a measured count rate that is lower than expected. The photon interaction processes are generally a function of atomic number (Z), mass density (g cm^{-3}), and photon energy. The probabilities for the different processes can be obtained from databases such as the XCOM database maintained by the United States National Institute of Standards and Technology [11].

The attenuation factor (AF) of photons starting from the emission point along a line can be described by

$$AF = e^{-(\mu/\rho)\cdot\rho\cdot d},\tag{13.4}$$

where μ/ρ is the mass-attenuation coefficient [11] for the current photon energy and material composition, ρ is the mass density and d is the distance from the source to the boundary of the object. For PET, which requires that both annihilation photons are detected to create a coincidence event, the AF is described by the following equation:

$$AF = e^{-(\mu/\rho)\cdot\rho\cdot d} \times e^{-(\mu/\rho)\cdot\rho\cdot(T-d)} = e^{-(\mu/\rho)\cdot\rho\cdot T}.\tag{13.5}$$

We can here see that for PET, the AF depends only on the total length, T, inside the object, and not on where the annihilation occurred. This effect makes it easier to correct for attenuation in PET when compared to SPECT, where the actual decay location is needed to obtain an AF.

Today, the correction for attenuation in SPECT and PET is primarily based on a CT study. Here, CT images are converted to attenuation maps, relevant for the proper photon energy. The calculated AFs are then included in the forward projection and sometimes also in the back projection (Figure 13.2). For PET, the attenuation correction can be applied directly on acquired sinograms. It should be noted that artifacts due to breathing can occur in regions of large attenuation differences if a fast CT acquisition has been used. Also, the attenuation images can be blurred to a spatial resolution representative of that of a SPECT/PET system to reduce absorbed dose artifacts, due to partial volume effects in boundaries between different attenuating compositions (lungs/tissue and tissue/bone). Due to the limited FOV of the CT, arms can be truncated in the CT images if these are not raised, which affects the attenuation correction. Streaks may appear in the image along projection angles of extensive attenuation (mostly in the lateral directions) resulting in large transmission ratios. Another potential problem is beam-hardening which increases the mean energy of the X-ray energy spectrum because of photons of lower energies being more attenuated along the beam path when compared to photons of higher energies.

13.4.2 SCATTER

As used here, the term "scatter" does not refer to the Compton and coherent scattering processes. It describes the unwanted contribution of events in the image formed by photons that have been scattered in the object and which, because of these processes, have changed directions. Due to the limited energy resolution in SPECT/PET systems, there is a need for a relatively wide energy window to maintain good counting statistics. Consequently, some events from scattered photons will obviously be detected and thus contribute to the image with false information about the origin of the emission. Scatter is thus an additive component that generally needs to be removed because it limits the possibility of activity measurement and decreases the image contrast. Since scatter originates from Compton and coherent scattering, the fraction of scatter in an image depends on the atomic number, Z, the mass density ρ and the photon energy $h\nu$. In addition, scatter depends on the energy resolution of the detector and energy window settings.

Two common and related methods for scatter correction often implemented in commercial image processing systems are the dual-energy window (DEW) method [12] and triple-energy window (TEW) method [13]. Both these methods are based on an estimation of the scatter contribution in the main photopeak energy window from data acquired in additional energy windows located near the main energy window. Here, it is assumed that the scatter in the main energy window can be described by scaling the data for DEW and TEW according to

$$p_{main}^{scatter\,(DEW)} = k \cdot p_{lower}, \tag{13.6}$$

$$p_{main}^{scatter\,(TEW)} = \left[\frac{p_{lower}}{w_{lower}} + \frac{p_{higher}}{w_{higher}} \right] \cdot \frac{w_{main}}{2}, \tag{13.7}$$

where p is the projection data recorded in an energy window with a width of w keV. Equations 13.6 and 13.7 are closely related. In the original publication concerning the DEW method, k was set to 0.5 and since the width of the scatter window here was equal to the width of the main window and only the lower scatter windows were used, Equations 13.6 and 13.7 would be the same. TEW can advantageously be used in cases where multiple photon emissions occur and downscatter from photons emitted with higher energies can appear in the main energy window.

The scatter estimate can be used either prior to reconstruction by subtracting it from the projection data of the main energy window or preferably by including it as an additive component in the forward-projection step in an iterative reconstruction procedure. It should be noted that scatter often refers to photon scattering in the patient but can also include scatter from the collimator, crystal, and the housing behind the crystal (backscatter).

Scatter also occurs in PET since a coincidence event can be generated by one or even two Compton-scattered annihilation photons. Compton scattering is the most probable interaction type for the first-order interaction of a 511 keV annihilation photon in tissue because of the low effective atomic number. Correction can be performed analytically by, for example, the single-scatter simulation (SSS) method that estimates the scatter contribution to LORs from a computation of the contribution to each detector pair from a grid of possible scatter points.

13.4.3 Spatial Resolution – SPECT

A parallel-hole collimator consists of many holes arranged symmetrically in a sheet of lead. The principle is that only those photons whose direction of travel is aligned with the axial direction of the hole will be able to pass through and interact in the crystal. The hole diameter cannot fulfill the related requirement of being infinitely small to match the above requirement of parallel projection lines because very few photons, if any, would then pass through. Selection of the hole diameter and length therefore needs to be a compromise so that reasonable counting statistics are obtained. This may increase the possibility of photons passing through adjacent collimator holes, which will result in an uncertainty in the position of the emission location. Since there are restrictions in administered activities arising from radiation dose considerations and the acquisition time, the hole dimensions are in practice such that the collimator resolution of a gamma camera is of the order of 8–10 mm, measured at 10 cm. Furthermore, if the source is located at greater distances away, then the spatial resolution will be even coarser. Within reasonable distances, the sensitivity (the count rate per unit of activity – cps/MBq) for a parallel-hole collimator is independent of the source-collimator distance and the number of registered counts therefore remains the same even if the spatial distribution of the counts changes as a function of the distance.

The degradation due to spatial resolution can in some part be compensated by modeling the distance-dependent resolution in the forward projection of an iterative reconstruction method [14]. Before summing up the values in the estimated projection, all voxels matching the same distance to the camera are separated into multiple images and the results are then filtered with a function describing the collimator resolution at each distance. For situations where no septal penetration in the collimator is expected, a Gaussian function can be used. To include septal penetration including star artifacts in the projection, Monte Carlo simulated functions can be used. When all multiple images are properly filtered, these are summed to the final estimated projection.

13.4.4 Spatial Resolution – PET

In a PET system, the spatial resolution depends mainly on the size of each individual detector because this defines the number of possible LORs (projection lines). Modern systems have crystals that are sliced into small channels, where the walls of each channel act as light guides so that the resolution can be improved above the limits of the physical size of the PMTs. In most PET systems, the detectors are long but with a small effective diameter to maximize the attenuation of photons entering in an orthogonal direction relative to the detector surface (sources in the center of the FOV). However, annihilation photons impinging in the tangential direction may enter a detector at an oblique angle. Since the photon energies are relatively large (511 keV), and the detector diameters are small, there is a probability that the photon will penetrate through the first detector and interact in an adjunct detector. Although it will be registered as a true coincidence, the spatial resolution will be affected because the LOR will be generated by the wrong detector pairs. This effect is often referred as depth-of-interaction (DOI).

A very important physical effect to remember is that the image reflects the distribution of annihilation locations and not the decay locations (i.e., the radiopharmaceutical). This is because the annihilation occurs when the positron has lost all of its kinetic energy at the end of its path. Since the actual track depends on the interactions of the positron with surrounding orbital electrons, the annihilation locations have a distribution around the decay and the resolution depends on the initial kinetic energy of the positron. The blurring, expressed as FWHM, due to positron travel can range from 0.54 mm for ^{18}F to 6.14 mm for ^{82}Rb [15].

Most positrons annihilate with electrons when they have come to rest (e.g., when they have lost all their kinetic energy). However, there is a finite chance that the annihilation occurs while the positron and electron are in motion. Due to the need for conservation of momentum, the emission angle between the two photons will therefore not be 180 degrees but a few degrees less. The result will be an inaccurate LOR that will affect and limit the spatial resolution of the PET system [15]. The impact of the effect depends on the radius of the FOV, and it is therefore larger for clinical systems than preclinical systems.

Spatial resolution in PET can be modeled in a similar way like described above for SPECT potentially also including models for positron range, noncollinearity, and DOI effects.

13.4.5 MISCELLANEOUS EFFECTS – PET

In PET, a false coincidence event may be registered from two annihilation photons that originated from positrons emitted from two separate decays but so close in time that they will be detected within the coincidence window. This will result in a false LOR. The probability of random coincidences increases with administered activity and the size of the coincidence window. To correct for random coincidences, the number of random events per LOR (R_{ab}) can be estimated from the measured singles count, detected in each crystal according to

$$R_{ab} = \frac{2\tau S_a S_b}{T},$$

(13.8)

where S_a and S_b are the number of singles measured on the two detector crystals spanning the LOR_{ab}, 2τ is the full coincidence timing window and T is the duration time of the measurement [16]. Coincidences can also occur between a single annihilation photon and a γ-photon, emitted at the same decay, that deposit energy detected within the energy window. This too will be a false LOR. Finally, multiple coincidences can occur where three or more LORs are possible. How these are handled (skip all or use all) may depend on the vendor.

13.4.6 DEAD TIME

When the rate of photons imping on a detector system increases, the electronics will at some point not be able to process the signals and the events correctly, resulting in a loss of detection events. The dead time, τ, is the time after each event during which the detector system is not able to record another event. In general terms, the behavior of a detector, when it is exposed to a high number of photons per second, is either paralyzable or non-paralyzable. A system is paralyzable when each detected event extends the dead time while the system is non-paralyzable when subsequent events that occur during the dead time of the detector are ignored. In diagnostic imaging with scintillation cameras, the activity levels are generally low and therefore the effects of dead time on the image data are of less importance. However, dead-time effects can be apparent in theranostic nuclear medicine applications where high activities are administered to provide a high absorbed dose to the treatment target at the same time as being used for imaging.

For a non-paralyzable system, a theoretical relationship between the expected count rate (R_t) and the measured count-rate (R_o) can be expressed as:

$$R_o = \frac{R_t}{(1 - R_t \tau)},$$

(13.9)

where τ is the dead time. For a paralyzable system, the relationship is instead described as:

$$R_o = R_t e^{-R_t \tau} \tag{13.10}$$

The measured count rates can be plotted as a function of expected count rates, calculated from a low count rate measurement of a system sensitivity (cps/MBq) for a particular camera system to determine if that camera system behaves as a paralyzable or non-paralyzable system. If the observed count rate increases and reaches its maximum value, then the system corresponds to a non-paralyzable model. However, if, after reaching its maximum, the curve then decreases in magnitude, then this behavior is a closer match to a paralyzable model. In a system with CZT-based detection, each anode acts as a single detector and consequently, the dead-time problem will be reduced compared to a camera system based on only one large detector. Furthermore, the coordinate of an event in a CZT system will not be affected by count rate because it is determined by the position of the anode pad rather than the center of gravity for a collection of signals from multiple PMTs.

In a PET, the count rate for singles is generally much higher than the rate for coincidences, which is the main information useful for imaging. Therefore, the timing properties of a PET crystal are of great importance and especially when including TOF information.

13.5   QUALITY CONTROL

To provide images that are not affected by the status of the camera, regular quality checks (QC) are performed on both gamma cameras, SPECT, and PET. These procedures are important for ensuring that system tuning is as good as possible but also for identifying malfunctions such as a broken PMT or damages to crystals and collimators. When installing a camera system, first an acceptance test is carried out to verify that the performance corresponds to that specified by the vendor. These acceptance tests include checks of system sensitivity, spatial resolution (intrinsic and system), energy resolution, linearity, and uniformity, and are carried out in a manner that is strictly regulated by National Electrical Manufacturers Association's (NEMA) protocols so that a correct comparison of the expected performance vis-à-vis the actual performance can be obtained.

To describe all tests in detail is beyond the scope of this chapter. However, the following paragraphs briefly describe some of the checks that need to be carried out on a regular basis. More information about QC and suggested procedures can be found in the publication of the International Atomic Energy Agency [17].

13.5.1   PLANAR IMAGING

One important parameter to check is the expected uniformity of an image when exposing the camera with a spatially uniform distribution of photons. This uniformity can reveal an unexpected difference in maximum and minimum count values and is calculated from the following equation:

$$Uniformity = 100 \frac{[c_{max} - c_{min}]}{[c_{min} + c_{min}]} \tag{13.11}$$

where c_{max} and c_{min} are the count values in the pixels located within a defined area on the camera. Due to the way scintillation cameras are designed, these areas can be categorized into (a) a geometrical FOV, (b) a useful field-of-view (UFOV) disregarding problems with counts detected at the edge of the FOV and (c) a central field-of-view (CFOV) where the main objects of interest are centered on. The integral uniformity determines non-uniformities on overall UFOV or CFOV, while the differential uniformity defines the non-uniformities at a more local level within the UFOV or CFOV.

Non-uniformities can occur if localized regions in the crystal do not emit scintillation light for a given absorbed energy as other parts of the crystal do. They can also be caused by non-linearities in the positioning of an event because of dead areas in between PMTs. For both, the result is a change in local sensitivity that can be very hard to detect in a clinical planar image. Corrections are made on a regular basis by specially designed flood-field measurements that are also the basis for correction matrices. Shorter uniformity checks are often part of the daily checking routine and easily reveal failures in PMTs or collimators.

13.5.2   SPECT

All the effects mentioned in Section 13.5.1 also hold true for SPECT imaging with a standard scintillation camera; therefore, a properly tuned camera for planar imaging is also a fundamental requirement here. The parameters used in the tomographic reconstruction can affect the noise levels and spatial resolution of the final image. Often, SPECT systems include noise-reducing low-pass filters such as Butterworth and Gaussian filters that are intended to balance the level of the increased image noise that results from the ramp filter in FBP or the use of multiple iterations in ML-EM/OS-EM. The application of a low-pass filter requires careful optimization because such filters generally also cause reduced spatial resolution in the reconstruction image. Differences in sensitivity due to non-homogeneities in the detector heads can cause ring-like image artifacts in the reconstructed image. They are most severe when they are located at the center of rotation that relates the matching of the reconstructed center in the tomographic images to the mechanical center of the camera's FOV. For each projection angle, the gravity can act differently on the camera heads and correction of these errors as a function of projection angle is therefore needed. A poor correction will provide insufficient or incorrect realignment, resulting in reduced spatial resolution and, in the worse cases, ring-type artifacts in the final reconstructed image.

Special phantoms are frequently used to test the image quality for SPECT. These can be phantoms constructed with rods of different diameters and arranged in a pie-shaped configuration for spatial resolution measurements. A common phantom for both SPECT and PET is the IQ phantom by the NEMA that can be used for noise evaluation, recovery-coefficient curves, activity quantitation and lesion detectability. The phantom includes six spherical inserts (10– 37 mm) and a low-density cylinder.

SPECT spatial resolution can also be measured using multiple line sources placed in air or in a water phantom. For example, line sources can be placed in the center, and in different off-center positions to allow for measurements of the variation in FWHM and FWTM within the FOVs. Although typically these are usually performed based on ^{99m}Tc measurements, other radionuclides could be useful for measurements, for example, to estimate collimator penetration effects.

13.5.3   PET

It is essential to assess the detector response in PET scanners to ensure the output is within expected limits. Individual detector blocks could fail at the level of the PMTs in analog PET systems or in the electronics when using digital Avalanche PhotoDiodes (APD) or SiPM. Energy peaking, coincidence timing, and crystal position maps could also become ineffective.

13.5.4   CT

Most CT systems have specific daily tests that must be performed. The X-ray tube is warmed up by a series of exposures as a very first step of the daily CT quality control process. Also, the system checks for objects in the FOV and potential contamination of CT contrast that could affect the CT detector outputs. During the standard daily QC, the scanner will acquire calibration scans using various tube and collimation settings to provide the "blank" data that are then used to form a patient CT scan. A specially designed CT phantom that includes various image quality assessment components is often used in these tests. The uniform section of this phantom should be scanned daily to assess possible non-uniformities due to detector malfunction.

Hybrid SPECT/CT and PET/CT assume alignment between the two types of images. However, since the position of the patient on the couch is different because of the side-by-side placement of the detector system, misalignment between the images may occur due to bending on the couch. Since CT is used for attenuation correction and sometimes for dosimetry calculation, the conversion from HU to the physical units used in these calculations needs to be verified. In both the attenuation correction and the radiation transport calculation, the type of material and voxel size are used to determine the track length of both photons and charged particles. Since HU units are based on an X-ray energy spectrum for a specific voltage setting, a conversion to proper photon energy used in the SPECT/PET study is needed. For attenuation correction, the energy corresponding to the mid-energy of the main energy window is often used and therefore a single AF is sufficient but when performing more sophisticated Monte Carlo-based radiation transport calculations with potential inclusion of multiple particle emissions, data relating to densities and attenuation coefficients/stopping powers need to be available for the whole energy range.

13.6   IMAGE QUALITY PARAMETERS

To quantify the quality of an image is not easy because its interpretation is very subjective. However, there are certain parameters that can be used to quantify the properties of an image.

13.6.1   SPATIAL RESOLUTION

Essentially, this describes a system's ability to display two objects as separate entities. No imaging system is perfect and as objects get closer to each other, there will eventually be a distance where a viewer interprets these two objects as one entity. The spatial resolution can be described as the FWHM measured from a measured point-spread function (PSF). The PSF is essentially an image of a point-like source where the shape of the image describes the degradation in the image. The system spatial resolution depends on the detector type (intrinsic spatial resolution), the collimator resolution (hole dimensions and length), the size of the image matrix and related pixel size, and the camera-source distance. As the FWHM is a somewhat rough and ready but still useful value, more information about the image characteristics can be obtained by calculating the modulation transfer function (MTF). The MTF describes the spatial frequency response of an imaging system and is calculated as the ratio of the output signal amplitude to the input signal amplitude for a given frequency. A perfect imaging system has an MTF(υ)=1 for all frequencies υ. This means that the input signal is not affected and that the image properly represents the object in all its details.

13.6.2   IMAGE CONTRAST

Image contrast describes the difference in signal in an area relative to the signals in the surrounding areas and is often used as a measure of the detectability. The contrast should be as close as possible to the object contrast, which in nuclear medicine applications is the true difference in activity or activity concentration. Image contrast is calculated using the following equation:

$$C = \frac{\bar{c}_{\text{voi}} - \bar{c}_{\text{bg}}}{\bar{c}_{\text{voi}}}. \qquad\qquad 13.12$$

Image contrast and spatial resolution are related because if the spatial resolution increases, the collected counts are concentrated into a smaller area of the image and consequently the contrast is also increased.

13.6.3 IMAGE NOISE

Due to the random nature of radioactive decay and subsequent photon interactions in the patient and detector, the images obtained from a scintillation camera or SPECT/PET images will always be subject to local variations, generally described as noise. Often, the noise can be characterized using the Poisson distribution. The magnitude of the noise is directly related to the activity of the source and the acquisition time used for the measurement (i.e., the total number of detected photons). Due to the required collimator, the count rate per unit activity is usually small, which implies that there will always be a noise problem in nuclear medicine studies. However, the scale of the noise problem depends on the application. For detection of small lesions of low uptake, noise can be a problem, while, for example, calculation of the average of counts in a larger VOI may average out the voxel-based noise.

Metrics to describe image quality for detection include the signal-to-noise ratio (SNR), defined according to

$$SNR = \frac{\bar{c}_{\text{VOI}}}{\sigma_{\text{VOI}}}, \tag{13.13}$$

where c_{voi} is the mean voxel count in a VOI and σ_{voi} is the standard deviation of the voxel values within that VOI. Another metric is the contrast-to-noise ratio (CNR) defined according to

$$CNR = \frac{\bar{c}_{\text{VOI}} - \bar{c}_{\text{bg}}}{\sigma_{\text{bg}}}, \tag{13.14}$$

where c_{bg} is the mean voxel value defined for a background VOI. The negative impact of noise can be reduced by post-filtering projections or reconstructed images with a low-pass filter applied in 2D on projection data or in 3D on reconstructed images. Here, higher frequencies in the images where noise is expected to appear are reduced by a function resulting in a smoother image. However, low-pass filtering also reduces high frequencies originating from the object, so the spatial resolution will also be affected.

13.7 ACTIVITY MEASUREMENT

Both scintillation cameras, SPECT, and PET systems generate "relative" results, that is, in terms of projections of measured counts or coincidence-based LORs. These relative values can then be reconstructed to form tomographic images, but they still show the activity distribution in relative values. To relate images to the underlying activity distribution, a calibration procedure is needed, which is often based on some measurement of a known activity in a specified geometry.

13.7.1 CAMERA CALIBRATION

The ratio of reconstructed count projections (or reconstructed coincidence LORs) per second measured by a source with a well-defined activity can be used as a calibration of image data to activity.

$$A(V) = \frac{\bar{c}_{\text{VOI}}}{t} \cdot \frac{1}{\left(\frac{cps}{MBq}\right)_{\text{system}}}. \tag{13.15}$$

If parallel-hole collimators are used, which is often the case, the system sensitivity (cps/MBq) within the cameras FOV is independent of source distance (for reasonable distances). Therefore, a single value of the system sensitivity can be used for calibration and activity determination (Equation 13.3). However, this requires that most of the above-described physical effects (photon attenuation, scatter, dead time, etc.) have been corrected for before obtaining c_{voi} from the images.

For SPECT, the planar sensitive in air at a specific distance, as specified by NEMA, can be used for calibration but this requires that the reconstruction program properly corrects for attenuation and scatter and normalizes the result based on the count rate. An alternative is to image a phantom with a known amount of activity using the same acquisition protocol as is used in a real patient study and obtain a calibration factor from the phantom study and images, reconstructed here with identical parameters to those used for the patient study. This means that unknown parameters in the tomographic image creation chain are assumed to cancel themselves out.

13.7.2 PARTIAL VOLUME CORRECTION

Due to the limited spatial resolution of nuclear medicine systems, the images from systems will not exactly represent the object being imaged. The spatial resolution depends not only on the inherent detector principles but also on the physical properties of the processes that generate the signals for the image. For PET systems, positron range, detector size, and noncollinearity are three effects that limit the spatial resolution, while for scintillation cameras and SPECT, the parallel-hole collimator and the source-to-detector distance are two major causes of poor resolution. In principle, a very narrow hole could be used that would result in a high spatial resolution, but this would require an unacceptably high administered activity. Thus, in some applications, the spatial resolution must be corrected for. One such application is determination of the activity in a well-defined volume (activity concentration) and the related absorbed dose. If the counts are determined based on a VOI defined from a registered high-resolution CT study and applied to SPECT/PET images, then some counts will be lost due to the spill-out of that VOI due to the limited spatial resolution. The outcome will then be a too-low activity concentration or related absorbed dose rate.

A common way of compensating for the spill-out is to use recovery factors that to some extent compensate for the spill-out. These factors are then implemented in the calculation according to

$$A(V) = \frac{\bar{c}_{VOI}}{t} \cdot \frac{1}{\left(\frac{cps}{MBq}\right)_{system}} \cdot \frac{1}{RC(V)} \tag{13.16}$$

where V is the delineated tissue volume. Figure 13.3 shows examples of recovery curves for different image spatial resolutions. Spherical count volumes were defined in an initial set of 256×256 images (voxel size 0.15 mm) and these images were then convolved with a Gaussian function of different FWHM values. The initial set of count images also defined the physical VOI and the fraction of counts remaining within these VOIs can then be calculated.

13.8 CONCLUSION

Activity quantification is today achievable for both SPECT and PET. Because of differences in the principles of data collections, PET has superior spatial resolution compared to SPECT, but both have partial volume effects for source dimensions close to their respective spatial resolution. The iterative reconstruction method ML-EM/OS-EM allows for accurate compensations of physical effects such as photon attenuation, scatter, and other effects. To achieve quantitative results in terms of activity, a calibration procedure is needed by a source with known activity in a well-defined geometry.

Recovery coefficients for various spatial resolutions (FWHM)

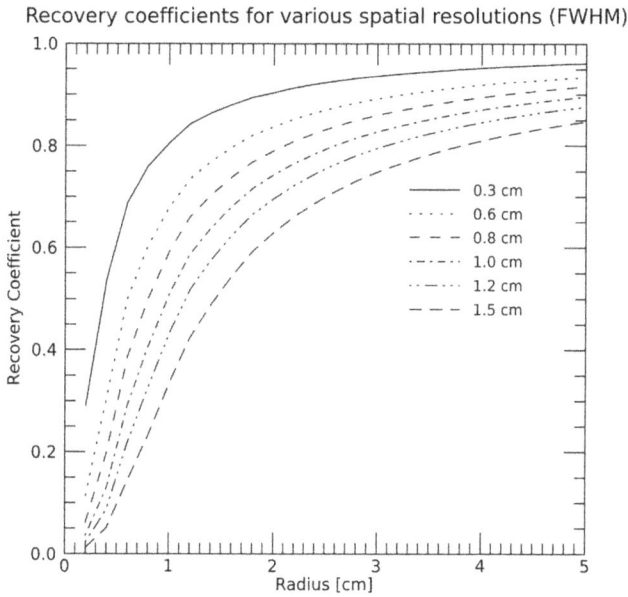

FIGURE 13.3 The figure shows the variation of recovery coefficients as a function of source radius for varying spatial resolutions expressed as FWHM from 0.3 to 1.5 cm. The recovery coefficients converge rapidly to unity as the source radius is increased, which means that the necessary correction for count losses within the volume will be less in magnitude. Note that these curves do not include effects from the camera, reconstruction methods or physical effects. They only serve as examples of how recovery curves might look.

REFERENCES

1. Anger HO. Scintillation camera. *Rev Sci Instrum*. 1958;29(1):27–33.
2. Anger HO. Scintillation camera with multichannel collimators. *J Nucl Med*. 1964;5(7):515–531.
3. Roth D, Larsson E, Sundlov A, Sjogreen Gleisner K. Characterisation of a hand-held CZT-based gamma camera for (177)Lu imaging. *EJNMMI Phys*. 2020;7(1):46.
4. Roth D, Larsson E, Ljungberg M, Sjogreen Gleisner K. Monte Carlo modelling of a compact CZT-based gamma camera with application to (177)Lu imaging. *EJNMMI Phys*. 2022;9(1):35.
5. Humm JL, Rosenfeld A, Del Guerra A. From PET detectors to PET scanners. *Eur J Nucl Med Mol Imaging*. 2003;30(11):1574–1597.
6. Sonni I, Baratto L, Park S, Hatami N, Srinivas S, Davidzon G, et al. Initial experience with a SiPM-based PET/CT scanner: influence of acquisition time on image quality. *EJNMMI Phys*. 2018;5(1):9-.
7. Erlandsson K, Buvat I, Pretorius PH, Thomas BA, Hutton BF. A review of partial volume correction techniques for emission tomography and their applications in neurology, cardiology and oncology. *Phys Med Biol*. 2012;57(21):R119–R159.
8. Ljungberg M, Erlandsson K. Single photon emission computed tomography (SPECT) and SPECT/CT hybrid imaging In: Ljungberg M, editor. *Handbook of Nuclear Medicine and Molecular Imaging for Physicists: Instrumentation and Imaging Procedures*. Vol. 1. Boca Raton, FL: CRC Press; 2022. pp. 297–314, ISBN 9781138593268.
9. S LA, Vardi Y. Maximum likelihood reconstruction for emission tomography. *IEEE Trans Med Imaging*. 1982;1(2):113–122.
10. Hudson HM, Larkin RS. Accelerated image reconstruction using ordered subsets of projection data. *IEEE Trans Nucl Sci*. 1994;13:601–609.
11. Berger MJ, Hubbell JH, Seltzer SM, J. C, Coursey JS, Sukumar R, et al. XCOM: Photon Cross Sections Database National Institute of Standards and Technology 2010 [Available from: https://www.nist.gov/pml/xcom-photon-cross-sections-database.
12. Jaszczak RJ, Greer KL, Floyd CE, Harris CC, Coleman RE. Improved SPECT quantification using compensation for scattered photons. *J Nucl Med*. 1984;25:893–900.

13. Ogawa K, Harata Y, Ichihara T, Kubo A, Hashimoto S. A practical method for position-dependent Compton-scatter correction in single photon emission CT. *IEEE Trans Med Imaging.* 1991;10:408–412.

14. Bronnikov AV, editor SPECT imaging with resolution recovery. 2011 2nd International Conference on Advancements in Nuclear Instrumentation, Measurement Methods and Their Applications; 2011 6–9 June 2011.

15. Moses WW. Fundamental limits of spatial resolution in PET. *Nucl Instrum Methods Phys Res A.* 2011;648 (Suppl 1):S236-S240.

16. Gallamini A, Zwarthoed C, Borra A. Positron emission tomography (PET) in oncology. *Cancers (Basel).* 2014;6(4):1821–1889.

17. *Quality Assurance for PET and PET/CT Systems.* Vienna: International Atomic Energy Agency; 2009.

Part 4

The Future

14 Human Resources

Multidisciplinary Team Education, Training, and Competence

Thomas N.B. Pascual, Gopinath Gnanasegaran, Diana Paez,
Kunthi Pathmaraj, and Somanesan Satchi

14.1 INTRODUCTION

With the increasing number of streamlined and emerging radiotheranostic (henceforth, theranostics) applications seen on the horizon of clinical practice, the cornerstone of the success of the implementation of these highly technical clinical interventions lies on a competent multidisciplinary team equipped with evidence-based knowledge and technical skills to ensure the success of this approach. In modern theranostics, this multidisciplinary team collectively consists of experts (1) directly involved in handling radiation: nuclear medicine physicians, radio-oncologists, nuclear medicine medical physicists, nuclear medicine technologists, nurses, health care assistants, radio pharmacists, and those (2) indirectly involved in handling radiation: oncologists, surgeons, oncology nurses, palliative care team, research practitioners, radiation protection/safety experts, and other professions related to medicine. With the gamut of new knowledge emerging from successful clinical trials and other research, there is a need to diffuse and mobilize this knowledge through curriculum innovation to inform the clinical practice of the multidisciplinary team. Central to this curriculum re-engineering process is an emphasis on the interdisciplinary [1] and transversality approach [2], highlighting the non-fragmented and non-linear teaching, learning and interaction expected within the community of multidisciplinary learners. Through this process, networking and collaboration of shared resources among emerging and expert theranostic practitioners are intended and enhanced, leading to communities of practice [3]. This approach is particularly advantageous since areas of expertise are limited worldwide, and the only way to facilitate research development and technology diffusion activities [4] is to ensure competence at a global level through local and international collaborations.

The following sections highlight technical and practical knowledge crucial for the learning and competence of the multidisciplinary team involved in theranostics. Focus is later given to the nuclear medicine physicians and other clinicians, nuclear medicine medical physicists, and nuclear medicine technologists. Since theranostics is already part of the approved training curriculum, additional learning activities and competency assessments are offered to provide more specialized training and instructional methodologies on how this knowledge can be mobilized more efficiently. Challenges that might impede adequate teaching and learning in the current context will also be discussed.

14.2 SCAFFOLDING THEMES IN MULTIDISCIPLINARY TEAM EDUCATION

Theranostics is gaining momentum and visibility in the world of clinical oncology. As introduced in Chapter 1, radionuclide theranostics is the pairing of radiolabeled diagnostic biomarkers with

DOI: 10.1201/9781003250913-18

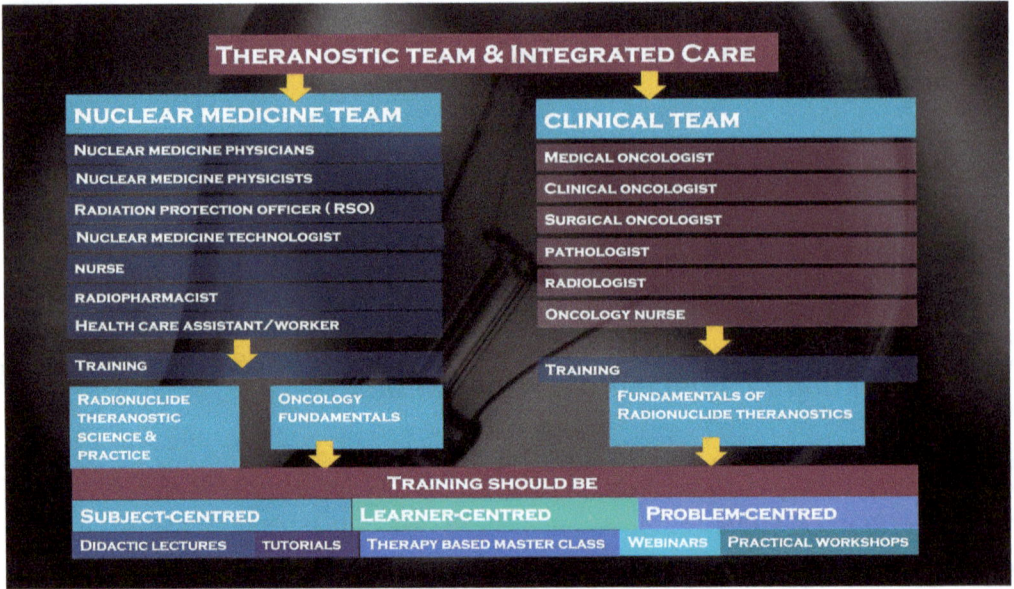

FIGURE 14.1 Multidisciplinary team approach in theranostics team education, training, and competence.

radiolabeled therapeutic agents that share a specific target in diseased cells or tissues [5]. The clinical indications are expanding, and evidence is evolving in several cancers. Incorporating theranostics in the management algorithm of cancer might improve patient selection, treatment response and toxicity prediction, and prognostication [5]. In the long run, it could avoid expensive and frequent diagnostic and therapeutic procedures.

Although there is significant growth in the science and technology related to theranostics, the workforce to implement and use them is limited [5–9]. There is an urgent need to provide a multidisciplinary framework for the practice of theranostics (Figure 14.1). The nuclear medicine team would consist of nuclear medicine physicians, nuclear medicine medical physicists, nuclear medicine technologists/radiographers, nurses, radiation protection/safety experts, health care assistants, and radiochemists/pharmacists. The clinical team would include oncologists, surgeons, radiotherapy specialists, oncology nurses, a palliative care team, research practitioners, and other medical professionals. The aim of a multidisciplinary theranostics program should focus on (a) developing high-quality education material; (b) recruiting the workforce; (c) getting funding; (d) standardizing training; and (e) promoting equal accessibility and opportunity [6–9].

14.3 GENERAL COMPETENCY REQUIREMENTS

The International Basic Safety Standards (BSS) lays the foundation of the required competencies of medical personnel involved in planned medical exposures [10] including theranostic procedures. As there are multidisciplinary teams involved in this developing practice, the regulatory bodies are tasked to ensure that those professionals directly involved in handling radiopharmaceuticals, especially the licensed users, need to comply with specific and specialized requirements for education, training, and competencies needed to be authorized to practice in this field. As such, they are tasked to assess competencies through verification of professional registration, accreditation, or certification as approved at the local setting, or if such mechanisms are not established yet, ensure that the qualifications of the theranostic team would subscribe to international best practices. This verification of appropriate education and training requirements can take the form of a formal assessment of general registration (or state licensing), specialized training, and certification of competencies or accreditation standards issued by the relevant local or international authorities.

14.4 GENERAL REGISTRATION, SPECIALIZED TRAINING, AND ACCREDITATION FOR MULTIDISCIPLINARY TEAM

Medical practitioners involved in the theranostic multidisciplinary team need, at minimum, to obtain a general registration or license (board certification) as a physician to practice the medical profession. This needs to be fulfilled based on the physician competencies' framework as their relevant authorities prescribe [11–15]. Further specialized training in postgraduate studies or clinical fellowships in different fields, such as oncology, urology, and nuclear medicine, can be undertaken. After successful completion, the physician would be qualified or accredited to practice the chosen field (specialist board certification). Additional subspecialty training may also be undertaken to have specific training in the field which requires skills. The accreditation process, which ensures high level standards of the educational program, is different for each country and typically takes guidance from international best practices [15,16]. The training curriculum for nuclear medicine physicians varies between countries, and efforts are underway to harmonize it on critical aspects of training necessary to acquire the competencies needed to provide adequate patient care and ensure the safety and quality of clinical practice [17]. Typical accrediting bodies for Nuclear Medicine physicians include the American Board of Nuclear Medicine for the United States [18], the European Board of Nuclear Medicine for select European countries [19–21], and equivalent local accrediting bodies for several countries in Asia, Australia, and the rest of the world [22–24]. Specific accreditation for the theranostic practice of nuclear medicine physicians varies, with some countries such as Australia requiring a specific number of theranostic procedures to be performed to be a recognized theranostic practitioner [7], while other experts emphasize theranostic fellowships or training on highly specialized centers as accepted by local or international nuclear medicine societies or organizations [25].

Radiographers and nuclear medicine technologists typically need to obtain an appropriate undergraduate degree followed by general registration or licensing if appropriate. They may undergo specialized training in their chosen tracks if resources are available [26,27]. Accreditation of nuclear medicine technologists is country-specific if present, such as the licensing exam sponsored in the United States by either the Nuclear Medicine Technology Certification Board or by the American Association of Radiology Technologists and by the Joint Review Committee on Educational Programs in Nuclear Medicine Technology (JRCNMT) in Canada [28,29]. Radiopharmacists or radiochemists ensure the safe and effective use of radioactive drugs for diagnosis and therapy and generally obtain undergraduate degrees in pharmacy or chemistry, followed by the needed general registration or licensing if appropriate. Subsequent specialized postgraduate training in radiopharmaceuticals and its preparation should be undertaken to be recognized practitioners in this field [30]. Accreditation is given by the Board of Pharmacy Certification for Nuclear Pharmacy in the United States [31] and by other countries' accreditation bodies when available.

Medical physicists undergo graduate degrees in medical physics, radiologic physics, physics, or other relevant physical science or engineering disciplines from an accredited institution. They need to be certified by the appropriate board thereafter [32–38]. International accrediting bodies for medical physicists include the International Medical Physics Certification Board [39], and guidelines were also developed to provide information on the establishment of certification schemes for clinically qualified medical physicists at the national or regional level when not available [40].

Radiation safety officers (RSO) or radiation protection officers (RPO) ensure the organization achieves and maintains compliance with applicable laws, regulations, and standards with regards to radiation practice [41]. With their expertise and knowledge of radiation protection obtained from their academic background and accredited certification courses, RSOs/RPOs are critical to implementing the licensees' radiation protection programs. They interact with and area member or the chair of the Radiation Safety Committee of a healthcare facility. They usually hold a bachelor's or graduate degree from an accredited college or university in physical science or engineering or biological science and have five or more years of professional experience in health physics, including at least three years in applied health physics [42–45].

14.5   THERANOSTICS CORE COMPETENCIES

The core of the theranostics multidisciplinary team training should focus on (a) patient selection and timing of radionuclide therapies, (b) performing radionuclide therapies, (c) cancer-specific diagnosis and management, (d) cancer-specific alternate surgical and medical treatment options or procedures, (e) management of side effects and complications, (f) short- and long-term follow-up of patients and cross training in clinical medicine (e.g., internal medicine, acute medicine, oncology, radiotherapy, palliative care) (Figure 14.2).

The training for the existing clinical and non-clinical staff involved in radionuclide therapies must be refined toward more practical applications. The extent and depth of topics discussed for each workforce category might differ depending on their level of involvement in clinical service. However, the main objective of multidisciplinary team learning should be to provide the best clinical service and outcomes. Innovative and effective teaching methodologies should be optimized to provide efficient training and achieve competence for the multidisciplinary team while utilizing many online educational resources within the community of practice.

14.6   ADVANCING THERANOSTICS COMPETENCE FOR NUCLEAR MEDICINE PHYSICIANS AND ONCOLOGISTS

The training should focus on immediate and long-term solutions. In addition to the incorporation of radionuclide therapy and the concept of theranostics into the curricula of the ongoing training programs for nuclear medicine and oncology residents, training and education of existing nuclear

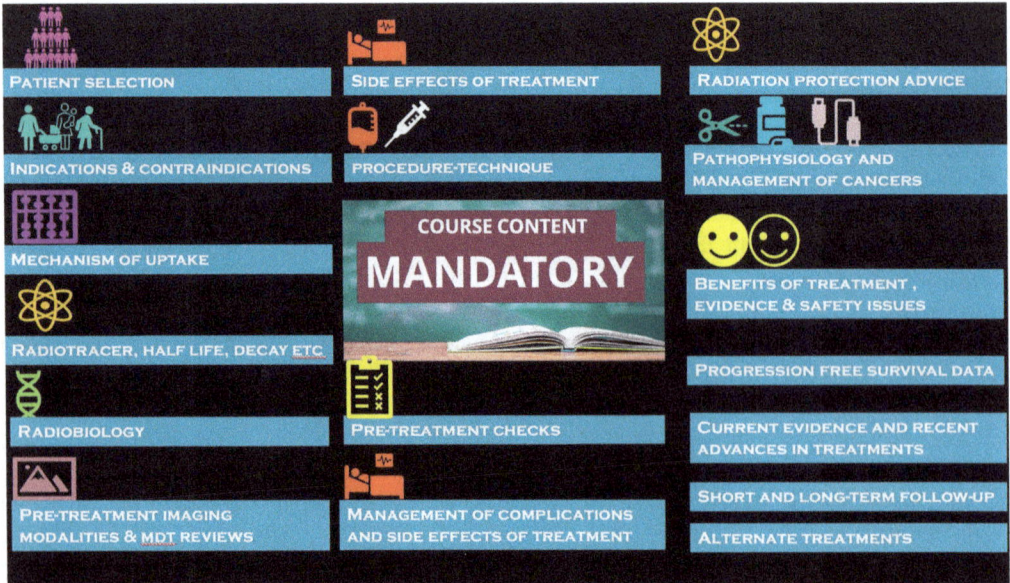

FIGURE 14.2   Core topics in multidisciplinary theranostics education and training.

TABLE 14.1

Radionuclide Theranostic Fellowship or Subspecialty Training for Nuclear Medicine Residents (Duration 12 Months)

Clinical and Medical Oncology (3–6 Months)	Nuclear Medicine Theranostics (6–12 Months)
Content:	Content:
Overview of indications, contraindications for surgery, chemotherapy, and radiotherapy	General principles of treatment using radiopharmaceuticals and unsealed radioactive sources
Pre-treatment clinical assessment on the day of treatment	Understanding indications, contraindications of radionuclide therapies for cancer subtypes
Overview of cancer-specific standard of care (surgical and medical) therapies for different cancer subtypes commonly referred for radionuclide therapies	Assessment of patient's suitability for radionuclide therapy (clinical assessment of the patient's medical condition, fitness, and co-morbidities)
Overview of side effects and complications related to surgery, chemotherapy, radiotherapy, immunotherapy for different cancer subtypes	Recommending and evaluating the appropriate radionuclide molecular imaging studies for radionuclide therapy
Knowledge of assessment of toxicities, interpretation of imaging, biochemical and pathology results relating to cancer subtypes	Knowledge of appropriate time frame for imaging and treatments
Overview of medical management of side effects and complications for different cancer subtypes	Understanding the potential side effects and complications related to specific radionuclide therapies
Prognosis of different cancer subtypes	Understanding the management of the side effects and long-term complications of specific radionuclide therapies
Follow-up	Understanding radiation protection
	Understanding dosimetry and individual dose planning for different radionuclide therapies.
	Understanding the informed consent process for radionuclide therapies
	Understanding of radiopharmaceutical production chain and local standard operating procedures (SOPs), equipment used in the manufacturing and quality control testing of radiopharmaceuticals
	Should observe and perform spectrum of radionuclide therapies and maintain a logbook

medicine specialists are vital [6–8]. The existing curricula should provide an overview of principles of theranostics for trainees with an option to subspecialize with more focused and extensive training (Tables 14.1 and 14.2).

14.7 ADVANCING THERANOSTICS COMPETENCE FOR MEDICAL PHYSICISTS

The roles and responsibilities of the nuclear medicine medical physicist in theranostics service delivery are diverse and demanding, as described in detail by the IAEA [32]. The higher therapeutic radioactivity in radionuclide therapy requires knowledge, skills, and training far more significant than in diagnostic nuclear medicine. The specifics of the training include internal dosimetry, image quality and dose optimization, research and teaching, radiation safety, quality assurance (QA), and equipment management. Nuclear medicine medical physicists apply their knowledge of mathematics, physics, and technology to establish, implement, and monitor processes that allow optimal theranostics service delivery, taking account of the radiation protection of the patients and others [33]. Medical physicist shall be responsible for overseeing the radiation safety program in the delivery of theranostic services, in coordination with the RSO/RPO, if (or when) the facility has one.

TABLE 14.2

Radionuclide Theranostic Advanced Training for Certified Nuclear Medicine Physicians (Duration 12 Months)

Curriculum for Certified Nuclear Medicine Physicians

Overview of indications, contraindications for surgery, chemotherapy, and radiotherapy

Principles of treatment using theranostic radiopharmaceuticals

Indications, contraindications of radionuclide therapies for cancer subtypes

Assessment of patient's suitability for radionuclide therapy

Recommending and evaluating the appropriate radionuclide molecular imaging studies for radionuclide therapy

Knowledge of appropriate time frame for imaging and treatments

Understanding the potential side effects and complications related to specific radionuclide therapies

Understanding the management of side effects and long-term complications of specific radionuclide therapies

Understanding the radiation protection and good radiation safety practice

Understanding dosimetry and individual dose planning for different radionuclide therapies

Understanding the informed consenting process for radionuclide therapies

Knowledge of assessment of toxicities, interpretation of imaging, biochemical andpathology results relating to cancer subtypes

Understanding of radiopharmaceutical production chain and local standard operating procedures (SOPs), equipment's used in the manufacturing and quality control testing of radiopharmaceuticals.

Should observe and perform spectrum of radionuclide therapies for benign and oncological conditions and maintain a logbook.

Nuclear medicine medical physicists involved in theranostics need to recognize and understand the sources of error in nuclear medicine procedures and are responsible for validating the techniques used. They should also be involved in the development, implementation, maintenance, quality control (QC), and QA of new theranostic processes and all training aspects.

The objective of the clinical training program in theranostic nuclear medicine is to produce an independent practitioner and a lifelong learner. They can work unsupervised within a multi-disciplinary team at a safe and highly professional standard. The 11 modules of the IAEA guide the clinical training of medical physicists specializing in nuclear medicine [33] and provide most of the knowledge and training experience needed for theranostic service delivery.

14.8 QUALITY ASSURANCE IN THERANOSTIC SERVICE DELIVERY

QA in theranostics is vital due to the accuracy needed to diagnose a condition and the personalized treatment with high-dose long-lived radionuclides to the patient. QA in theranostics refers to the correct use of equipment, such as radionuclide calibrators, gamma cameras and SPECT/CT and PET/CT scanners, and the unique acquisition protocols that account for the radiopharmaceutical being used. An example would be selecting the ^{68}Ga acquisition protocol versus ^{18}F for a PET/CT patient undergoing a ^{68}Ga radiopharmaceutical scan, as there are specific acquisition and pre-processing algorithms unique to the radionuclide.

The medical physicist, together with the other members of the nuclear medicine team, plays a crucial role in establishing clinical standards, protocols, consistent techniques, and methods in the clinical setting for each theranostic pair (e.g. ^{68}Ga-PSMA-11 for diagnosis and ^{177}Lu-PSMA-617 for therapy). While this is a task undertaken by a team, the responsibilities of each task member shall be defined clearly in the standard operating procedure (SOP). In summary, medical physicists are responsible for ensuring that the equipment, systems, and processes used for theranostics service delivery are always working optimally. A QA program exists to ensure dependable performance of safe, accurate, and reproducible equipment operation and application of radio-pharmaceuticals [46–50]. Medical physicists must be able to recognize common artifacts in clinical images and undertake remedial action to correct the problem. A medical physicist should be involved in cooperation with nuclear medicine physicians/radiologists and nuclear medicine technologists/radiographers in:

- Supporting the setup and monitoring of routine QA programs
- Evaluati newly installed radiological equipment with the determination of fundamental parameters for routine QC
- Training of staff on basic QA procedures and radiation safety
- Designing protocols for new theranostic procedures.

14.9 RADIATION SAFETY IN THERANOSTIC SERVICE DELIVERY

The RSO/RPO is, according to the BSS [10], a person technically competent in radiation protection matters relevant to a given type of practice designated by the regulator, licensee, or employer to oversee the application of regulatory requirements. They interact with and is a member or the chair of the Radiation Safety Committee of a healthcare facility. An RSO/RPO is also a multi-disciplinary team member in theranostic service delivery. In many facilities, the medical physicist functions as an RSO/RPO, but in others is a separate individual with proficiency in radiation protection. Whichever the case, the medical physicist shall oversee the radiation safety program in delivering theranostic services in coordination with the RSO/RPO if (or when) the facility has one. The roles of RPO/RSO include the following [42–45]:

- Ensure radiation safety procedures for staff, patients, carers, the general public, and the environment.
- Manage new radionuclide therapy procedures.
- Ensure facility or site planning for new radionuclide therapy.
- Provide expertise in imaging, personalized internal dosimetry, and accurate radioactivity determination, ensuring patient dose optimization.
- Provide protocol internal audits and review of QC data to ensure scanner and other equipment's optimization.
- Provide radiation dose estimation based on imaging parameters, as well as the amount of radioactivity used.
- Understand trends and potential problems that may arise and assist in troubleshooting and mitigating to find solutions.
- Oversee the training and supervision of personnel in radiation safety aspects.
- Supervise the radioactive spill management and decontamination of personnel and environment.
- Undertake a local risk assessment in theranostic service delivery.
- Ensure all diagnostic and therapeutic procedures follow relevant local legislation and international best practice.
- Oversee the patient discharge, instructions, and mitigation of any incidents and accidents, including management of the untimely death of a patient with radionuclides.
- Monitor personal staff exposure to ensure no breach of dose limits.
- Ensure that an environmental radiation monitoring program is in place.

This list is not exhaustive. However, it should provide a starting point for determining how to modify current existing medical physics residency training programs and training for practicing medical physicists, considering the exciting expansion in theranostic service provision.

14.10 ADVANCING THERANOSTICS COMPETENCE FOR THE NUCLEAR MEDICINE TECHNOLOGIST (NMT)

NMTs participating in theranostics must be formally qualified in nuclear medicine (e.g., a Degree program in Nuclear Medicine, Medical Radiations Sciences equivalent, or relevant Graduate Diploma) and should have at least five years of experience in conventional nuclear medicine and PET imaging. Qualifications in CT imaging would also be of benefit. NMTs should be well trained in the scanners ofthe department and must have an intimate knowledge of common problems encountered with the scanners so that they can troubleshoot effectively.

Theranostics is a maturing field in nuclear medicine, and it would be highly desirable for NMTs to have a valid and up-to-date Good Clinical Practice (GCP) certificate. GCP is an international ethical and scientific quality standard for the design, conduct, performance, monitoring, auditing, recording, analyses, and reporting of clinical trials [50,51]. Being cognizant of the principles of GCP will enable an NMT to adhere to the rigor, details, and expectations of performing radio-nuclide therapy safely, ensuring optimal patient care. There are many resources on the web for training on GCP and obtaining appropriate certification [50,51].

The NMT should be familiar with the radiation protection program of the department and the radiation management plan of the facility. Since theranostics deals with high amounts of unsealed radioactivity, the safe practice of radiation handling is paramount. NMTs should adhere to the As Low As Reasonable (ALARA) principles when drawing up radiopharmaceuticals, when dealing with patients who have received radionuclide therapy, and when performing post-therapy imaging. The radiation dose to staff must also be monitored and their occupational exposure reviewed regularly to ensure that internal limits are adhered to, and ICRP recommended levels are not exceeded.

The role of the NMT can be at multiple levels and will vary within departments, states, and countries depending on the staffing structures within a particular nuclear medicine department. For NMTs to be competent in the theranostics space, they must have the appropriate education and training for the various tasks they may be responsible for, with continuous education programs for skill development, and dissemination of best practice principles. This includes both the diagnostic and therapeutic aspects of this service. It also requires close liaison with the medical practitioners referring the patients, the medical practitioners reporting the diagnostic scans and administering the treatment, medical physicists, radiopharmaceutical scientists, nurses, and coordinators within the department.

There must be a strong, established SOP within a department, which provides a basic under-standing of the roles and responsibilities of NMTs, and how they fit into the framework of the theranostic service delivery in that department. The SOPs should be crafted by theranostics spe-cialists, NMTs, medical physicists, nurses, and other relevant parties involved in the provision of this service. Consideration of a mentor program that identifies the experts in the field who may be able to advise when issues are encountered, would also be strategically appropriate for ongoing training.

14.11 CONCLUSION

There is increasing demand for theranostics procedures. However, the prime challenges are infrastructure and appropriately skilled professional staff.

In addition, there is significant global variation in the training, regulatory aspects, financial, reimbursement, and medical landscapes [2–5]. The workforce shortage is related to multiple factors such as education and training, limited funding, awareness, and limited partnership with clinical teams. However, providing regular teaching and training for professionals is often chal-lenging. The onus is not only on local departments but also on the responsibility of national and international societies. Networking and collaboration of shared resources should be encouraged and enhanced, leading to communities of practice in the field of theranostics.

REFERENCES

1. Pharo, E., Davison, A., McGregor, H., Warr, K., & Brown, P. (2014). Using communities of practice to enhance interdisciplinary teaching: lessons from four Australian institutions. *Higher Education Research & Development, 33*(2), 341–354.

2. Cole, D. R., & Bradley, J. P. (2018). Principles of transversality in globalization and education. In *Principles of Transversality in Globalization and Education* (pp. 1–15). Springer, Singapore.

3. Engel-Hills, P., & Chhem, R. K. (2012). The nature of professional expertise. In *Radiology Education* (pp. 3–9). Springer, Berlin, Heidelberg.

4. Pareja Roblin, N., & McKenney, S. (2019). Classic design of curriculum innovations: investigation of teacher involvement in research, development, and diffusion. In *Collaborative Curriculum Design for Sustainable Innovation and Teacher Learning* (pp. 19–34). Springer, Cham.

5. Gomes Marin, J., Nunes, R., Coutinho, A., Zaniboni, E., Costa, L., Barbosa, F., Queiroz, M., Cerri, G., & Buchpiguel, C. (2020). Theranostics in nuclear medicine: emerging and re-emerging integrated imaging and therapies in the era of precision oncology. *RadioGraphics, 40*(6), 1715–1740.

6. Herrmann, K., Giovanella, L., Santos, A., Gear, J., et al. (2022). Joint EANM, SNMMI and IAEA enabling guide: how to set up a theranostics centre. *European Journal of Nuclear Medicine and Molecular Imaging, 11*, 2306.

7. Lee, S. T., Emmett, L. M., Pattison, D. A., Hofman, M. S., Bailey, D. L., Latter, M., Francis, R. J., & Scott, A. (2022). The importance of training, accreditation and guidelines for the practice of theranostics: the Australian perspective. *Journal of Nuclear Medicine, 7*, 82–821:numed.122.263996.

8. Herrmann, K., Schwaiger, M., Lewis, J. S., et al. (2020). theranostics: a roadmap for future development. *Lancet Oncology, 21*(3), e146–e156.

9. Gnanasegaran, G., Paez, D., Sathekge, M., Giammarile, F., Fanti, S., Chiti, A., Bom, H., Vinjamuri, S., Pascual, T. N., & Bomanji, J. (2022 Jan). Coronavirus (COVID-19) pandemic mediated changing trends in nuclear medicine education and training: time to change and scintillate. *European Journal of Nuclear Medicine and Molecular Imaging, 49*(2), 427–435.

10. European Commission, Food and Agriculture Organization of the United Nations, International Atomic Energy Agency, International Labour Organization, OECD Nuclear Energy Agency, Pan American Health Organization, United Nations Environment Programme, World Health Organization, Radiation Protection and Safety of Radiation Sources: International Basic Safety Standards, IAEA Safety Standards Series No. GSR Part 3, IAEA, Vienna (2014).

11. Pascual, T. N., Ros, S., Engel-Hills, P., & Chhem, R. K. (2012). Medical competency in postgraduate medical training programs. In *Radiology Education* (pp. 29–45). Springer, Berlin, Heidelberg.

12. Patel, M. (2016). Changes to postgraduate medical education in the 21st century. *Clinical Medicine (London, England), 16*(4), 311–314. doi:10.7861/clinmedicine.16-4-311

13. Ten Cate, O. (2017). Competency-based postgraduate medical education: past, present and future. *GMS Journal for Medical Education, 34*(5), 1–2.

14. International Atomic Energy Agency, Nuclear Medicine Resources Manual 2020 Edition, IAEA Human Health Series No. 37, IAEA, Vienna (2020).

15. Weggemans, M. M., Van Dijk, B., Van Dooijeweert, B., Veenendaal, A. G., & Ten Cate, O. (2017). The postgraduate medical education pathway: an international comparison. *GMS Journal for Medical Education, 34*(5), 2–3.

16. Karle, H. (2006). Global standards and accreditation in medical education: a view from the WFME. *Academic Medicine, 81*(Suppl):S43–S48. doi:10.1097/01.acm.0000243383.71047.c4

17. International Atomic Energy Agency, Training Curriculum for Nuclear Medicine Physicians, IAEA-TECDOC-1883, IAEA, Vienna (2019).

18. American Board of Nuclear Medicine American Board of Nuclear Medicine: An ABMS member board. American Board of Medical Specialties. https://www.abms.org/board/american-board-of-nuclear-medicine/. Published August 17, 2022. Accessed October 27, 2022.

19. European Union of Medical Specialists (UEMS) European Standards in Medical Training. Main UEMS – European Standards in Medical Training – ETRs. https://www.uems.eu/areas-of-expertise/postgraduate-training/european-standards-in-medical-training. Accessed October 27, 2022.

20. Muylle, K., & Maffioli, L. (2017). Nuclear medicine training in Europe: "all for one, one for all." *Journal of Nuclear Medicine, 58*(12), 1904–1905. doi:10.2967/jnumed.117.201012

21. Stefanoyiannis, A. P., Prigent, A., Bakalis, S., et al. (2014). Structured intercomparison of nuclear medicine physicians' education and training programs in 12 EANM member-affiliated member countries. *Médecine Nucléaire, 38*(6), 456–468. doi:10.1016/j.mednuc.2014.09.004

22. Durr-E-Sabih. (2013 Fall). The Asian Nuclear Medicine Board (ANMB); why do we need it? *Asia Oceania Journal of Nuclear Medicine and Biology.*, *1*(2), 1–3. PMID: 27408843; PMCID: PMC4927045.
23. Royal Australasian College of Physicians Physicians TRAC of The Royal Australasian College of Physicians. www.racp.edu.au. Accessed October 27, 2022. https://www.racp.edu.au/trainees/advanced-training/advanced-training-programs/nuclear-medicine
24. Arevalo-Perez, J., Paris, M., Graham, M. M., Osborne, J. R. (2016). A perspective of the future of nuclear medicine training and certification. *Seminars in Nuclear Medicine*, *46*(1), 88–96. doi:10.1053/j.semnuclmed.2015.10.003
25. Herrmann, K., Giovanella, L., Santos, A., Gear, J., Kiratli, P. O., Kurth, J., … & Kunikowska, J. (2022). Joint EANM, SNMMI and IAEA enabling guide: how to set up a theranostics centre. *European Journal of Nuclear Medicine and Molecular Imaging*, 1–10.
26. Lass, P. (2002). Nuclear medicine technologist training in European countries. *European Journal of Nuclear Medicine and Molecular Imaging*, *29*(8), 1083–1090.
27. Patterson, H. E., Nunez, M., Philotheou, G. M., & Hutton, B. F. (2013, May). Meeting the challenges of global nuclear medicine technologist training in the 21st century: The IAEA Distance Assisted Training (DAT) program. In *Seminars in Nuclear Medicine* (Vol. 43, No. 3, pp. 195–201). WB Saunders.
28. Lass, P. (2001). Nuclear medicine technologists' training in different countries – a comparison. *Nuclear Medicine Review*, *4*(2), 65–68.
29. Nuclear Medicine Technology Certification Board I NMTCB. www.nmtcb.org. Accessed October 27, 2022. https://www.nmtcb.org/#section-1
30. Schwarz, S. W. (2007). *Issues on Training of Radiochemists/Radiopharmacists* (No. IAEA-CN--157).
31. BPS Board Certification in the Real World. Board of Pharmacy Specialties. Accessed October 27, 2022. https://www.bpsweb.org/impact-of-bps-certification/bps-board-certification-in-the-real-world/
32. International Atomic Energy Agency, Roles and Responsibilities, and Education and Training Requirements for Clinically Qualified Medical Physicists, IAEA Human Health Series No. 25, IAEA, Vienna (2013).
33. International Atomic Energy Agency, Clinical Training of Medical Physicist Specialising in Nuclear Medicine, Training Course Series No. 50, IAEA Vienna (2011)
34. International Atomic Energy Agency, Clinical Training of Medical Physicists Specializing in Nuclear Medicine, Training Course Series No. 50, IAEA, Vienna (2011)
35. Clements, J. B., Baird, C. T., de Boer, S. F., Fairobent, L. A., Fisher, T., Goodwin, J. H., … & Wingreen, N. (2018). AAPM medical physics practice guideline 10.a.: scope of practice for clinical medical physics. *Journal of Applied Clinical Medical Physics*, *19*(6), 11–25.
36. Caruana, C. J., Tsapaki, V., Damilakis, J., et al. (2018). EFOMP policy statement 16: the role and competences of medical physicists and medical physics experts under 2013/59/EURATOM. *Physica Medica*, *48*, 162–168. doi:10.1016/j.ejmp.2018.03.001
37. European Board for Accreditation in Medical Physics (EBAMP) – Just another WordPress site. Accessed October 27, 2022. https://www.ebamp.eu/
38. AFOMP Revised Constitution – Asia-Oceania Federation of Organizations for Medical Physics. Accessed October 27, 2022. https://afomp.org/afomp-revised-constitution/
39. Accreditation – International Organization for Medical Physics. Published March 28, 2018. Accessed October 27, 2022. https://www.iomp.org/accreditation/
40. International Atomic Energy Agency, Guidelines for the Certification of Clinically Qualified Medical Physicists, Training Course Series No. 71, IAEA, Vienna (2021).
41. Canadian Nuclear Safety Commission. (2019). Role of the Radiation Safety Officer. Final Evaluation Report. http://nuclearsafety.gc.ca/eng/resources/publications/reports/internal-audit-and-evaluation/role-of-the-rso-final-evaluation-report.cfm?pedisable=true
42. Morgan, T. L., & Konerth, S. (2021). The role of the radiation safety officer in patient safety. In *Contemporary Topics in Patient Safety – Volume 1*. IntechOpen.
43. Berry, K., Elder, D., Kroger, L. (2018). The evolving role of the medical radiation safety officer. *Health Physics*, *115*(5), 628–636. 10.1097/hp.0000000000000949
44. Morgan, T. L., & Konerth, S. (2021). The role of the radiation safety officer in patient safety. In S. P. Stawicki, & M. S. Firstenberg (Eds.), *Contemporary Topics in Patient Safety – Volume 1*. IntechOpen, London, Uk. 10.5772/intechopen.97058
45. Baes, F. hps.org. Health Physics Society. https://hps.org/publicinformation/ate/faqs/rso.html#

46. American Association of Physicists in Medicine. (2012). The Selection, Use, Calibration, and Quality Assurance of Radionuclide Calibrators Used in Nuclear Medicine. *Maryland, United States: AAPM Report*, (181).

47. International Atomic Energy Agency, Quality Assurance for Radioactivity Measurement in Nuclear Medicine, Technical Reports Series No. 454, IAEA, Vienna (2006).

48. Busemann Sokole, E., Płachcínska, A., Britten, A., Lyra Georgosopoulou, M., Tindale, W., & Klett, R. (2010). Routine quality control recommendations for nuclear medicine instrumentation. *European Journal of Nuclear Medicine and Molecular Imaging*, 37(3), 662–671.

49. Busemann Sokole, E., Płachcínska, A., & Britten, A. (2010). Acceptance testing for nuclear medicine instrumentation. *European Journal of Nuclear Medicine and Molecular Imaging*, 37(3), 672–681.

50. Guideline, I. H. T. (2001). Guideline for good clinical practice. *Journal of Postgraduate Medicine*, 47(3), 199–203.

51. Guideline, I. H. (2015). Integrated addendum to ICH E6 (R1): guideline for good clinical practice E6 (R2). *Current Step*, 2, 1–60.

15 Theranostics Today

Looking Backwards to Tomorrow

Dale L. Bailey

15.1 THE CURRENT ROLE OF MOLECULAR RADIONUCLIDE THERAPY AND THERANOSTICS

Incidence rates for cancer continue to increase globally, while at the same time knowledge of and strategies to deal with cancer are also making great advances. The latest figures available from the US CDC in 2019 showed that cancer was the second leading cause of death in the USA after heart disease. The most effective cancer management is prevention based on modifying lifestyle factors such as exercise, diet, vaccinations, and reducing exposure to carcinogens. Increasing longevity, however, means that high levels of cancer will exist into the future. Deeper knowledge of genetic predisposition to cancer and somatic alterations provides optimism for targeted treatments so that cancer may become, at worst, a disease that the individual dies *with* rather than dies *from*. Examples of cancer targeting that have made a dramatic impact include the identification of somatic mutations in the BRAF, PIK3CA and EGFR oncogenes, among others.

Once cancer is established in an individual, there are a limited number of approaches to attempt to cure or control the cancer process depending on the status of the disease. These approaches range from highly invasive methods such as surgical excision with curative intent through to managing widespread disseminated malignancy with less invasive systemic medical therapies to achieve disease control or palliation. The major tools available and their application domains are summarized in Figure 15.1. This shows that, generally, as cancer becomes more widespread throughout the body, the treatments also become more systemic and less invasive: surgery, the most invasive approach, has limited regional extent and attempts predominantly to control localized disease, whereas radiotherapy can be applied to a number of regions of the body but is generally used to treating a limited number of sites (≤5), while the management of widespread metastatic disease is the domain of medical therapies and, increasingly, molecular radionuclide therapy (RNT).

As discussed in depth throughout this book, the theranostic[1] approach of modern molecular RNT offers the attraction of targeted systemic treatment for disseminated disease, including microscopic disease, combined with the ability to image the delivery and subsequent fate of the therapeutic compound with either a SPECT (Single Photon Emission Computed Tomography) or PET (Positron Emission Tomography) camera. The theranostic approach is not a new one, however, as theranostics has been in use in nuclear medicine in the form of radioiodine treatment of thyroid conditions for over 75 years [1,2], the practice predating the introduction of the term by more than 50 years. In fact, theranostic management of thyroid disease has proven so effective since its introduction that little has changed in its use in that period, a remarkable feature given the stunning advances in medicine in that time. Radioiodine therapy even predates the discovery of the double-helical structure of DNA [3], which ushered in the era of molecular biology on which much of current theranostic developments are based, and has set an extremely high standard for all

DOI: 10.1201/9781003250913-19

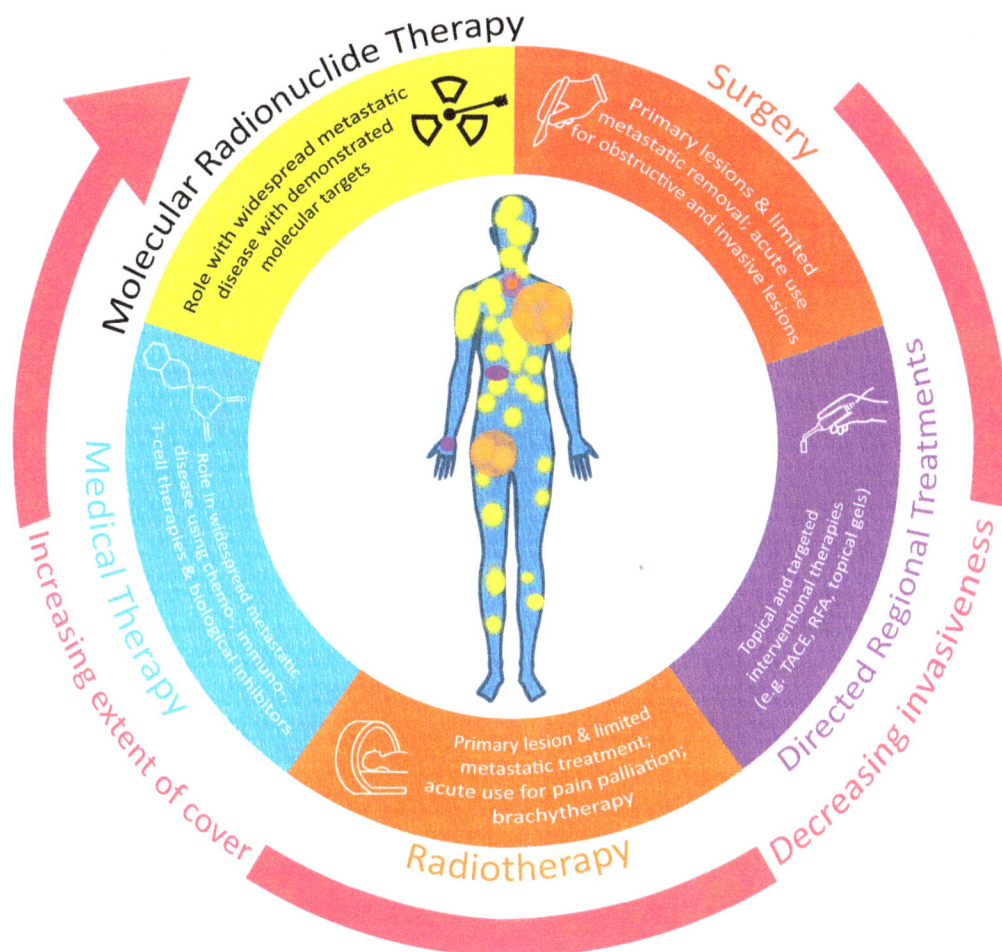

FIGURE 15.1 Current cancer control options are shown. The colors used in the wheel surrounding the subject are shown in the figure to demonstrate their application. Surgery is the most invasive approach and has the most limited coverage. If complete local resection of the cancerous tissue is achieved, however, it offers the best option for a complete cure. With a decreasing level of invasiveness follows directed targeted treatments such as interventional radiological procedures and topical applications. Radiotherapy is, in general, minimally invasive but can only treat limited extent of disease. When disease is more widespread, a systemic approach is required with medical therapies such as chemo-, immuno-, and biological therapies. Molecular radionuclide therapy is a systemic approach that offers the advantage of being able to assess targeting prior to treatment and can monitor therapy as it is delivered using whole-body SPECT or PET imaging.

subsequent theranostic treatments to match. The test for any new theranostic strategy could well be "*Is it as good as radioiodine?*".

Today, the imaging methodologies SPECT and PET can be quantitative whereby the degree of uptake of the radioactivity in the tissues is proportional to the amount of the compound present, and from this the radiation dose delivered to the tissues can be determined. This permits personalized treatment planning prior to therapy commencing and monitoring of retention subsequent to therapy delivery.

With the increasing ability to identify targets and chemically engineered molecules, peptides, antibodies, and other designer moieties with increased specificity for the cancers' characteristics, it is anticipated that molecular RNT will enjoy an increasing role in modern cancer management over the next few decades. However, we have much still to learn to optimize this form of radiation therapy such as how best to measure biological dose, the effect of the type and energy of the radiation, dose rate effects, the impact of tumor and molecular RNT delivery heterogeneity, dose fractionation strategies and the optimal timing for delivery of therapy. In this chapter, we will consider some of the issues related to improving molecular RNT.

15.2 TYPES OF RADIATION AND THERANOSTIC RADIONUCLIDE PAIRS

15.2.1 β⁻ PARTICLES

Traditionally, beta-minus (β^-) particles emitted from unstable nuclei have been the preferred radiation used in RNT. Common examples include ^{131}I (0.19 MeV average energy of emission, 90% branching ratio, 8.02 d half-life), ^{90}Y (0.93 MeV, 100%, 64 h), ^{188}Re (0.79 & 0.73 MeV, 70% and 26%, 17 h) and ^{177}Lu (0.15 MeV, 79%, 6.7 d). Beta-minus particles typically have a range of millimeters in tissue, and this is seen as advantageous as DNA breaks can be affected without the need to have the β^- particle internalized in the cancer cell or even on the surface of the cell – being in the vicinity can be sufficient. It is suggested that this extended path length is particularly useful in the case of heterogeneous disease which is infiltrating normal tissues. The downside of this, though, is that normal tissues can be damaged as well. In particular, the bone marrow can be impacted in the case of treating skeletal metastatic disease. Another desirable feature of β^- decay is that it is often accompanied by the emission of gamma (γ) radiation, subsequent to the β^- emission, which can be imaged using the gamma camera although this must be balanced against the radiation exposure hazard created by the γ-radiation. This allows the biodistribution of the targeted therapy to be monitored after the treatment has been administered. For therapeutic radionuclides such as ^{67}Cu and ^{177}Lu, the γ photons emitted are suitable for imaging on the gamma camera with a medium energy collimator and have reasonably good imaging properties given that large amounts of the radiopharmaceutical (~GBqs) are typically administered. Radioiodine (^{131}I) emits a higher energy γ photon of 0.364 MeV which can also be imaged with the gamma camera using appropriate high-energy collimation.

15.2.2 α PARTICLES

It is only in relatively recent times that therapy with alpha (α) particles has been accepted clinically [4]. Due to their greater mass compared with the β^- particle (over 7,000 times greater) alpha particles are able to deposit large amounts of energy in a very short range (~80 keV/μm). This short range however necessitates having the nucleus of the decaying radionuclide which is emitting the alpha particle in close proximity to the DNA of the cancer cell. Ideally, it will be internalized within the cell. The typical range of an alpha particle in tissue is of the order of tens of microns. Therapy with alpha particles on a commercial scale was introduced only a decade or so ago using [^{223}Ra]RaCl$_2$ (5.5–5.7 MeV, 97%, 11.4 d) (Xofigo®, Bayer), a bone-seeking agent to treat skeletal metastases from prostate cancer. While alpha particles are very effective and highly toxic to cancer cells, the same is also true for any non-target cells that take up the radionuclide under normal physiological conditions, such as the salivary glands with radiolabeled Prostate-Specific Membrane Antigen (PSMA) in prostate cancer. Alpha particles attached to highly specific radiopharmaceuticals that are highly selective for cancer cell targeting hold great promise in controlling disease as long as the off-target effects can be adequately managed. In the near future, it is expected that a number of alpha-emitting radionuclides will emerge as potential therapies including ^{149}Tb, ^{213}Bi, ^{210}Pb, ^{212}Pb/^{212}Bi, ^{225}Ac, and ^{227}Th (parent of ^{223}Ra). One potential limitation of the use of α particles for therapy is when the molecular target is not the cancer cell, but an associated cell overexpressed in the tumor microenvironment and hence potentially some distance from the cancer cell itself. One such example could be targeting cancer-associated fibroblasts such as fibroblast activation protein inhibitors that form part of the tumor micro-environment in the stroma of many epithelial cancers but are not the actual cancer cell. Here, the short range of the α particle could be a limitation in delivering sufficient radiation dose to the cancer cells.

15.2.3 AUGER ELECTRONS

Auger electrons are very low-energy electrons that arise from radionuclides that decay by electron capture. Auger electrons are emitted as a consequence of the vacancy that is created after electron capture, typically leaving the atom with an inner shell vacancy. Any inner shell vacancy is rapidly filled by an electron transition from a higher orbital, thereby resulting in a characteristic X-ray of energy equal to the difference between the binding energies of the two electron shells ($E_{b1}-E_{b2}$). However, instead of being emitted from the atom as an X-ray, this same energy can be instantaneously transferred to an additional outer shell orbiting electron of binding energy E_{b3}, which is ejected with energy equal to ($E_{b1}-E_{b2}$) − E_{b3}. Electrons emitted from the atom in this way are referred to as either Auger electrons, or Coster–Kronig electrons if the ejected electron emanates from a higher subshell of the same orbital as the electron involved in the transition to fill the initial inner shell vacancy. Since Auger and Coster-Kronig electrons are the consequence of transitions between electron orbitals, they have discrete energies unlike β⁻ particles that are emitted with a continuum of energies up to a maximum value for each radionuclide. The energies of Auger and Coster–Kronig electrons range from a value just below the characteristic X-ray energies to a few electron volts. The path lengths of these electrons are mostly sub-micronic. Auger electron emitters have been used in clinical studies in order to selectively exploit the high Linear Energy Transfer (LET) of these particles when targeted to cancer cells. Examples include the use of [^{125}I]-thymidine precursors as well as ^{125}I-labeled antibodies. Auger electrons are often produced as part of the decay process by what are thought of as pure "gamma-emitting" radionuclides such as ^{67}Ga, ^{99m}Tc, ^{111}In, ^{123}I and ^{125}I.

15.2.4 POSITRONS (β⁺)

Finally, our group has been exploring the potential of positrons (β⁺) for therapy [5]. Compared to β⁻ particles, β⁺s have a shorter range (for the same emitted energy) and higher LET at sub-keV energies than β⁻-emitting radionuclides due to their positive charge. The secondary electrons and ions generated along the β⁺ track are within each other's Coulomb electrostatic field resulting in higher localized energy deposition compared to β⁻ particles. Finally, they are likely to create orbital vacancies when they annihilate with an atomic electron which can lead to Auger electron production. Many β⁺-emitters are already used as radiopharmaceuticals for diagnostic imaging in PET and would not require further radiochemistry developments prior to use as a radiotherapeutic. This could provide a radically different approach to RNT: instead of using a radionuclide with a relatively long half-life delivering the treatment over weeks, the therapy might be given as a series of "fractionated" doses as is done in external beam radiation therapy (EBRT) as an outpatient. In radiation-based therapies, the rate of DNA breakages is dependent on the dose rate and is being recognized as an increasingly important factor in delivering effective RNTs. The shorter half-lives of some β⁺-emitting radionuclides, particularly radiometals, might have some attractive properties for addressing this issue by delivering large amounts of radiation with the associated high dose rate (rate of emission of the β⁺s) that decays rapidly. Copper-61, for example, with a 3.3 hr half-life and over 50% β⁺ branching ratio could be an ideal candidate. Using a radionuclide with a short half-life would also have the advantage that the radiopharmaceutical would not need to be radiochemically stable and remain bound in vivo to the target for a number of days as the bulk of the radiation dose would be delivered in a few hours.

15.2.5 IDEAL THERANOSTIC RADIONUCLIDE PAIRS

When considering theranostic radionuclide pairs, three different combinations can be employed. These are:

- *same radionuclide* for imaging and therapy (e.g., ^{131}I);
- different radioisotopes of the *same element* for imaging and therapy (e.g., ^{123}I (SPECT) / ^{131}I (RNT), ^{64}Cu (PET) / ^{67}Cu (RNT));
- radionuclides of *different elements* for imaging and therapy (e.g., ^{68}Ga (PET) / ^{177}Lu (RNT)).

The first option, using the same radionuclide for imaging and therapy, has the downside of potentially imparting a significant radiation dose as part of any diagnostic imaging procedure. This can have detrimental effects such as the so-called "stunning" of ^{131}I and ^{124}I when imaging thyroid cancer prior to treatment, which can reduce the subsequent uptake of the therapy. The second option, using the same element for both imaging and therapy, would appear to be the ideal combination, where the imaging radionuclide delivers a very small radiation dose to the target organ which is followed by the radiation dose from the larger LET therapeutic radionuclide using the same element. The third option of different radioactive elements for imaging and therapy is potentially problematic as the different radiolabeling required for the different elements will likely change the chelation chemistry of the targeting agent in some way and thereby change the uptake and biodistribution compared to the imaging radiopharmaceutical. There are already examples where the compound used for imaging with a radiometal is unsuitable when radiolabeled with a therapeutic radiometal (e.g., PSMA-11). Due to these issues, there has been increasing research interest in the use of radioisotopes of the same element such as scandium (^{43}Sc, ^{44}Sc, ^{47}Sc) and terbium (^{149}Tb, ^{152}Tb, ^{155}Tb, ^{161}Tb) as they each have a number of radionuclides suitable for both imaging and therapy. Table 15.1 shows a number of "same element" radionuclides suitable for theranostic applications.

TABLE 15.1
Examples of Some "Same Element" Radiotheranostics

Element	Radionuclide	Use	t-half (hr)
Copper	Cu-61	PET	3.3
	Cu-64	PET	12.7
	Cu-67	RNT/SPECT	61.8
Iodine	I-123	SPECT	13.0
	I-124	PET	101
	I-125	RNT	1416
	I-131	RNT/SPECT	192
Scandium	Sc-43	PET	3.9
	Sc-44	PET	4.0
	Sc-47	RNT/SPECT	80.4
Terbium	Tb-149	RNT/PET	4.1
	Tb-152	PET	17.5
	Tb-155	SPECT	128
	Tb-161	RNT	165
Yttrium	Y-86	PET	14.7
	Y-90	RNT/PET	64.0

In addition to these radiochemical considerations, a number of other factors related to production mode, radiochemical yield, half-life and transport issues, particle energy/range and radiopharmaceutical "escape" after decay of the parent radionuclide (especially for α-emitters that decay via a long, cascading series of intermediary radionuclides) will determine which radionuclide combinations will find wider acceptance. Radionuclide generators such as the ^{188}W/^{188}Re system (^{188}W $t_{1/2}$ = 69.4 d) [6] provide for a convenient "on demand" on-site local supply of the β$^-$-emitting ^{188}Re which might otherwise not find widespread use due to the relatively short half-life (17.0 h). It is a convenient and relatively inexpensive system. Conversely, a biologically near-ideal therapeutic radionuclide such as ^{67}Cu with a half-life of 61.8 h, produced using high-energy X-ray accelerators, is currently only made in few locations globally, which presents challenges for worldwide supply.

15.3   THE MEDICAL PHYSICS TOOLKIT FOR RADIOTHERANOSTICS

The general tools for performing theranostics include the imaging and therapeutic radionuclide pair, the appropriate molecularly targeted construct (e.g., molecule, peptide, antibody, nanoparticle) and the imaging equipment for monitoring. For the medical physicist, there are a number of further tools that can be employed to provide greater insights into the theranostic process. These include:

- image data acquisition and reconstruction optimization to produce quantitative maps of the biodistribution of the theranostic pairs;
- software to extract the temporal course of the biodistribution over time;
- the ability to generate time-activity curves (TACs) for different organs and tissues or at the voxel level;
- dosimetry software that takes into account the physics of the radionuclides used;
- the modeling of cell survival based on the Linear Quadratic (LQ) model [7] with additional factors to account for effects such as radioactive decay, tissue proliferation rate, and dose rate effects;
- the dosimetry methodology framework such as provided by the MIRD and RADAR committees [8];
- the ability to generate Biologically Effective Dose (BED) estimates which will relate more directly to outcomes.

One factor that should be further investigated in the future is a deeper understanding of the radiobiological effects on living cells of slowly decaying, particle-emitting radiation. The majority of textbooks that deal with clinical applications of radiation therapy and clinical radiobiology are mostly based on data and experience obtained from EBRT. Some of the contrasting features of EBRT and RNT are summarized in Table 15.2.

15.4   THE NEXT CHALLENGE: PRECISION THERANOSTICS

Most theranostic practice today is being delivered using standardized amounts of RNT with little, if any, adjustment for factors such as patient size and weight, burden of disease, histological grading of the cancer and the biodistribution uptake and retention of the theranostic compound over time. Further, a number of treatments ("cycles") are usually administered at fixed intervals (e.g., 6–12 weeks apart). Again, this does not necessarily reflect the individual's trajectory of disease and response to each cycle of treatment and is just as likely dictated by the schedule of outpatient clinic visits. This approach follows in the footsteps of the highly successful "one-size-fits-all" regime that has been in general used for treating thyroid cancer for nearly 70 years. An approach such as this will necessarily undertreat some patients and overtreat others. As the

TABLE 15.2

Differences between EBRT and RNT. Most of our recent knowledge about the cellular effects of radiation is based on EBRT

External Beam Radiotherapy (EBRT)	Radionuclide Therapy (RNT)
High dose rate	Low dose rate
Acute irradiation (secs)	Continuous irradiation (days/weeks)
Fractionation (early vs late effects)	Single dose (or one very long continuous dose)
Dose rate: 60–120+ Gy/hr	Dose rate: <0.1–1 Gy/hr
Ionizing MV X-ray photons	Ionizing particles
Mostly homogeneous dose distribution in target	Likely highly heterogeneous distribution of radiation in the target
Likely cellular effect – necrosis/mitotic catastrophe/cell death	Likely cellular effect – inducing apoptosis/loss of clonogenic potential

theranostic paradigm possesses the unique capability of being able to visually map in three dimensions the treatment over the entire body in a quantitative manner, it would seem inevitable that within the next 5–10 years we should be moving from the one-size-fits-all approach to one where each treatment is individually planned: that is, delivering on the promise of *precision theranostics*.

To achieve the goal of a precision-guided approach in the individual subject, the medical physicist will need to address a number of current limitations. These include:

- accurate spatial alignment of the organs and tissues of the body imaged over multiple timepoints. The motion of internal organs (e.g., liver due to diaphragmatic movement) and changes in conformation (e.g., bladder, stomach, bowel) will require further elastic registration techniques to be implemented in a largely unsupervised way, where an artificial intelligence approach may be a solution;
- automated segmentation of predefined organs based on a combination of morphological and functional imaging to readily extract TACs;
- automated segmentation of lesions and metastatic disease based on the theranostic pre-treatment imaging;
- the limitations of measuring small-volume disease with our existing imaging equipment due to the limited spatial resolution and hence the partial volume effect (PVE) [9,10]. As theranostics are mostly reserved for the metastatic setting, we often encounter tens or hundreds of sites of disease spread throughout the body of which many will be affected by the PVE. This leads to an underestimation of the degree of uptake of the theranostic agent and hence an underestimation in the dose of radiation that is delivered to the tissue. Methods to mitigate this effect are being developed and the need is most acute with gamma camera (SPECT) imaging of the post-treatment distribution of medium-energy γ-emitting therapeutic radionuclides such as ^{177}Lu and ^{67}Cu;
- the development of more sophisticated LQ models that incorporate factors that will give more accurate predictions of the efficacy of low dose rate RNT such as individualized radiobiological parameters (α/β, etc.) and the Lea–Catcheside dose protraction factor (G) [11], which incorporates dose rate into the dosimetry calculations, tissue proliferation rate and the DNA repair rate;

- an improved understanding of the relationship between radiation dose delivered to tissue (J/kg) and the actual BED that this will achieve [12];
- the effect of dose heterogeneity on the BED;
- defining non-toxic safe limits for organs of risk that are not based on EBRT but have been derived for RNT;
- an improved understanding of the differences in dose delivery between the short-lived diagnostic agent and the usually longer-lived therapeutic agent in the theranostic pair.

A further limitation is the demand from regulators and reimbursement providers to generate high-level evidence to support implementing new practices such as is generated via randomized controlled trials (RCTs). As it is possible with theranostics to directly image dose delivered and monitor response with functional imaging, it is hoped that in the future these techniques will be an acceptable surrogate for demonstrating early efficacy and will replace the need for large, expensive RCTs that are often difficult to recruit to the required level in rare cancers and where there is unmet need. In addition, more flexible dose administration regimes could be investigated and monitored with functional imaging for an early assessment of metabolic or cellular response.

15.5   THE FUTURE

It has been predicted that by the middle of the next decade, molecular RNT will account for more than 50% of all radiation treatments as our knowledge base of molecular targets and cancer phenotypes increases along with the ability to engineer a variety of chemical entities to direct at the targets. To achieve this, we will need to build our knowledge of how to use the radiation to a level similar to that of EBRT today. External beam treatments deliver a highly homogeneous flux of photons or particles under extremely precise conditions that are thoroughly planned beforehand. Contrast this with in vivo RNT with its less well-controlled dynamic physiological environment of constantly changing biodistribution, spatially heterogeneous targeting and less well understood interaction of the various radiations with living cells.

Beta-minus particles are likely to remain the first-line radiation of choice for delivering RNT. Many potential β^- emitting radionuclides are extremely convenient to use with respect to factors such as half-life, which allows for transport from the site of production to the treatment clinic, selectable energy of the β^- particles, and the coexistence of imageable photons (γ or annihilation) with which to map the distribution of the RNT and potentially monitor it over time. Beta-minus emitting radionuclides are convenient to use, and the radiation is relatively easy to shield in most cases. The range of energies of the emitted β^- particles also allows tailoring of the radiation dose delivery to be adjusted from lower energy, short range (e.g., ^{177}Lu) to relatively higher energy and longer path lengths (e.g., ^{90}Y). The conjugation chemistry of many of the β^- emitters is extremely robust and stable in vivo. Many of the beta-emitting radionuclides have a sufficiently low external photon emission that the subjects being treated can be done so on an outpatient basis, thereby minimizing cost and inconvenience.

Alpha particles have emerged in recent years as holding great promise to deliver very large amounts of radiation over a very small range. However, these are not without their challenges such as often the presence of a number of radioactive daughters that are produced in a cascading decay chain and which are chemically distinct from the therapeutic parent, the need to ideally have the alpha-emitting RNT taken up within the cancer cell rather than targeting a surface receptor or a nearby component of the tumor microenvironment, and the logistical challenges of global supply and demand. It is possible that alpha particle RNT will find its main role as a second-line treatment where β^- RNT has failed to contain the disease due to intrinsic radio-resistance.

Other particles, such as Auger electrons or positrons, are likely to find niche roles; however, the radionuclides delivering these particles are likely to have high external photon flux rates which may limit their use due to the need to isolate the treated individual from the community for a period of time due to high external radiation exposure rates.

Beyond oncology, the role of RNT is relatively underdeveloped. In the past, RNT has been used to treat a range of conditions such as the bone marrow disorder *polycythæmia rubra vera* (using ^{32}P), for articular joint "radiation synovectomy" (^{90}Y) and, of course, hyperthyroidism (^{131}I). In principle, any cells of the body which are behaving in an "overactive" manner physiologically that are not amenable to pharmacological or hormonal control and contain a suitable target could be treated using RNTs. Further, RNT has the potential for expanded uses in interventional procedures, such as radioembolization as an alternative to chemoembolization, and intra-cavity administration (e.g., post neuro-oncological resection) and should generally have less side effects than systemic chemotherapies.

It is also highly likely in the future that RNT will evolve to be used as part of a combination therapy regime rather than a monotherapy as is often done at present. With the introduction in the past decade of immunotherapy in oncology, we will need to consider how to use systemic RNT not just in combination with, but synergistically with, other chemical, biological and immunological treatment approaches where the effect of either or both modalities is enhanced by the simultaneous delivery. An example that is already being investigated is the use of PARP inhibitors to prevent DNA repair after radiation-induced single-strand breaks [13].

Improved therapeutic strategies will be the product of a multidisciplinary approach involving numerous health professionals from different fields including the medical physicist who must be able to understand and speak the same "language" as they do to have the best understanding of not only the clinical problem at hand but also to discern ways to develop better techniques to improve patient outcomes. Coupled with this, a deeper understanding of how different radiations interact with living cells and the ability of the medical physicist to determine how best to deliver a lethal dose of radiation to the target while sparing the normal tissues of the body is the future that we should all embrace.

NOTE

1 The first use of the term "theranostic" is attributed to the American John Funkhouser in a press release from the company *Cardiovascular Diagnostics* in August 1998.

REFERENCES

1. Hertz S, Roberts A. Radioactive iodine in the study of thyroid physiology: the use of radioactive iodine therapy in Graves' disease. *West J Surg Obstet Gynecol.* 1946;54:474–486.
2. Hertz S, Roberts A. Radioactive iodine in the study of thyroid physiology: the use of radioactive iodine therapy in hyperthyroidism. *J Am Med Assoc.* 1946;131:81–86.
3. Watson JD, Crick FH. Molecular structure of nucleic acids: a structure for deoxyribose nucleic acid. *Nature.* 1953;171:737–738.
4. Parker C, Nilsson S, Heinrich D, et al. Alpha emitter radium-223 and survival in metastatic prostate cancer. *N Engl J Med.* 2013;369:213–223.
5. Hioki T, Gholami YH, McKelvey KJ, et al. Overlooked potential of positrons in cancer therapy. *Sci Rep.* 2021;11:2475.
6. Argyrou M, Valassi A, Andreou M, Lyra M. Rhenium-188 production in hospitals, by W-188/Re-188 generator, for easy use in radionuclide therapy. *Int J Mol Imaging.* 2013;2013:290750.
7. McMahon SJ. The linear quadratic model: usage, interpretation and challenges. *Phys Med Biol.* 2018;64:01TR01.
8. Stabin MG, Siegel JA. Physical models and dose factors for use in internal dose assessment. *Health Phys.* 2003;85(3):294–310.
9. Hoffman EJ, Huang SC, Phelps ME. Quantitation in positron emission tomography: 1. Effect of object size. *J Comput Assist Tomogr.* 1979;3:299–308.

10. Soret M, Bacharach SL, Buvat I. Partial-volume effect in PET tumor imaging. *J Nucl Med.* 2007;48:932–945.

11. Lea DE, Catcheside DG. The mechanism of the induction by radiation of chromosome aberrations in *Tradescantia. J Genet.* 1942;44:216–245.

12. Abbott EM, Falzone N, Lee BQ, et al. The impact of radiobiologically-informed dose prescription on the clinical benefit of yttrium-90 SIRT in colorectal cancer patients. *J Nucl Med.* 2020;61:1658–1664.

13. Nonnekens J, van Kranenburg M, Beerens CE, et al. Potentiation of peptide receptor radionuclide therapy by the PARP inhibitor olaparib. *Theranostics.* 2016;6:1821–1832.

Index

Note: *Italicized* and **bold** page numbers refer to figures and tables.

For Product Safety Concerns and Information please contact our EU
representative GPSR@taylorandfrancis.com
Taylor & Francis Verlag GmbH, Kaufingerstraße 24, 80331 München, Germany